Female Pelvic Medicine and Reconstructive Surgery

Guest Editor

JOSEPH I. SCHAFFER, MD

OBSTETRICS AND GYNECOLOGY CLINICS OF NORTH AMERICA

www.obgyn.theclinics.com

Consulting Editor
WILLIAM F. RAYBURN, MD, MBA

September 2009 • Volume 36 • Number 3

SAUNDERS an imprint of ELSEVIER, Inc.

W.B. SAUNDERS COMPANY

A Division of Elsevier Inc.

Elsevier, Inc. • 1600 John F. Kennedy Blvd. • Suite 1800 • Philadelphia, PA 19103-2899

http://www.theclinics.com

OBSTETRICS AND GYNECOLOGY CLINICS OF NORTH AMERICA Volume 36, Number 3
September 2009 ISSN 0889-8545, ISBN-13: 978-1-4377-1249-0, ISBN-10: 1-4377-1249-5

Editor: Carla Holloway
Developmental Editor: Donald Mumford

Obstetrics and Gynecology Clinics (ISSN 0889-8545) is published quarterly by Elsevier Inc., 360 Park Avenue South, New York, NY 10010-1710. Months of issue are March, June, September, and December. Periodicals postage paid at New York, NY, and additional mailing offices. Subscription price per year is $257.00 (US individuals), $431.00 (US institutions), $130.00 (US students), $309.00 (Canadian individuals), $544.00 (Canadian institutions), $191.00 (Canadian students), $376.00 (foreign individuals), $544.00 (foreign institutions), and $191.00 (foreign students). To receive student/resident rate, orders must be accompanied by name of affiliated institution, date of term, and the signature of program/residency coordinator on institution letterhead. Orders will be billed at individual rate until proof of status is received. Foreign air speed delivery is included in all *Clinics* subscription prices. All prices are subject to change without notice. POSTMASTER: Send address changes to *Obstetrics and Gynecology Clinics*, Elsevier Health Sciences Division, Subscription Customer Service, 3251 Riverport Lane, Maryland Heights, MO 63043. **Customer Service: Telephone: 1-800-654-2452 (U.S. and Canada); 314-447-8871 (outside U.S. and Canada). Fax: 314-447-8029. E-mail: journals customerservice-usa@elsevier.com (for print support); journalsonlinesupport-usa@elsevier.com (for online support).**

Reprints. For copies of 100 or more of articles in this publication, please contact the Commercial Reprints Department, Elsevier Inc., 360 Park Avenue South, New York, New York 10010-1710. Tel.: 212-633-3818; Fax: 212-462-1935; E-mail: reprints@elsevier.com.

Obstetrics and Gynecology Clinics of North America is also published in Spanish by McGraw-Hill Interamericana Editores S.A., P.O. Box 5-237, 06500, Mexico; in Portuguese by Reichmann and Affonso Editores, Rio de Janeiro, Brazil; and in Greek by Paschalidis Medical Publications, Athens, Greece.

Obstetrics and Gynecology Clinics of North America is covered in MEDLINE/PubMed (Index Medicus), Excerpta Medica, Current Concepts/Clinical Medicine, Science Citation Index, BIOSIS, CINAHL, and ISI/BIOMED.

Printed and bound by CPI Group (UK) Ltd, Croydon, CR0 4YY

Transferred to Digital Print 2011

GOAL STATEMENT

The goal of *Obstetrics and Gynecology Clinics of North America* is to keep practicing physicians up to date with current clinical practice in OB/GYN by providing timely articles reviewing the state of the art in patient care.

ACCREDITATION

The *Obstetrics and Gynecology Clinics of North America* is planned and implemented in accordance with the Essential Areas and Policies of the Accreditation Council for Continuing Medical Education (ACCME) through the joint sponsorship of the University of Virginia School of Medicine and Elsevier. The University of Virginia School of Medicine is accredited by the ACCME to provide continuing medical education for physicians.

The University of Virginia School of Medicine designates this educational activity for a maximum of 15 AMA PRA Category 1 Credits™ for each issue, 60 credits per year. Physicians should only claim credit commensurate with the extent of their participation in the activity.

The American Medical Association has determined that physicians not licensed in the US who participate in this CME activity are eligible for a maximum of *15 AMA PRA Category 1 Credits*™ for each issue, 60 credits per year.

Category 1 credit can be earned by reading the text material, taking the CME examination online at: http://www.theclinics.com/home/cme, and completing the evaluation. After taking the test, you will be required to review any and all incorrect answers. Following completion of the test and evaluation, your credit will be awarded and you may print your certificate.

FACULTY DISCLOSURE/CONFLICT OF INTEREST

The University of Virginia School of Medicine, as an ACCME accredited provider, endorses and strives to comply with the Accreditation Council for Continuing Medical Education (ACCME) Standards of Commercial Support, Commonwealth of Virginia statutes, University of Virginia policies and procedures, and associated federal and private regulations and guidelines on the need for disclosure and monitoring of proprietary and financial interests that may affect the scientific integrity and balance of content delivered in continuing medical education activities under our auspices.

The University of Virginia School of Medicine requires that all CME activities accredited through this institution be developed independently and be scientifically rigorous, balanced and objective in the presentation/discussion of its content, theories and practices.

All authors/editors participating in an accredited CME activity are expected to disclose to the readers relevant financial relationships with commercial entities occurring within the past 12 months (such as grants or research support, employee, consultant, stock holder, member of speakers bureau, etc.). The University of Virginia School of Medicine will employ appropriate mechanisms to resolve potential conflicts of interest to maintain the standards of fair and balanced education to the reader. Questions about specific strategies can be directed to the Office of Continuing Medical Education, University of Virginia School of Medicine, Charlottesville, Virginia.

The faculty and staff of the University of Virginia Office of Continuing Medical Education have no financial affiliations to disclose.

The authors/editors listed below have identified no professional or financial affiliations for themselves or their spouse/partner:

Lily A. Arya, MD, MS; Shanna D. Atnip, MSN,WHNP-BC; Marlene M. Corton, MD; Carla Holloway (Acquisitions Editor); William Irvin, MD (Test Author); Colleen D. McDermott, MD, FRCSC; Sujatha Pathi, MD; David D. Rahn, MD; William F. Rayburn, MD, MBA (Consulting Editor); Shayzreen M. Roshanravan, MD; Emily K. Saks, MD; Vivian W. Sung, MD, MPH; Clifford Wai, MD; Cecilia K. Wieslander, MD; and R. Ann Word, MD.

The authors/editors listed below identified the following professional or financial affiliations for themselves or their spouse/partner:

Kathryn L. Burgio, PhD is a consultant and investigator for Pfizer, and serves on the Advisory Committee for Astellas.

Charles W. Butrick, MD is an industry funded research/investigator for Ortho McNeil and Boston Scientific and serves on the Advisory Committee for Ortho McNeil, Astellas, Pfizer, and Novartis.

Jeffrey B. Garris, MD, MS serves on the Speakers Bureau for Pfizer and Gynecure.

Kimberly A. Gerten, MD is an industry funded research/investigator for Pfizer, Inc.

Douglass S. Hale, MD, FACOG, FACS is an industry funded research/investigator for Allergan and Women's Health and Urology.

Brittany Star Hampton, MD is a consultant for Ethicon Women's Health and Urology.

Miles Murphy, MD, MSPH is an industry funded research/investigator for Ethicon Women's Health and Urology and serves on the Advisory Committee for Ethicon Women's Health and Urology, American Medical Systems, and Bard.

Tola B. Omotoshi, MD serves in an investigator initiated study for Pfizer.

Rebecca G. Rogers, MD is an industry funded research/investigator and consultant for Pfizer, and serves on the Speakers Bureau and Advisory Committee for Pfizer.

Joseph I. Schaffer, MD (Guest Editor) serves on the Speakers Bureau and Advisory Committee for Astellas/GlaxoSmithKline.

Marc R. Toglia, MD is a consultant for Astellas Pharma and Ethicon Women's Health, is an industry funded research/investigator and serves on the Advisory Committee for Astellas Pharma, and serves on the Speakers Bureau for Astellas Pharma, Ethicon Women's Health, and Ortho McNeil Pharmaceuticals.

Thomas L. Wheeler, II, MD, MSPH serves on the Speakers Bureau for Pfizer.

Stephen B. Young, MD is a consultant for Mpathy Medical, Inc.

Disclosure of Discussion of non-FDA approved uses for pharmaceutical products and/or medical devices:

The University of Virginia School of Medicine, as an ACCME provider, requires that all faculty presenters identify and disclose any off-label uses for pharmaceutical and medical device products. The University of Virginia School of Medicine recommends that each physician fully review all the available data on new products or procedures prior to clinical use.

TO ENROLL

To enroll in the Obstetrics and Gynecology Clinics of North America Continuing Medical Education program, call customer service at 1-800-654-2452 or visit us online at: www.theclinics.com/home/cme. The CME program is available to subscribers for an additional fee of $195.00.

Contributors

CONSULTING EDITOR

WILLIAM F. RAYBURN, MD, MBA
Randolph Seligman Professor and Chair, Department of Obstetrics and Gynecology;
Chief of Staff, University Hospital, University of New Mexico Health Science Center,
Albuquerque, New Mexico

GUEST EDITOR

JOSEPH I. SCHAFFER, MD
Professor of Obstetrics and Gynecology, Chief of Gynecology/Urogynecology, and
Director, Division of Female Pelvic Medicine and Reconstructive Surgery, University
of Texas Southwestern Medical Center, Dallas, Texas

AUTHORS

LILY A. ARYA, MD, MS
Associate Professor and Division Director, Department of Obstetrics and Gynecology,
Division of Urogynecology and Pelvic Reconstructive Surgery, University of Pennsylvania
School of Medicine, Philadelphia, Pennsylvania

SHANNA D. ATNIP, MSN, WHNP-BC
Women's Health Nurse Practitioner, Division of Female Pelvic Medicine and
Reconstructive Pelvic Surgery, University of Texas Southwestern Medical Center;
Director, Continence and Urodynamic Services, Parkland Health and Hospital System,
Dallas, Texas

KATHRYN L. BURGIO, PhD
Professor of Medicine, University of Alabama at Birmingham; Associate Director
for Research, Department of Veterans Affairs, Birmingham/Atlanta Geriatric Research,
Education, and Clinical Center, Birmingham, Alabama

CHARLES W. BUTRICK, MD
Director, The Urogynecology Center, Overland Park; Assistant Clinical Professor,
Department of Obstetrics and Gynecology, Kansas University Medical School, Kansas
City, Kansas

MARLENE M. CORTON, MD
Associate Professor and Associate Residency Program Director, Department of
Obstetrics and Gynecology, Division of Female Pelvic Medicine and Reconstructive
Pelvic Surgery, University of Texas Southwestern Medical Center, Dallas, Texas

JEFFREY B. GARRIS, MD, MS
Clinical Associate Professor, Division of Female Pelvic Medicine and Reconstructive
Pelvic Surgery, University of South Carolina, Greenville Campus, Greenville, South
Carolina

KIMBERLY A. GERTEN, MD
Private Practice, Park Nicollet Urogynecology and Reconstructive Pelvic Surgery,
St. Louis Park, Minnesota

DOUGLASS S. HALE, MD, FACOG, FACS
Fellowship Director, Female Pelvic Medicine and Reconstructive Surgery, Urogynecology
Associates, Indiana University Methodist Hospital; Associate Professor, Department of
Obstetrics and Gynecology, Division of Urogynecology, Indiana University, Indianapolis,
Indiana

BRITTANY STAR HAMPTON, MD
Assistant Professor, Department of Obstetrics and Gynecology, Division of
Urogynecology and Reconstructive Pelvic Surgery, Women and Infants Hospital of Rhode
Island and Alpert Medical School at Brown University, Providence, Rhode Island

COLLEEN D. McDERMOTT, MD, FRCSC
Fellow, Female Pelvic Medicine and Reconstructive Surgery, Urogynecology Associates,
Indiana University Methodist Hospital, Indianapolis, Indiana

MILES MURPHY, MD, MSPH
Chief, Department of Obstetrics and Gynecology, Division of Urogynecology, Abington
Memorial Hospital, Abington; Assistant Clinical Professor, Department of Obstetrics/
Gynecology and Reproductive Sciences, Temple University School of Medicine; Institute
for Female Pelvic Medicine and Reconstructive Surgery, North Wales, Pennsylvania

TOLA B. OMOTOSHO, MD
Assistant Professor, Department of Gynecology and Obstetrics, Johns Hopkins
University School of Medicine, Women's Center for Pelvic Health, Baltimore, Maryland

SUJATHA PATHI, MD
Department of Obstetrics and Gynecology, Division of Female Pelvic Medicine
and Reconstructive Surgery, University of Texas Southwestern Medical Center, Dallas,
Texas

DAVID D. RAHN, MD
Assistant Professor, Department of Obstetrics and Gynecology, Division of Female Pelvic
Medicine and Reconstructive Surgery, University of Texas Southwestern Medical Center,
Dallas, Texas

REBECCA G. ROGERS, MD
Director, Department of Obstetrics and Gynecology, Division of Female Pelvic Medicine
and Reconstructive Surgery; Professor, University of New Mexico, Albuquerque, New
Mexico

SHAYZREEN M. ROSHANRAVAN, MD
Fellow, Department of Obstetrics and Gynecology, Division of Female Pelvic Medicine
and Reconstructive Surgery, University of Texas Southwestern Medical Center, Dallas,
Texas

EMILY K. SAKS, MD
Fellow, Department of Obstetrics and Gynecology, Division of Urogynecology and Pelvic
Reconstructive Surgery, University of Pennsylvania School of Medicine, Philadelphia,
Pennsylvania

JOSEPH I. SCHAFFER, MD
Professor of Obstetrics and Gynecology, Chief of Gynecology/Urogynecology, and
Director, Division of Female Pelvic Medicine and Reconstructive Surgery, University
of Texas Southwestern Medical Center, Dallas, Texas

VIVIAN W. SUNG, MD, MPH
Assistant Professor, Department of Obstetrics and Gynecology, Division
of Urogynecology and Reconstructive Pelvic Surgery, Women and Infants Hospital
of Rhode Island and Alpert Medical School at Brown University, Providence,
Rhode Island

MARC R. TOGLIA, MD
Director, Division of Urogynecology and Reconstructive Pelvic Surgery, Urogynecology
Associates of Philadelphia, Wynnewood; Assistant Clinical Professor, Department
of Obstetrics and Gynecology, Thomas Jefferson University School of Medicine,
Philadelphia, Pennsylvania

CLIFFORD Y. WAI, MD
Associate Professor and Fellowship Director, Department of Obstetrics and Gynecology,
Division of Female Pelvic Medicine and Reconstructive Surgery, University of Texas
Southwestern Medical Center, Dallas, Texas

THOMAS L. WHEELER II, MD, MSPH
Clinical Assistant Professor, Division of Female Pelvic Medicine and Reconstructive
Pelvic Surgery, University of South Carolina, Greenville, South Carolina

CECILIA K. WIESLANDER, MD
Assistant Professor, Department of Obstetrics and Gynecology, Division of Female Pelvic
Medicine and Reconstructive Surgery, David Geffen School of Medicine at University
of California Los Angeles, Los Angeles; Department of Obstetrics and Gynecology, Olive
View-University of California Los Angeles Medical Center, Sylmar, California

R. ANN WORD, MD
Department of Obstetrics and Gynecology, Division of Female Pelvic Medicine
and Reconstructive Surgery, University of Texas Southwestern Medical Center,
Dallas, Texas

STEPHEN B. YOUNG, MD
Director and Professor of Obstetrics & Gynecology, Department of Obstetrics
and Gynecology, Division of Urogynecology and Reconstructive Pelvic Surgery,
University of Massachusetts Memorial Medical Center, Worcester, Massachusetts

ILLUSTRATOR

LINDSAY OKSENBERG, MA, BFA
Medical Illustrator, Dallas, Texas

Contents

> Normal physiologic function of the pelvic organs depends on the anatomic
> integrity and proper interaction among the pelvic structures, the pelvic
> floor support components, and the nervous system. Pelvic floor dysfunc-
> tion includes urinary and anal incontinence; pelvic organ prolapse; and
> sexual, voiding, and defecatory dysfunction. Understanding the anatomy
> and proper interaction among the support components is essential to di-
> agnose and treat pelvic floor dysfunction. The primary aim of this article
> is to provide an updated review of pelvic support anatomy with clinical cor-
> relations. In addition, surgical spaces of interest to the gynecologic sur-
> geon and the course of the pelvic ureter are described. Several
> concepts reviewed in this article are derived and modified from a previous
> review of pelvic support anatomy.

> The epidemiology of female pelvic floor disorders, including urinary incon-
> tinence, pelvic organ prolapse, anal incontinence, and interstitial cystitis/
> painful bladder syndrome is reviewed. The natural history, prevalence,
> incidence, remission, risk factors, and potential areas for prevention are
> considered.

> Pelvic floor disorders are common health issues for women and have
> a great impact on quality of life. These disorders can present with a wide
> spectrum of symptoms and anatomic defects. This article reviews the clin-
> ical approach and office evaluation of patients with pelvic floor disorders,
> including pelvic organ prolapse, urinary dysfunction, anal incontinence,
> sexual dysfunction, and pelvic pain. The goal of treatment is to provide
> as much symptom relief as possible. After education and counseling,
> patients may be candidates for non-surgical or surgical treatment, and
> expectant management.

Urinary incontinence and voiding dysfunction are common forms of pelvic floor dysfunction affecting women. The complex interactions between the nervous system and lower urinary tract anatomy allow for the coordinated functions of urine storage and evacuation. A thorough understanding of these components and their interactions is the foundation for the diagnosis and treatment of pathologic conditions affecting urine storage or evacuation. These components include changes in neurologic or muscular function, alterations in anatomy, and the deleterious effects of many common comorbid conditions on the lower urinary tract.

Behavioral treatments have been used for several decades to treat urinary incontinence, overactive bladder, and other lower urinary tract symptoms. The spectrum of behavioral treatments includes those that target voiding habits and life style, as well as those that train pelvic floor muscles to improve strength and control. What they all have in common is that they improve symptoms by teaching skills and by changing the patient's behavior. Most patients are not cured through behavioral intervention, but the abundance of literature tells us that most patients experience significant reductions in symptoms and improvements in quality of life. Behavioral treatments should be a mainstay in the care of women of all ages with incontinence or other lower urinary tract symptoms.

Most drugs used in the treatment of urinary incontinence and voiding dysfunction in women modulate neuromuscular transmission in the urethra and bladder. Pharmacotherapy is the mainstay of treatment for overactive bladder. Although several different antimuscarinic medications are available for the treatment of overactive bladder, most have similar efficacy and tolerability. Pharmacotherapy has a limited role in the management of stress incontinence and voiding dysfunction in women. Newer drugs that target different mechanisms of action are being developed for the treatment of urinary incontinence and voiding dysfunction in women.

Surgical management for urinary incontinence is appropriate when conservative treatment is unsuccessful or not desired. Although many operations have been developed for the treatment of incontinence, there is no consensus on which is the single 'best' treatment and therapy should be individualized for each patient. This review will mainly focus on stress urinary incontinence, discuss some of the theories behind the pathophysiology of this condition, and provide some rationale for selecting a particular surgical procedure for incontinence.

The pathophysiology of pelvic organ prolapse is believed to be multifactorial. Several risk factors, such as childbirth and aging, have been identified. Suspected aberrations in the structure and function of the connective tissue, muscles, and nerves of the pelvic floor are still under investigation. In this article, the cellular, biochemical, and molecular basis of pelvic organ prolapse is discussed with a focus on the new theory of elastinopathy as an etiology of prolapse.

Pessary is a low-risk and effective non-surgical treatment option for pelvic organ prolapse. Indications for pessary include symptomatic prolapse, if surgery is not desired or recommended, and use as a diagnostic tool to predict surgical outcomes. Evidence for pessary selection and management is incomplete so trial and error, expert opinion, and experience remain the best guides for use and management of the pessary. With proper training and understanding of pessary management, most patients can be successfully fitted and taught to manage the pessary either for short- or long-term relief of symptoms. Patient satisfaction is high making pessary an important tool in treating prolapse.

The vaginal approach to pelvic organ prolapse repair has been a mainstay of surgical therapy since the beginning of modern gynecologic surgery. In this article, the major vaginal procedures are reviewed with emphasis on techniques of pelvic reconstruction. Vaginal hysterectomy, apical suspension, repair of the anterior and posterior compartments, and perineal repair are covered in detail.

Abdominal correction of pelvic organ prolapse remains a viable option for patients and surgeons. The transition from open procedures to less invasive laparoscopic and robotic-assisted surgeries is evident in the literature. This article reviews the surgical options available for pelvic organ prolapse

Charles W. Butrick

The pelvic floor represents the neuromuscular unit that provides support and functional control for the pelvic viscera. Its integrity, both anatomic and functional, is the key in some of the basic functions of life: storage of urine and feces, evacuation of urine and feces, support of pelvic organs, and sexual function. When this integrity is compromised, the results lead to many of the problems seen by clinicians. Pelvic floor dysfunction can involve weakness and result in stress incontinence, fecal incontinence, and pelvic organ prolapse. Pelvic floor dysfunction can also involve the development of hypertonic, dysfunctional muscles. This article discusses the pathophysiology of hypertonic disorders that often result in elimination problems, chronic pelvic pain, and bladder disorders that include bladder pain syndromes, retention, and incontinence. The hypertonic disorders are very common and are often not considered in the evaluation and management of patients with these problems.

Charles W. Butrick

Patients with hypertonic pelvic floor disorders can present with pelvic pain or dysfunction. Each of the various syndromes will be discussed including elimination disorders, bladder pain syndrome/interstitial cystitis (BPS/IC), vulvodynia, vaginismus, and chronic pelvic pain. The symptoms and objective findings on physical examination and various diagnostic studies will be reviewed. Therapeutic options including physical therapy, pharmacologic management, and trigger point injections, as well as botulinum toxin injections will be reviewed in detail.

THE CLINICS ARE NOW AVAILABLE ONLINE!

Access your subscription at:
www.theclinics.com

Foreword

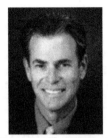

William F. Rayburn, MD, MBA
Consulting Editor

This issue, guest edited by Joseph Schaffer, MD, provides a comprehensive overview of pelvic floor dysfunction. As Dr. Schaffer mentions in the Preface, the field of female pelvic medicine and reconstructive surgery has undergone remarkable evolution in the past decade.

Pelvic floor dysfunction is a descriptor of support disorders in which the organs have lost their normal support and descend through the urogenital hiatus. Approximately half of multiparous women have some degree of pelvic floor dysfunction and many seek help for relief. Symptoms include urinary or fecal loss or retention; vaginal pressure or heaviness; abdominal low back or perineal pain; a mass sensation; difficulty sitting, lifting, or walking; and difficulty with sexual relations. Life-threatening symptoms, such as ureteral obstruction, systemic infection, incarceration, and evisceration, are, fortunately, uncommon.

Examples of pelvic floor dysfunction reviewed in this issue include uterine prolapse, voiding dysfunction, defectory dysfunctions, and pelvic floor hypertonic disorder. As described in several articles about epidemiology and pathophysiology, these defects result from neuromuscular and connective tissue injuries to the pelvic floor. Childbirth injury is the most common condition predisposing to the development of pelvic support disorders. Other injury mechanisms, such as aging, estrogen deficiency, congenital connective tissue weakness, constipation, obesity, chronic coughing, and vigorous physical activity, contribute to pelvic support dysfunction.

With the advancing age of the population, obstetrician-gynecologists are likely to encounter more women with pelvic floor dysfunction. For example, the lifetime risk for a woman undergoing surgery for uterine prolapse or urinary incontinence is estimated at 11%. Approximately 200,000 inpatient procedures for uterine prolapse are now performed annually in the United States, with prolapse the most common indication for hysterectomy in women aged 55 years and older.

This issue provides readers with data-driven, up-to-date information about the nonsurgical and surgical management of women with pelvic floor dysfunction. Nonsurgical management of urinary incontinence, voiding dysfunction, and overactive

Obstet Gynecol Clin N Am 36 (2009) xv–xvi
doi:10.1016/j.ogc.2009.09.005
0889-8545/09/$ – see front matter © 2009 Elsevier Inc. All rights reserved.

bladder consists of behavioral and pharmacologic management. Patients with pelvic support defects should be evaluated on an individual basis to determine the most appropriate approach to surgery. Conditions that influence a surgeon's choice include patient age, body habitus, medical comorbidities, and patient desire to preserve sexual function. Therapeutic decisions are also based on surgeon experience with various vaginal, abdominal, laparoscopic, and robotic operative techniques.

It is my desire that this issue both inspires and activates attention to issues of pelvic floor dysfunction for a vast array of physicians. On behalf of Dr. Schaffer and his excellent group of knowledgeable contributors, I hope that the practical information provided herein will aid in the implementation of evidence-based and well-planned approaches to evaluating and treating women with these common maladies.

William F. Rayburn, MD, MBA
Randolph Seligman Professor and Chair
Department of Obstetrics and Gynecology
University of New Mexico School of Medicine
MSC10 5580, 1 University of New Mexico
Albuquerque, NM 87131-0001, USA

E-mail address:
wrayburn@salud.unm.edu (W.F. Rayburn)

Preface

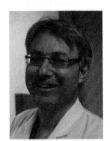

Joseph I. Schaffer, MD
Guest Editor

Since the last urogynecology issue of *Obstetrics and Gynecology Clinics of North America* (December 1998), there has been rapid growth in understanding of the epidemiology, anatomy, pathophysiology, evaluation, and treatment of pelvic floor disorders. This growth has been driven by high-quality clinical research from groups, such as the National Institutes of Health–sponsored Urinary Incontinence Treatment Network and the Pelvic Floor Disorders Network, and a surge of activity in urogynecologic basic and translational research. Additionally, the American Board of Obstetrics and Gynecology and the American Board of Urology initiative to accredit and standardize training in female pelvic medicine and reconstructive surgery has produced a cadre of highly trained physicians and researchers specializing in the care of women with pelvic floor disorders. Thus, the availability of high-quality data in conjunction with skilled practitioners has provided a setting for a new focus on the practice of evidence-based female pelvic medicine and reconstructive surgery. This new focus is providing great improvements in the evaluation and treatment of women with pelvic floor disorders.

The aim of this volume is to provide gynecologists, urogynecologists, urologists, colorectal surgeons, nurse practitioners, physical therapists, and other pelvic floor health care practitioners with a clinically useful update of the epidemiology, anatomy, pathophysiology, evaluation, and treatment of pelvic floor disorders. It is hoped that practitioners will use the information in this issue to provide high-level evidence-based care for the patients they serve.

Joseph I. Schaffer, MD
Professor of Obstetrics and Gynecology
Chief of Gynecology/Urogynecology
Director, Division of Female Pelvic Medicine and Reconstructive Surgery
University of Texas Southwestern Medical Center
5323 Harry Hines Boulevard
Dallas, Texas 75390-9032, USA

E-mail address:
joseph.schaffer@utsouthwestern.edu (J.I. Schaffer)

Obstet Gynecol Clin N Am 36 (2009) xvii
doi:10.1016/j.ogc.2009.09.006
0889-8545/09/$ – see front matter © 2009 Elsevier Inc. All rights reserved.

obgyn.theclinics.com

Anatomy of Pelvic Floor Dysfunction

Marlene M. Corton, MD

KEYWORDS

- Pelvic floor • Levator ani muscles • Pelvic connective tissue
- Ureter • Retropubic space • Prevesical space

NORMAL PELVIC ORGAN SUPPORT

The main support of the uterus and vagina is provided by the interaction between the *levator ani (LA) muscles* (**Fig. 1**) and the *connective tissue* that attaches the cervix and vagina to the pelvic walls (**Fig. 2**).[1] The relative contribution of the connective tissue and levator ani muscles to the normal support anatomy has been the subject of controversy for more than a century.[2–5] Consequently, many inconsistencies in terminology are found in the literature describing pelvic floor muscles and connective tissue. The information presented in this article is based on a current review of the literature.

LEVATOR ANI MUSCLE SUPPORT

The LA muscles are the most important muscles in the pelvic floor and represent a critical component of pelvic organ support (see **Fig. 1**). The normal levators maintain a constant state of contraction, thus providing an active floor that supports the weight of the abdominopelvic contents against the forces of intra-abdominal pressure.[6] This action is thought to prevent constant or excessive strain on the pelvic "ligaments" and "fascia" (**Fig. 3**A). The normal resting contraction of the levators is maintained by the action of type I (slow twitch) fibers, which predominate in this muscle.[7] This baseline activity of the levators keeps the urogenital hiatus (UGH) closed and draws the distal parts of the urethra, vagina, and rectum toward the pubic bones. Type II (fast twitch) muscle fibers allow for reflex muscle contraction elicited by sudden increases in abdominal pressure (**Fig. 3**B). The levators can also be voluntarily contracted as with Kegel exercises. Relaxation of the levators occurs only briefly and intermittently during the processes of evacuation (voiding, defecation) and parturition.

The LA muscle is a complex unit that consists of several muscle components with different origins and insertions, and therefore, different functions. Knowing the precise

Division of Female Pelvic Medicine and Reconstructive Pelvic Surgery, Department of Obstetrics and Gynecology, University of Texas Southwestern Medical Center 5323 Harry Hines Boulevard, Dallas, Texas 75390 9032, USA
E-mail address: marlene.corton@utsouthwestern.edu

Obstet Gynecol Clin N Am 36 (2009) 401–419
doi:10.1016/j.ogc.2009.09.002
0889-8545/09/$ – see front matter © 2009 Elsevier Inc. All rights reserved.

obgyn.theclinics.com

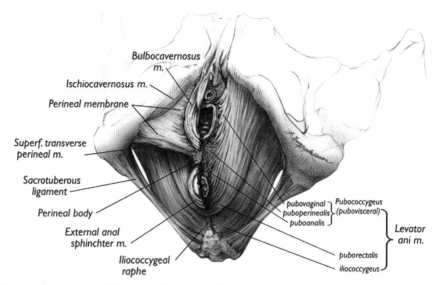

Fig. 1. Inferior view of the pelvic floor. Superficial perineal muscles and perineal membrane have been removed on the left to show attachments of the levator ani (LA) muscles to distal vagina, anus, perineal body, and perineal membrane. Note the absence of direct attachments of LA to urethra. (*Courtesy of* Lianne Kruger Sullivan, Dallas, TX; with permission.)

attachments, function, and innervation of each LA component allows better understanding of the various clinical manifestations that may result from specific injuries (ie, anterior vaginal wall prolapse and stress urinary incontinence with injury to the pubovaginal muscle).

The pubococcygeus, puborectalis, and iliococcygeus are the three components of the muscle recognized in the *Terminologia Anatomica* (see **Fig. 1**).[8] The pubococcygeus is further divided into the pubovaginalis, puboanalis, and puboperineal muscles according to fiber attachments. Because of the significant attachments of the pubococcygeus to the walls of the pelvic viscera, the term pubovisceral muscle is frequently used to describe this portion of the levator ani muscle.[9,10] In a magnetic resonance imaging (MRI) study of 80 nulliparous women with normal pelvic support, the subdivisions of the levator ani muscles were clearly visible on MR scans.[11]

The anterior ends of the pubococcygeus or pubovisceral muscle arise on either side from the inner surface of the pubic bone. The *pubovaginalis* refers to the medial fibers that attach to the lateral walls of the vagina. Although there are no direct attachments of the levator ani muscles to the urethra in females, those fibers of the muscle that attach to the vagina are responsible for elevating the urethra during a pelvic muscle contraction and hence may contribute to urinary continence (**Fig. 4**).[12] The *puboperinealis* refers to the fibers that attach to the perineal body and draw this structure toward the pubic symphysis. The *puboanalis* refers to the fibers that attach to the anus at the intersphincteric groove between the internal and external anal sphincter. These fibers elevate the anus and along with the rest of the pubococcygeus and puborectalis fibers keep the UGH closed.

The *puborectalis* fibers of the LA muscle also arise on either side from the pubic bone and form a U-shaped sling behind the anorectal junction, just above the external anal sphincter muscle. The action of the puborectalis draws the anorectal junction

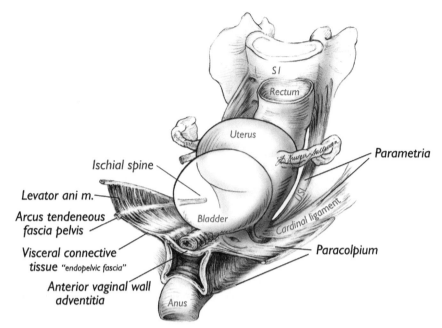

Fig. 2. Schematic representation of connective tissue support of uterus and upper two thirds of vagina. Urethra and vagina were transected just above the pelvic floor muscles. Note the continuity of the connective tissue at the level of the lower cervix. (*Courtesy of* Lianne Kruger Sullivan, Dallas, TX; with permission.)

toward the pubis, contributing to the anorectal angle (**Fig. 3**). This muscle is considered part of the anal sphincter complex; however, its role in maintenance of fecal continence remains controversial (see "Pathophysiology of Anal Incontinence, Constipation, and Defecatory Dysfunction" by Drs Marc R. Toglia and "Evaluation and Treatment of Anal Incontinence, Constipation and Defecatory Dysfunction" by Drs Tola Omotosho and Rebecca G. Rogers, also in this issue).

The *iliococcygeus*, the most posterior and thinnest part of the levators, has a primarily supportive role. It arises laterally from the arcus tendenius levator ani (ATLA) and the ischial spines, and muscle fibers from one side join those from the opposite side at the iliococcygeal (anococcygeal) raphé and the coccyx.

Levator Plate

The *levator plate* is the clinical term used to describe the region between the anus and the coccyx formed primarily by the insertion of the iliococcygeus muscles (iliococcygeal raphé) (see **Fig. 3**). This portion of the levators forms a supportive shelf upon which the rectum, the upper vagina, and the uterus rest away from the urogenital hiatus. A consequence of Berglas and Rubin[13] 1953 landmark radiographic levator myography study has been the prevailing theory that in women with normal support, the levator plate lies almost parallel to the horizontal plane in the standing position. A recent supine dynamic MRI study during Valsalva showed that the levator plate in women with normal support has a mean angle of 44.3° relative to a horizontal reference line.[14] In this study, women with prolapse had a modest but significantly greater vertical inclination (9.1°) of the levator plate during Valsalva compared with those with

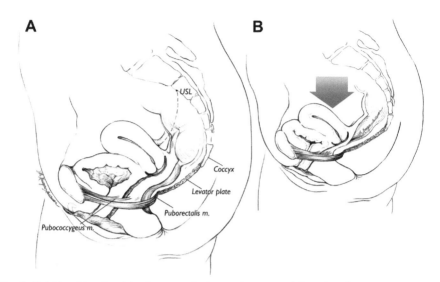

Fig. 3. Relationship of pelvic viscera and LA muscles at rest (*A*) and with increases in intra-abdominal pressure (*B*). Note anorectal angle. (*Courtesy of* Lianne Kruger Sullivan, Dallas, TX; with permission.)

normal support; they also had larger levator hiatus lengths and more inferior perineal body displacements.

Levator Ani Muscle Injury

Another existing theory suggests that neuromuscular injury to the levators may lead to eventual sagging or vertical inclination of the levator plate and lengthening of the UGH.[13,15] Consequently, the vaginal axis becomes more vertical and the cervix is oriented over the opened hiatus (**Fig. 5**). The mechanical effect of this change is to increase strain on the connective tissue "ligaments" and "fasciae" that supports the pelvic viscera. This concept does not preclude primary connective tissue damage as a potential cause of prolapse, but explains how injury to the pelvic floor muscles can eventually lead to disruption of the connective tissue component of support. However, whether vertical inclination of the levator plate or widening or lengthening of the urogenital hiatus occurs first is not known. A recent MRI study showed that 20% of primiparous women had defects in the levator ani muscles, whereas no defects were identified in nulliparous women.[16] Importantly, most defects (18%) were identified in the pubovisceral portion of the levators; only 2% involved the iliococcygeal portion of the muscle, which is the portion of the muscle that forms the levator plate. It is possible that birth-related neuromuscular injury to the pubovisceral portion of the muscle eventually leads to alterations of the iliococcygeal portion, as all muscle components are interrelated and form part of the same complex unit. Further studies are needed that correlate anatomic location of the injuries with clinical manifestations later in life.

Recent data obtained from 2-dimensional (2D) and 3D computer models of cystocele formation support clinical findings that levator ani muscle impairment as well as connective tissue impairment play a critical role in cystocele formation.[17,18]

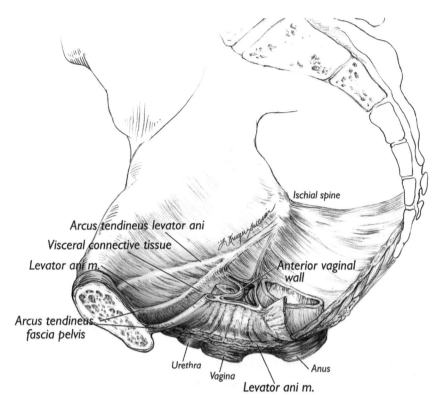

Fig. 4. Lateral view of the pelvic sidewall and floor. Pelvic organs were transected at the level of the proximal urethra. Note the anterior vaginal wall and its connective tissue connections to the ATFP provide a tissue platform that supports the urethra. The attachments of the anterior vaginal wall to the medial portion of the levator ani muscles at this level account for elevation of the urethra with increases in intra-abdominal pressure. (*Courtesy of* Lianne Kruger Sullivan, Dallas, TX; with permission.)

Levator Ani Muscle Innervation

Traditionally, a dual innervation of the levators has been described where the pelvic or superior surface of the muscles is supplied by direct efferents from the second through the fifth sacral nerve roots and the perineal or inferior surface is supplied by pudendal nerve branches. Recent literature suggests the pudendal nerve does not contribute to levator muscle innervation.[19,20] The pudendal nerve does, however, innervate parts of the striated urethral sphincter and external anal sphincter by way of separate branches (**Fig. 6**). Different innervation of the levators and the striated urethral and anal sphincters may explain why some women develop pelvic organ prolapse and others develop urinary or fecal incontinence.

Other Pelvic Floor Structures

The muscles that span the pelvic floor are collectively known as the pelvic diaphragm. This diaphragm consists of the LA and coccygeus muscles along with their superior and inferior investing layers of fasciae. Inferior to the pelvic diaphragm, the perineal membrane and perineal body also contribute to the pelvic floor (see **Fig. 1**).

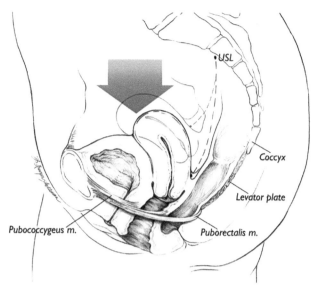

Fig. 5. Levator plate, urogenital hiatus (UGH), and vaginal axis in the presence of levator ani muscle dysfunction. Note the more vertical orientation of the levator plate and vaginal axis and the opened UGH. (*Courtesy of* Lianne Kruger Sullivan, Dallas, TX; with permission.)

Perineal Membrane (Urogenital Diaphragm)

Another area where debate has persisted for decades relates to the anatomy and function of the perineal membrane. The perineal membrane, previously known as the urogenital diaphragm,[8,21] has recently been shown to consist of two histologically, and probably functionally, distinct portions that span the opening of the anterior pelvic

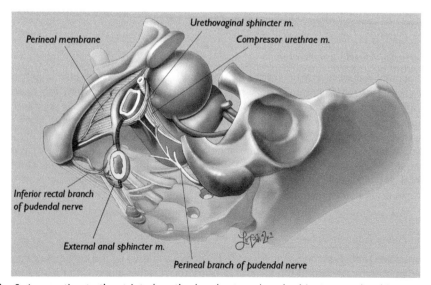

Fig. 6. Innervation to the striated urethral and external anal sphincter muscles. (*Courtesy of* Lindsay Oksenberg, Dallas, TX; with permission.)

outlet.[22] The *dorsal* or posterior portion consists of a sheet of dense fibrous tissue that attaches laterally to the ishiopubic rami and medially to the distal third of the vagina and to the perineal body (see **Fig. 1**). The *ventral* or anterior portion of the perineal membrane is intimately associated with the compressor urethra and urethrovaginal sphincter muscles, previously called the deep transverse perineal muscles in the female.[21] In addition, the *ventral* portion of the perineal membrane is continuous with the insertion of the arcus tendineus fascia pelvis. In the previously mentioned histology study, the deep or superior surface of the perineal membrane was shown to have direct connections to the levator ani muscles and the superficial or inferior surface of the membrane was fused with the vestibular bulb and clitoral crus. A follow-up MR image study showed that many of the distinct anatomic features of the perineal membrane described previously can be seen with MR.[23] In summary, the perineal membrane provides support to the distal vagina and urethra by attaching these structures to the bony pelvis. In addition, its attachments to the levator ani muscles suggest that the perineal membrane may play a more active role in support than what was previously thought.

Perineal Body

The perineal body is a mass of dense connective tissue found between the distal third of the posterior vaginal wall and the anus below the pelvic floor (see **Fig. 1**). It is formed primarily by the midline connection between the halves of the perineal membrane.[24] Distal or superficial to the perineal membrane, the medial ends of the bulbocaverno-sus and superficial transverse perineal muscles also contribute to the perineal body. Superior of deep to the perineal membrane, fibers of the pubovisceral portion of the levator ani attach to the perineal body. The perineal body has direct attachments to the posterior vaginal wall anteriorly and the external anal sphincter posteriorly. In the sagittal plane, the perineal body is triangular in shape with a base that is much wider than its apex. The apex or superior extent of the perineal body extends 2 to 3 cm above the hymeneal ring. Clinical assessment of perineal body length takes into account the anterior portion of the external anal sphincter and the vaginal and anal wall thickness. The perineal body contributes to support the distal vagina and rectum; therefore, during episiotomy repairs and perineal reconstructive procedures emphasis should placed on reapproximation of the torn ends of the anatomic structures that form the perineal body. The relationships of the perineal body in reference to posterior compartment anatomy were demonstrated in a recent MRI study.[25]

Pelvic Connective Tissue ("Ligaments" and "Fascia")

Pelvic ligaments

The term ligament is most often used to describe dense connective tissue that connects two bones. However, the "ligaments" of the pelvis are variable in composition and function. They range from connective tissue structures that contribute to support the bony pelvis and pelvic organs to smooth muscle, fibrous tissue, and loose areolar tissue structures that have no significant role in support. The sacrospinous, sacrotuberous, and anterior longitudinal ligaments of the sacrum consist of dense connective tissue that joins bony structures and contributes to the stability of the bony pelvis. The sacrospinous and anterior longitudinal ligaments serve as suture fixation sites in suspensory procedures used to correct pelvic organ prolapse. The iliopectineal (Cooper) ligament, a thickening in the periosteum of the pubic bone, is used to anchor the sutures in the Burch retropubic bladder neck suspension. The round ligaments consist of smooth muscle and fibrous tissue and the broad ligaments consist of loose areolar tissue. Although the round and broad ligaments connect the uterus and adnexa to the pelvic walls, they do not contribute to the support of these organs. The uterine "ligaments" that contribute to pelvic organ orientation and support are discussed in the following sections.

Parietal fascia

The connective tissue that invests striated muscles is termed *parietal fascia*. Histologically, this tissue consists of regular arrangements of collagen. Pelvic parietal fascia provides muscle attachment to the bony pelvis and serves as anchoring points to the visceral connective tissue known as endopelvic fascia. The *arcus tendineous levator ani (ATLA)*, a condensation of fascia covering the medial surface of the obturator internus muscle, serves as the point of origin for parts of the levator ani muscles (see **Fig. 4**). The *arcus tendineous fascia pelvis (ATFP)*, a condensation of fascia covering the medial aspect of the obturator internus and LA muscles, represents the lateral point of attachment of the anterior vaginal wall. It expands from the inner surface of the pubic bones to the ischial spines. The average length of the ATFP is 9 cm.[26]

Visceral (endopelvic) fascia

The questionable existence of a separate layer of vaginal fascia and the role of this tissue in supporting the urethra and bladder anteriorly and the rectum posteriorly has been another area where controversy has persisted for more than a century. The subperitoneal perivascular connective tissue and loose areolar tissue that exists throughout the pelvis and connects the pelvic viscera to the pelvic walls is known as endopelvic (visceral) fascia (see **Fig. 2**). This visceral "fascia," however, differs anatomically and histologically from parietal fascia, the connective tissue that invests the striated muscles of the body. Histologically, visceral fascia consists of loose arrangements of collagen, elastin, and adipose tissue, whereas parietal fascia is characterized by organized arrangements of collagen. Although parietal fascia provides attachment of muscles to bones, visceral fascia allows for expansion and contraction of the pelvic organs and encases blood vessels, lymphatics, and nerves. This tissue is intimately associated with the walls of the viscera and cannot be dissected in the same fashion that parietal fascia (ie, rectus fascia) can be separated from the corresponding skeletal muscle. Therefore, designation of this tissue as fascia has led to significant confusion.

Anterior vaginal wall

The terms pubocervical fascia and paravesical fascia are commonly used to describe the layers that support the bladder and urethra and the tissue that is used for reconstructive pelvic surgeries. However, histologic examination of the anterior vaginal wall has failed to demonstrate a separate layer of fascia between the vagina and the bladder.[3,5,27] The anterior vaginal wall has been shown to consist of three layers: a mucosal layer consisting of nonkeratinized squamous epithelium overlying a lamina propia; a muscular layer consisting of smooth muscle, collagen, and elastin; and an adventitial layer consisting of collagen and elastin. The vagina is separated from the bladder anteriorly by the vaginal adventitia (see **Fig. 2**). The tissue that attaches the lateral walls of the vagina to the ATFP is a condensation of connective tissue that contains blood vessels, lymphatics, and nerves. This paravaginal tissue attaches to the vaginal wall muscularis and adventitia on each side of the vagina and is responsible for the appearance of the anterior vaginal sulci. The vagina and bladder are not invested in their own separate layer of connective tissue capsule. Based on the histologic absence of a true "fascial" layer between the vagina and the bladder, it has been appropriately recommended that when describing the anterior vaginal wall tissue and support, terms such as "pubocervical fascia" or "paravesical fascia" be abandoned, and replaced by more accurate descriptive terms such as *vaginal muscularis* or *fibromuscular wall*.

Posterior vaginal wall

Another topic of ongoing controversy is the debatable presence of one or two separate fascial layer(s) between the vagina and the rectum.[3,4,28–30] These layers are often indiscriminately referred to as the rectovaginal septum (RVS) or rectovaginal fascia (RVF). The RVS is similar to the rectovesical septum originally described by Denonvilliers and it is believed to be a peritoneal remnant.[31] It is described as extending for 2 to 3 cm proximal to the perineal body and being absent superior to the level of the rectovaginal pouch.[4,30] However, many have failed to demonstrate a separate layer of fascia between the vagina and the rectum on histologic examination of this region.[3,32] On histologic examination of the posterior vaginal wall, DeLancey[24] showed that the paravaginal connective tissue that attaches the posterior vaginal wall to the pelvic walls attaches primarily to the lateral wall of the posterior vagina on either side; only a few connective tissue fibers were found to cross the midline between the posterior vaginal wall and rectum. Thus, similar to the anterior vaginal wall, the tissue labeled as "fascia," and the plane dissected surgically includes portions of the vaginal muscularis.

The lateral attachments of the posterior vaginal walls are to the pelvic sidewalls at another condensation of connective tissue called the ascus tendineus fascia rectovaginalis (see **Fig. 4**).[33] The apex of the posterior wall is attached to the uterosacral ligaments, which extend down to the level of the cul-de-sac peritoneum and the inferior wall has direct connections to the perineal body and the levator ani muscles.[25]

CONNECTIVE TISSUE SUPPORT

Although the visceral connective tissue in the pelvis is continuous and interdependent, DeLancey[34] has described three levels of vaginal connective tissue support that help understand various clinical manifestations of pelvic support dysfunction.

Cervical and Upper Vaginal Support

The connective tissue that attaches lateral to the uterus is called the parametria and consists of what is clinically known as the cardinal and uterosacral ligaments (see **Fig. 2**). These "ligaments" are condensations of visceral connective tissue that have assumed special supportive roles. The *cardinal (transverse cervical or Mackenrodt's) ligaments* consist primarily of perivascular connective tissue. They attach to the posterolateral pelvic walls near the origin of the internal iliac artery, and surround the vessels supplying the uterus and vagina.[35] The *uterosacral ligaments* attach to a broad area of the sacrum posteriorly and form the lateral boundaries of the posterior cul-de-sac of Douglas. They consist primarily of smooth muscle and contain some of the pelvic autonomic nerves.[36] The parametria continues down the vagina as the paracolpium. This tissue attaches the upper part of the vagina to the pelvic wall, suspending it over the pelvic floor. These attachments are also known as level I support or the suspensory axis and provide the connective tissue support to the vaginal apex after a hysterectomy.[34] In the standing position, level I support fibers are mainly vertically oriented (see **Fig. 2**). Clinical manifestations of parametrial and level I support defects include cervical and post-hysterectomy apical prolapse respectively (**Fig. 7**). In addition, recent data describe the clinical correlation between anterior and apical compartment support and the important contribution of apical support to development and size of cystoceles.[17,18,37,38]

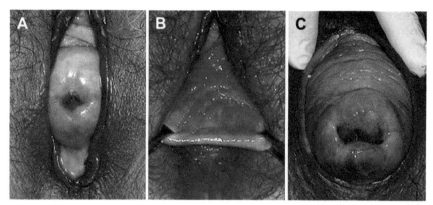

Fig. 7. Clinical manifestations of apical support defects: cervix (A), vaginal apex (B), and anterior wall prolapse (C).

Mid-Vaginal Support

The lateral walls of the mid portion of the vagina are attached to the pelvic walls on each side by visceral connective tissue (see **Fig. 3**). These lateral attachments of the anterior vaginal wall are to the ATFP and to the medial aspect of the LA muscles (see **Fig. 7**). Attachment of the anterior vaginal wall to the levators is responsible for the bladder neck elevation noted with cough or Valsalva. Therefore, these attachments may have significance for stress urinary continence.[39] The midvaginal attachments are referred to as level II support or the attachment axis.[34]

   Clinical manifestations of level II support defects include anterior vaginal wall prolapse and stress urinary incontinence (**Fig. 8**).

Distal Vaginal Support

The distal third of the vagina is directly attached to its surrounding structures. Anteriorly, the vagina is fused with the urethra, laterally it attaches to the pubovaginalis muscle and perineal membrane, and posteriorly to the perineal body (see **Fig. 1**). These vaginal attachments are referred to as level III support or fusion axis[34] and they are considered the strongest of the vaginal support components. Failure of this

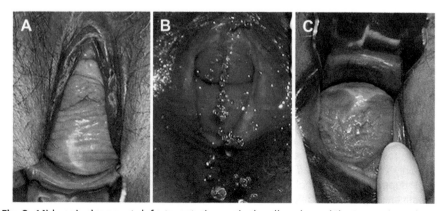

Fig. 8. Mid-vaginal support defects: anterior vaginal wall prolapse (A), stress urinary incontinence (B), and posterior wall prolapse (C).

level of support can result in distal rectoceles or perineal descent. Anal incontinence may also result if the perineal body is absent from obstetric trauma (**Fig. 9**).

VAGINAL WALL SUPPORT

Although recent studies indicate that there are altered histomorphologic features in the vaginal walls of women with pelvic organ prolapse and incontinence and that these features are accompanied by changes in the ratio of collagen subtypes and in elastic fiber homeostasis, it is currently not well understood whether these changes are the result of stretch or mechanical distention induced by the prolapse or if they contribute to the pathogenesis of prolapse and incontinence.[40–46] A recent study has challenged the theory that enteroceles are a result of defects in the fibromuscular tube of the vagina, which allows the peritoneum to come in contact with the vaginal wall epithelium. Histologic examination of the vaginal wall in patients with enteroceles showed a well-developed vaginal wall muscularis with no focal defects.[47] These findings challenge the role of vaginal wall tissue in pelvic organ support. Further investigation in this area is warranted.

The etiology of pelvic floor prolapse is complex and multifactorial. It likely includes a combination of acquired dysfunction of pelvic floor muscles and/or connective tissue as well as genetic predisposition. However, the interaction between the pelvic floor muscles and connective tissue is essential for normal pelvic organ orientation and support.

LOWER URINARY TRACT AND NERVE SUPPLY TO THE PELVIC VISCERA

The anatomy of the bladder and urethra and autonomic nerve plexuses is described in "Pathophysiology of Urinary Incontinence, Voiding Dysfunction, and Overactive Bladder" by Drs David D. Rahn and Shayzreen M. Roshanravan, also in this issue. The course of the ureter is described under the section "Surgical spaces and clinical correlations."

RECTUM AND ANAL SPHINCTER COMPLEX

The anatomy of the rectum and anal sphincter complex is described in "Evaluation and Treatment of Anal Incontinence, Constipation and Defecatory Dysfunction" by Drs Tola Omotosho and Rebecca G. Rogers, also in this issue.

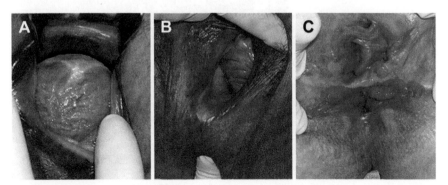

Fig. 9. Distal support defects: distal rectocele (*A*), perineal descent (*B*), and absent perineal body (*C*).

SURGICAL SPACES AND CLINICAL CORRELATIONS
Pelvic Sidewall

The retroperitoneal space of the pelvic sidewalls contains the internal iliac vessels and pelvic lymphatics, pelvic ureter, and the obturator nerve (see the following section "Retropubic Space"). Entering this space is especially useful for identifying the ureter and for ligation of the uterine or internal iliac arteries in the setting of hemorrhage.

Pelvic Ureter

The ureter enters the pelvis by crossing over the bifurcation of the common iliac artery just medial to the ovarian vessels (**Fig. 10**). It descends into the pelvis attached to the medial leaf of the pelvic sidewall peritoneum. Along this course, the ureter lays medial to the internal iliac branches and anterolateral to the uterosacral ligaments. The ureter then traverses the cardinal ligament approximately 1 cm to 2 cm lateral to the cervix. Near the level of the uterine isthmus it courses below the uterine artery ("water under the bridge"). It then travels anteromedially toward the base of the bladder, and in this path, it is in close proximity to the upper third of the anterior vaginal wall. Finally, the ureter enters the bladder and travels obliquely for approximately 1.5 cm before opening at the ureteral orifices. The pelvic ureter receives blood supply from the

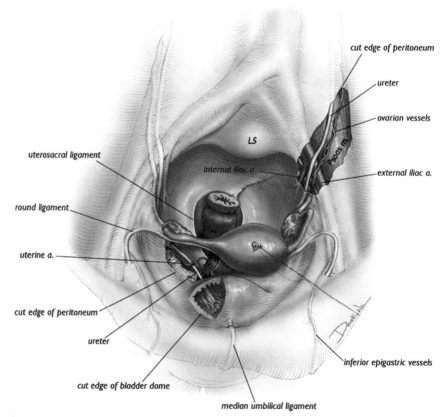

Fig. 10. Course of the pelvic ureter. (*Courtesy of* Derek Wu, Dallas, TX; with permission.)

vessels it passes: the common iliac, internal iliac, uterine, and vesicals. Vascular anastomoses on the connective tissue sheath enveloping the ureter form a longitudinal network of vessels.

Clinical correlations

Most ureteral injuries occur during gynecologic surgery for benign disease. More than 50% of these injuries are not diagnosed intraoperatively. In a study that used universal cystoscopy, the rate of ureteral injury during benign gynecologic procedures was reported to be 1.7%.[48] In the same study, a 7.3% ureteral injury rate was reported in patients undergoing concomitant procedures for urinary incontinence or pelvic organ prolapse.

The most common sites of ureteral injury include the pelvic brim area while clamping the infundibulopelvic ligament, the isthmic region while ligating the uterine vessels, and the vaginal apex while clamping or suturing the vaginal cuff. In a recent study that evaluated urinary tract injury during hysterectomy based on universal cystoscopy, the ureteral injury rate was 1.8%; the most common site of ureteral injury in this study was at the level of the uterine artery.[49] In pelvic reconstructive procedures, the ureter is especially vulnerable at the pelvic sidewall during placement of the uterosacral ligament suspension (USLS) sutures. Ureteral injury rates of up 11% have been reported during USLS.[50] The ureter can also be injured during plication of the anterior vaginal wall or placement of the apical sutures in a paravaginal defect repair. A 2% rate of ureteral injury during anterior colporrhaphy has been reported.[51] A ureteral obstruction rate of 5.1% was recently reported during vaginal surgery for anterior and/or apical pelvic organ prolapse.[52] Because of the pelvic ureter's proximity to many structures encountered during gynecologic surgery, emphasis should be placed on its precise intraoperative identification. Several cadaver dissection studies have recently described the relationship of the ureter to the uterosacral ligaments and upper third of the vagina.[53–55]

Presacral Space

The presacral space is a retroperitoneal space located between the sacrum posteriorly and the rectosigmoid and posterior abdominal wall peritoneum anteriorly (**Fig. 11**). It begins below the aortic bifurcation and extends inferiorly to the pelvic floor. The internal iliac vessels and branches and the ureters constitute the lateral boundaries of this space. Contained within the loose areolar and connective tissue in this space are the superior hypogastric plexus, hypogastric nerves, and portions of the inferior hypogastric plexus (see the article, Pathophysiology of Urinary Incontinence, Voiding Dysfunction, and Overactive Bladder by Rahn and Roshanravan, also in this issue). The vascular anatomy of the presacral space is complex and includes an extensive and intricate venous plexus (sacral venous plexus) formed primarily by the anastomoses of the middle and lateral sacral veins on the anterior surface of the sacrum. The middle sacral vein commonly drains into the left common iliac vein, whereas the lateral sacral vein opens into the internal iliac. Ultimately, these vessels drain into the caval system. The sacral venous plexus also receives contributions from the lumbar veins of the posterior abdominal wall and from the basivertebral veins that pass through the pelvic sacral foramina. The median sacral artery, which courses in proximity to the median sacral vein, arises from the posterior and distal part of the abdominal aorta. In a recent study that looked at the vascular anatomy of the presacral space in unembalmed female cadavers, the left common iliac vein was the closest major vessel identified both cephalad and lateral to the midsacral promontory.[56]

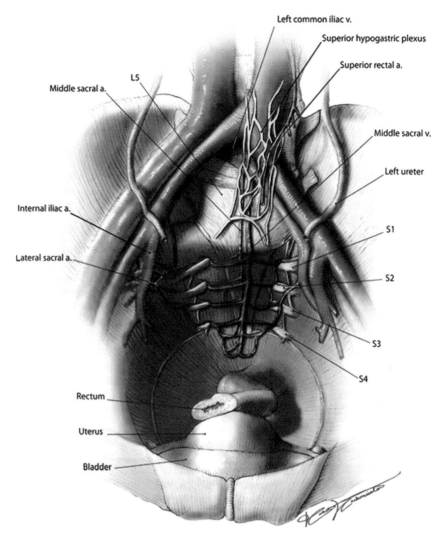

Fig. 11. Presacral space. (*Courtesy of* Robert Werkmeister, Dallas, TX; with permission.)

The average distance of the left common iliac vein to the midsacral promontory in this study was 2.7 cm (range 0.9 to 5.2 cm).

Clinical correlation

The presacral space is most commonly entered to perform abdominal sacral colpopexies and presacral neurectomies. The proximity of the left common iliac vein to the sacral promontory makes this vessel especially vulnerable to injury during entrance and dissection in this space. Additionally, bleeding from the sacral venous plexus may be difficult to control, as the veins often retract into the sacral foramina. Therefore, careful dissection and knowledge of the presacral space vascular anatomy is essential to prevent or minimize potentially life-threatening vascular complications.

Retropubic Space

This space is also called the prevesical space or space of Retzius (**Fig. 12**). It can be entered by perforating the transversalis fascial layer of the anterior abdominal wall. This space is bounded by the bony pelvis and muscles of the pelvic wall anteriorly and laterally and by the anterior abdominal wall superiorly. The bladder and proximal urethra lie posterior to this space. Attachments of the paravaginal connective tissue to the arcus tendineus fascia pelvis constitute the posterolateral limit of the space and separate it from the vesicovaginal and vesicocervical spaces. There are a number of vessels and nerves in this space. The dorsal vein of the clitoris passes under the lower border of the pubic symphysis and drains into the vesical venous plexus, also termed the plexus of Santorini. The obturator neurovascular bundle courses along the lateral pelvic walls and enters the obturator canal to reach the medial compartment of the thigh. Additionally, in most women, accessory obturator vessels that arise from the inferior epigastric or external iliac vessels are found crossing the superior pubic rami and connecting with the obturator vessels near the obturator canal.[57]

Clinical correlations

Injury to the obturator neurovascular bundle or accessory obturator vessels is most often associated with pelvic lymph node dissections and paravaginal defect repair procedures. Thus, knowledge of the approximate location of these vessels and of the obturator canal is critical when this space is dissected. The obturator canal is found approximately 5 to 6 cm from the midline of the pubic symphysis and 1 to 2 cm below the upper margin of the iliopectineal (Cooper) ligament.[57] Bleeding from the vesical venous plexus is often encountered while placing the sutures or passing

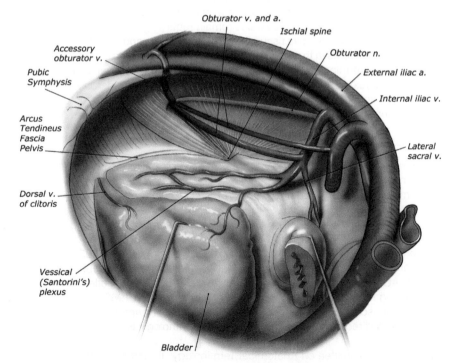

Fig. 12. Retropubic space. (*Courtesy of* Genevra Garrett, Dallas, TX; with permission.)

the needles into this space during retropubic bladder neck suspensions and midurethral retropubic procedures, respectively. This venous bleeding usually stops when pressure is applied or the sutures are tied.

With the advent of midurethral slings, anti-incontinence procedures once requiring entry and direct visualization of the retropubic space have declined. In addition, several transvaginal mesh devices have recently been developed and marketed as minimally invasive approaches to pelvic floor repair. Of these, procedures aimed to correct anterior compartment defects involve the blind passage of needles and trocars through the retropubic space. As a result, pelvic surgeons are growing increasingly less familiar with the 3D anatomic relationships within this space. In a recent cadaver study that evaluated the anatomic relationships of clinically relevant structures in the retropubic space, the obturator vein was the closest of the obturator neurovascular structures to the ischial spine, median distance 3.4 cm.[58] The vesical venous plexus included two to five rows of veins that coursed within the paravaginal tissue parallel to the bladder and drained into the internal iliac veins. The internal iliac vein was formed cephalad to the level of the ischial spine; the closest distance between these structures was 3.8 (1.6 to 6.2) cm.

The retropubic space is a richly vascular potential space with considerable variation of its vascular structures. A thorough understanding of the relationship of bony landmarks to neurovascular structures within this space becomes increasingly important as the popularity and widespread use of procedures that rely on blind placement of trocars increases.

SUMMARY

Significant contributions recently made to the area of pelvic support anatomy have led to our better understanding of pelvic organ dysfunction and the role of parturition on pelvic floor injury. However, controversies remain regarding the precise anatomy and function of the pelvic connective tissue, levator ani muscles, and vaginal walls, and the specific role that defects in these structures play in the genesis of pelvic floor dysfunction. Inconsistent terminology is commonly found, and incorrect terminology is perpetuated in classic texts and publications. Efforts to clarify and standardize terminology as well as techniques to analyze the interactive role of the supporting structures in their 3D environment should continue.

REFERENCES

1. Corton MM. Anatomy of the pelvis: how the pelvis is built for support. Clin Obstet Gynecol 2005;48:611–26.
2. Paramore RH. The supports-in-chief of the female pelvic viscera. J Obstet Gynaecol Br Emp 1908;13:391–409.
3. Ricci JV, Thom CH. The myth of a surgically useful fascia in vaginal plastic reconstructions. Q Rev Surg Obstet Gynecol 1954;2:253–61.
4. Uhlenhuth E, Nolley GW. Vaginal fascia, a myth? Obstet Gynecol 1957;10:349–58.
5. Weber AM, Walter MD. What is vaginal fascia? AUGS Quart Rep 1995;13 [report].
6. Parks AG, Porter NH, Melzak J. Experimental study of the reflex mechanisms controlling muscles of the pelvic floor. Dis Colon Rectum 1962;5:407–14.
7. Heit M, Benson T, Russell B, et al. Levator ani muscle in women with genitourinary prolapse: indirect assessment by muscle histopathology. Neurourol Urodyn 1996; 15:17–29.
8. Federative Committee on Anatomical Terminology. Terminologia anatomica. New York: Thieme; 1998. Stuttgart (Germany).

9. Lawson JO. Pelvic anatomy. I. Pelvic floor muscles. Ann R Coll Surg Engl 1974;54: 244–52.
10. Kerney R, Sawhney R, DeLancey JOL. Levator ani muscle anatomy evaluated by origin-insertion pairs. Obstet Gynecol 2004;104:168–73.
11. Margulies RU, Hsu Y, Kearney R, et al. Appearance of the levator ani muscle subdivisions in magnetic resonance images. Obstet Gynecol 2006;107(5): 1064–9.
12. DeLancey JOL, Starr RA. Histology of the connection between the vagina and levator ani muscles: implications for the urinary function. J Reprod Med 1990; 35:765–71.
13. Berglas B, Rubin IC. The study of the supportive structures of the uterus by levator myography. Surg Gynecol Obstet 1953;97:677–92.
14. Hsu Y, Summers A, Hussain HK, et al. Levator plate angle in women with pelvic organ prolapse compared to women with normal support using dynamic MR imaging. Am J Obstet Gynecol 2006;194:1427–33.
15. Smith ARB, Hosker GL, Warrel DW. The role of partial denervation of the pelvic floor in the etiology of genitourinary prolapse and stress incontinence of urine: a neurophysiologic study. Br J Obstet Gynaecol 1989;96:24–8.
16. DeLancey JOL, Kearney R, Chou Q, et al. The appearance of levator ani muscle abnormalities in magnetic resonance images after vaginal deliveries. Obstet Gynecol 2003;101:46–53.
17. Chen L, Ashton-Miller JA, Hsu Y, et al. Interaction among apical support, levator ani impairment, and anterior vaginal wall prolapse. Obstet Gynecol 2006;108: 324–32.
18. Chen L, Ashton-Miller JA, Delancey JOL. A 3D finite element model of anterior vaginal wall support to evaluate mechanisms underlying cystocele formation. J Biomech 2009;42:1371–7.
19. Barber MD, Bremer RE, Thor KB, et al. Innervation of the female levator ani muscles. Am J Obstet Gynecol 2002;187:64–71.
20. Pierce LM, Reyes M, Thor KB, et al. Innervation of the levator ani muscles in the female squirrel monkey. Am J Obstet Gynecol 2003;188:1141–7.
21. Oelrich TM. The striated urogenital sphincter muscle in the female. Anat Rec 1983;205:223–32.
22. Stein TA, DeLancey JO. Structure of the perineal membrane in females: gross and microscopic anatomy. Obstet Gynecol 2008;111:686–93.
23. Brandon CJ, Lewicky-Gaupp C, Larson KA, et al. Anatomy of the perineal membrane as seen in magnetic resonance images of nulliparous women. Am J Obstet Gynecol 2009;200:583.e1–6.
24. DeLancey JOL. Structural anatomy of the posterior pelvic compartment as it relates to rectocele. Am J Obstet Gynecol 1999;180:815–23.
25. Hsu Y, Lewicky-Gaupp C, DeLancey JO. Posterior compartment anatomy as seen in magnetic resonance imaging and 3-dimensional reconstruction from asymptomatic nulliparas. Am J Obstet Gynecol 2008;198:651.e1–7.
26. Albright TS, Gehrich AP, Davis GD, et al. Arcus tendineus fascia pelvis: a further understanding. Am J Obstet Gynecol 2005;193:677–81.
27. Weber AM, Walters MD. Anterior vaginal prolapse: review of anatomy and techniques of surgical repair. Obstet Gynecol 1997;89:311–8.
28. Milley PS, Nichols DH. A correlative investigation of the human rectovaginal septum. Anat Rec 1969;163:443–51.
29. Richardson AC. The rectovaginal septum revisited: its relationship to rectocele and its importance in rectocele repair. Clin Obstet Gynecol 1993;36:976–83.

30. Kuhn RJP, Hollyock VE. Observations of the anatomy of the rectovaginal pouch and rectovaginal septum. Obstet Gynecol 1982;59:445.

31. Denonvilliers CP. Propositions et observation d'anatomie, de physiologie at de pathologie. These de l'Ecole de Medicine 1837;285:23 [in French].

32. Kleeman SD, Westermann C, Karram MM. Rectoceles and the anatomy of the posteriorvaginal wall: revisited. Am J Obstet Gynecol 2005;193(6):2050–5.

33. Leffler KS, Thompson JR, Cundiff GW, et al. Attachment of the rectovaginal septum to the pelvic sidewall. Am J Obstet Gynecol 2001;185:41–3.

34. DeLancey JOL. Anatomic aspects of vaginal eversion after hysterectomy. Am J Obstet Gynecol 1992;166:1717.

35. Range RL, Woodburne RT. The gross and microscopic anatomy of the transverse cervical ligaments. Am J Obstet Gynecol 1964;90:460–7.

36. Campbell RM. The anatomy and histology of the sacrouterine ligaments. Am J Obstet Gynecol 1950;59:1–12.

37. Rooney K, Kenton K, Mueller ER, et al. Advanced anterior vaginal wall prolapse is highly correlated with apical prolapse. Am J Obstet Gynecol 2006;195:1837–40.

38. Summers A, Winkel LA, Hussain HK, et al. The relationship between anterior and apical compartment support. Am J Obstet Gynecol 2006;194:1438–43.

39. DeLancey JOL. Structural support of the urethra as it relates to stress urinary incontinence: the Hammock hypothesis. Am J Obstet Gynecol 1994;170:1713–20.

40. Falconer C, Ekman G, Malmström A, et al. Decreased collagen synthesis in stress-incontinent women. Obstet Gynecol 1994;84:583–6.

41. Fitzgerald MP, Mollenhauer J, Hale DS, et al. Urethral collagen morphologic characteristics among women with genuine stress incontinence. Am J Obstet Gynecol 2000;182:1565–74.

42. Boreham MK, Wai CY, Miller RT, et al. Morphometric analysis of smooth muscle in the anterior vaginal wall of women with pelvic organ prolapse. Am J Obstet Gynecol 2002;187:56–63.

43. Boreham MK, Wai CY, Miller RT, et al. Morphometric properties of the posterior vaginal wall in women with pelvic organ prolapse. Am J Obstet Gynecol 2002;187:1501–8.

44. Wong MY, Harmanli OH, Agar M, et al. Collagen content of nonsupport tissue in pelvic organ prolapse and stress urinary incontinence. Am J Obstet Gynecol 2003;189:1597–9.

45. Drewes PG, Yanagisawa H, Starcher B, et al. Pelvic organ prolapse in fibulin-5 knockout mice: pregnancy changes in elastic fiber homeostasis in mouse vagina. Am J Pathol 2007;170:578–9.

46. Rahn DD, Ruff MD, Brown SA, et al. Biomechanical properties of the vaginal wall: effect of pregnancy, elastic fiber deficiency, and pelvic organ prolapse. Am J Obstet Gynecol 2008;198:590.e1–6.

47. Tulikangas PK, Walters MD, Brainard JA, et al. Enterocele: is there a histologic defect. Obstet Gynecol 2001;98:634–7.

48. Vakili B, Chesson RR, Kyle BL, et al. The incidence of urinary tract injury during hysterectomy: a prospective analysis based on universal cystoscopy. Am J Obstet Gynecol 2005;192:1599–604.

49. Ibeanu OA, Chesson RR, Echols KT, et al. Urinary tract injury during hysterectomy based on universal cystoscopy. Obstet Gynecol 2009;113:6–10.

50. Barber MD, Visco AG, Weidner AC, et al. Bilateral uterosacral ligament vaginal vault suspension with site-specific endopelvic fascia defect repair for treatment of pelvic organ prolapse. Am J Obstet Gynecol 2001;185:1009.

51. Kwon CH, Goldberg RP, Koduri S, et al. The use of intraoperative cystoscopy in major vaginal and urogynecologic surgeries. Obstet Gynecol 2002;187:1466–72.

52. Gustilo-Ashby AM, Jelovsek JE, Barber MD, et al. The incidence of ureteral obstruction and the value of intraoperative cystoscopy during vaginal surgery for pelvic organ prolapse. Am J Obstet Gynecol 2006;194:1478–85.
53. Buller JR, Thompson JR, Cundiff GW, et al. Uterosacral ligament: description of anatomic relationships to optimize surgical safety. Obstet Gynecol 2001;97: 873–9.
54. Rahn DD, Bleich AT, Wai CY, et al. Anatomic relationships of the distal third of the pelvic ureter, trigone, and urethra in unembalmed female cadavers. Am J Obstet Gynecol 2007;197:668.e1–4.
55. Wieslander CK, Roshanravan SM, Wai CY, et al. Uterosacral ligament suspension sutures: anatomic relationships in unembalmed female cadavers. Am J Obstet Gynecol 2007;197:672.e1–6.
56. Wieslander CK, Rahn DD, McIntire DD, et al. Vascular anatomy of the presacral space in unembalmed female cadavers. Am J Obstet Gynecol 2006;195: 1736–41.
57. Drewes PG, Marinis SI, Schaffer JI, et al. Vascular anatomy over the superior pubic rami in female cadavers. Am J Obstet Gynecol 2005;193:2165–8.
58. Pathi SD, Castellanos ME, Corton MM. Variability of the retropubic space anatomy in female cadavers. Am J Obstet Gynecol. September 19, 2009 [Epub ahead of print].

Epidemiology of Pelvic Floor Dysfunction

Vivian W. Sung, MD, MPH*, Brittany Star Hampton, MD

KEYWORDS

- Pelvic floor disorders • Urinary incontinence • Pelvic prolapse
- Anal incontinence • Epidemiology • Prevalence

Female pelvic floor dysfunction includes urinary incontinence, pelvic organ prolapse, anal incontinence, sensory abnormalities of the lower urinary tract, defecatory dysfunction, and chronic pain syndromes related to the pelvic organs. Epidemiologic data for some of these conditions have significantly increased in the past decade. This article updates the previous review[1] and focuses on the epidemiology of urinary incontinence, pelvic organ prolapse, anal incontinence, and painful bladder conditions.

EPIDEMIOLOGY
Urinary Incontinence

Prevalence rates
The definition of urinary incontinence is highly variable among clinicians, epidemiologists, and patients. The International Continence Society (ICS) defines urinary incontinence as "the complaint of any involuntary leakage of urine," providing a good clinical definition for patient evaluation.[2] However, the generalized lack of agreement on an epidemiologic definition of incontinence has limited the ability to obtain precise and consistent estimates of prevalence, incidence, and remission rates. In addition, differences in target populations, study and survey methodology, and questionnaire design increase the variability of estimates between studies.[3]

Table 1 demonstrates the variation in definitions of urinary incontinence and estimates of prevalence, incidence, and remission rates in the literature. Prevalence rates reflect the total number of cases of disease in the population at a given time. A review of 21 studies by Thom[4] revealed that the pooled mean prevalence for older women was 34% for any incontinence and 12% for daily incontinence. Among middle-aged and younger adults, the pooled mean prevalence was 25%. Stress incontinence was more common in younger women, whereas urge and mixed incontinence was more common in older women.

Using a more strict definition of "at least weekly leakage or monthly leakage more than drops," Nygaard and colleagues[5] reported a 15.7% prevalence in the United

Department of Obstetrics and Gynecology, Division of Urogynecology and Reconstructive Pelvic Surgery, Women and Infants Hospital of Rhode Island and Alpert Medical School at Brown University, 695 Eddy Street, lower level, Providence, RI 02903, USA
* Corresponding author.
E-mail address: vsung@wihri.org (V.W. Sung).

Obstet Gynecol Clin N Am 36 (2009) 421–443
doi:10.1016/j.ogc.2009.08.002
0889-8545/09/$ – see front matter © 2009 Elsevier Inc. All rights reserved.

Table 1
Definitions and prevalence rates of urinary incontinence

Study	Definition	Population	Prevalence (%)
Hannestad et al[12]	Any involuntary loss of urine	Norway >20 years of age	25
Melville et al[9]	At least monthly incontinence	United States (Washington State) 30–90 years	45
Irwin et al[14]	Any involuntary loss of urine	Sweden, Germany, Italy, Canada, UK >18 years of age	13.1
Waetjen et al[7]	At least monthly incontinence	United States 42–52 years of age	46.7
Dooley et al[6]	Incontinence past 12 months	United States >20 years of age	49.6
Nygaard et al[5]	At least weekly leakage or monthly leakage more than drops	United States >20 years	15.7

States in women 20 years of age or older. In contrast, Dooley and colleagues[6] reported a higher prevalence of 49.6%, using the definition of any amount of incontinence during the past 12 months. Waetjen and colleagues[7] reported that, in middle-aged women, changing the definition from at least monthly to at least weekly incontinence decreased the prevalence estimates in the same population from 46.7% to 15.3%, respectively.

Prevalence rates also vary depending on the severity of symptoms. Melville and colleagues[8] measured urinary incontinence severity based on the Sandvik Severity Index, which incorporates the frequency and amount of urine loss.[9] In this study, the prevalence of slight incontinence was 9%, moderate was 15%, and severe was 18%. The prevalence also varies depending on the type of incontinence (**Fig. 1**). The prevalence of stress incontinence ranges from 12% to 25%,[6,10] urge incontinence ranges from 1.6% to 9.9%,[10,11] and mixed incontinence ranges from 9% to 17%.[6,12]

Another aspect of incontinence severity that deserves mention is how bothered a woman is by her symptoms. Large-scale epidemiologic studies can be limited in the rigor with which patient bother is assessed to limit the burden of a lengthy questionnaire. In addition, many women who suffer from lower urinary tract symptoms are extremely bothered even if they do not have urinary incontinence. In 3 large, multinational, population-based studies, the prevalence of lower urinary tract symptoms ranged from 59.2% to 76.3%, but the prevalence of actual incontinence ranged from 9.3% to 14.8%.[13–15] A large epidemiologic study of community-dwelling women in the United States by Lukacz and colleagues[16] reported that women with frequent daytime or nighttime voiding had twofold higher bother scores compared with unaffected women, and that increases in voiding frequency incrementally increased patient bother. This finding highlights the point that many women have bothersome symptoms even though they do not have incontinence.

Race and age on incontinence prevalence Most epidemiologic studies have included predominantly white populations, with conflicting results about the effect of race or ethnicity on incontinence. Nygaard and colleagues[5] found no differences in prevalence rates between Hispanic, non-Hispanic whites, non-Hispanic blacks, and other

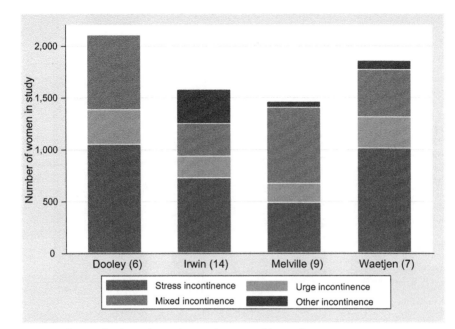

Fig. 1. Prevalence of urinary incontinence by type of incontinence.

races, whereas Dooley and colleagues[6] found that white and Mexican American women had almost double the prevalence rates for stress incontinence compared with blacks, but blacks had a higher rate of urge incontinence (11% compared with 7.5% for white and Mexican American women).

Thom and colleagues[17] specifically evaluated differences in incontinence prevalence among major race and ethnic groups in the Reproductive Risks of Incontinence Study at Kaiser (RRISK) and found that the prevalence for all types of incontinence was highest in Hispanic women (36%), followed by white (30%), black (25%) and Asian American (19%) women. After adjusting for other covariates, including age, the risk of weekly incontinence was higher among Hispanic women, but lower in Asian American and black women compared with white women. Additional analysis from the RRISK suggests that incontinence is significantly associated with a decrease in quality of life, and this effect does not vary significantly by race.[18]

The Establishing the Prevalence of Incontinence (EPI) study focused on comparing incontinence prevalence between white and black women. In this study, Fenner and colleagues[19] reported that a significantly higher proportion of white women reported stress incontinence compared with black women (39.2% vs 25%, respectively), whereas a greater proportion of black women reported urge incontinence compared with white women (23.8% vs 11%, respectively). This study also found that half of black incontinent women reported losing urine to the point of wetting their pad or underwear, whereas only a third of white women reported this degree of severity. In contrast to previous studies,[20] the EPI study showed that, other than race, risk factors for incontinence were similar between black and white women, including increased age, mobility impairment, constipation, obesity, and depressive symptoms.

The prevalence of incontinence increases with age (**Fig. 2**).[5,9,14,21] Nygaard and colleagues[5] reported that the prevalence of incontinence in women in the United States over the age of 80 years was 31.7% compared with women aged 40 to 59 years

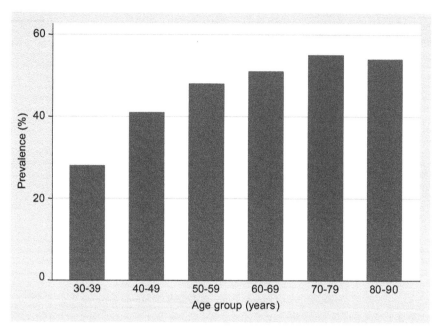

Fig. 2. Prevalence of urinary incontinence by decade of life. (*Data from* Melville JL, Katon W, Delaney K, et al. Urinary incontinence in US women. Arch Intern Med 2005;165:537–42.)

with a prevalence of 17.2%. Other reported risk factors for incontinence include co-morbidities such as diabetes mellitus, obesity, parity, and prior hysterectomy.[7,22–24]

Incidence, remission, improvement and progression rates
Urinary incontinence is a dynamic condition and many factors may contribute to the incidence, progression, improvement, or even remission of symptoms. Rates are summarized in **Table 2**. Incidence rates reflect the number of new cases of disease in the population during a specified period of time. In general, young to middle-aged women have reduced incidence rates compared with older women. The average 1-year incidence is estimated to range from 6.9%[25] to 11.1%[7] in the United States in women younger than 55 years. In older women 54 to 79 years, the annual incidence is 13.8% for developing any incontinence.[26] In a study by Komesu and colleagues,[21] the 4-year cumulative incidence of women 50 years or older ranged from 12.7% to 33.8%.

Data on remission, improvement, and progression of incontinence are more limited. Average 1-year remission rates (resolution of symptoms) range from 4.6% to 9.1%.[21,25–27] Annual improvement rates in symptom severity range from 4.5% to 16%[25,26] and 1 estimate of symptom progression is 16%.[26] Many of these large epidemiologic studies are unable to control for ongoing or previous treatments of incontinence, which may affect remission and improvement rate estimates.

Urinary incontinence costs
The financial burden of incontinence includes direct and indirect costs. Direct costs include routine care (absorbent products and laundry), medical visits and treatments, and treatment complications or failures. Indirect costs are more difficult to estimate, and include loss of productivity and costs of paid or unpaid caregivers.

Table 2
Incidence and remission rates of urinary incontinence

Study	Population	Incidence	Remission/Progression
Townsend et al[25]	United States 36–55 years of age	Any incontinence: 13.7%/2 years Monthly incontinence: 10.1%/2 years Weekly incontinence: 3.7%/2 years	Remission: 13.9%/2 years Improvement: 32.8%/2 years
Lifford et al[26]	United States 54–79 years of age	Any incontinence: 27.6%/2 years Monthly incontinence: 9.2%/2 years Severe incontinence: 1.4%/2 years	Remission: 10.3%/2 years Progression: 32.1%/2 years Improvement: 8.9%/2 years
Waetjen et al[7]	United States 42–52 years of age	Monthly incontinence: 11.1%/1 year	–
Komesu et al[21]	United States >50 years of age	Any incontinence: 15.8%/4 years	Remission: 36.3%/4 years Progression: 6.7%/4 years Improvement: 45.8%/4 years

In 2001, Wilson and colleagues[28] estimated the annual direct cost of incontinence (including routine care, diagnostics, evaluations, treatments, and complications) in women to be $12.4 billion, with the largest cost category being routine care (70% of all costs), followed by nursing home admissions (14%), treatment (9%), complications (6%), and diagnosis and evaluations (1%). Surgical therapy accounted for 88% of treatment costs in this study. In 2005, Thom and colleagues[29] estimated the economic impact of incontinence using multiple national databases, and found that medical expenditures for inpatient and outpatient care for Medicare beneficiaries 65 years of age or older doubled from $128.1 million in 1992 to $234.4 million in 1998. Although unable to estimate a cost associated with loss of productivity, the study showed that 23% of incontinent women missed an average of 28.7 hours of work for inpatient and outpatient care. It is estimated that for stress incontinence, direct costs of medical care for surgical patients without comorbidities was $13,212 per patient.[30] Another study estimated that, for community women, the total economic cost of overactive bladder was $7.4 billion in 2000 dollars.[31]

Subak and colleagues[32–34] provided more accurate estimates of the individual economic costs for routine incontinence care. The annual direct cost of routine care ranged from $250 to $900 in 2005 dollars per woman.[31–34]

Pelvic Organ Prolapse

Prevalence

Pelvic organ prolapse is defined by the ICS as the descent of 1 or more of: the anterior vaginal wall, the posterior vaginal wall, and the apex of the vagina or vault.[2] Currently, most epidemiologic studies define prolapse based on examination or patient symptom report, but not both (**Table 3**). Two studies from the Women's Health

Table 3
Prevalence, incidence, and remission rates of pelvic organ prolapse

Study	Definition	Prevalence	Incidence	Remission/Progression
Swift et al[127]	Pelvic organ prolapse quantification	6.4% stage 0 43.3% stage 1 47.7% stage 2 2.6% stage 3		
Hendrix et al[36]	Women's Health Initiative grading system (grades 1, 2 or 3)	Any prolapse: 41.1% Cystocele: 34.3% Uterine: 14.2% Rectocele: 18.6%		
Handa et al[35]	Women's Health Initiative grading system (grades 1, 2 or 3)	Cystocele: 24.6% Uterine: 3.8% Recocele: 12.9%	(Grades 1, 2, or 3) Cystocele: 9.3/100 women-years Uterine: 1.5/100 women-years Rectocele: 5.7/100 women-years	Remission: Rectocele: 3%/1 year Cystocele: 9%/1 year Progression: Rectocele: 14%/1 year Cystocele: 9.5%/1 year Uterine: 1.9%/1 year
Nygaard et al[39]	Pelvic organ prolapse quantification	2.3% stage 0 33% stage 1 63% stage 2 1.9% stage 3 25.6% based on leading edge ≥ 0		
Bradley et al[38]	Pelvic organ prolapse quantification	23.5%–49.4%	26%/1 year 40%/3 years	1-year remission: 21% 3-year remission: 19%
Rortveit et al[41]	Patient symptoms past 12 months (not confirmed by examination)	5.7%		
Nygaard et al[5]	Affirmative to "Do you experience bulging or something falling out you can see or feel in the vaginal area?"	2.9%		

Initiative (WHI) including women in the United States aged 50 to 79 years reported the prevalence of any degree of prolapse (grades 1–3) based on examination to be 41.1%.[35,36] The prevalence of cystocele was 24.6% to 34.3%, rectocele was 12.9% to 18.6%, and uterine prolapse was 3.8% to 14.2%. Two ancillary studies from a midwestern site for the WHI measured prolapse based on the Pelvic Organ Prolapse Quantification (POPQ)[37] examination and used a more clinically useful definition of prolapse at or beyond the hymen.[38,39] They reported the prevalence of prolapse to be 23.5% to 49.4% during a 4-year follow-up period. These studies did not consider patient symptoms.

Other studies have defined prolapse solely based on patient symptoms, most commonly as an affirmative response to the question: "Do you experience bulging or something falling out that you can see or feel in the vaginal area?" Using this definition, the prevalence of prolapse symptoms ranges from 2.9% to 5.7% in the United States.[5,40,41] An ancillary study of the WHI by Bradley and colleagues[40] using patient examination and symptoms reported that obstructive urinary symptoms and seeing/feeling a bulge were symptoms most commonly associated with prolapse on examination.

Risk factors for prolapse cited in the literature include age, body mass index (BMI, calculated as weight in kilograms divided by the square of height in meters), and higher vaginal parity.[5,35,36,38,41] Two studies have reported that African American women are at lower risk for prolapse compared with white women.[36,41]

Incidence and remission

There are limited data regarding the natural history of pelvic organ prolapse (see **Table 3**). A study by Handa and colleagues[35] using data from a 2 to 8-year time period from one WHI site reported the incidence of grades 1 to 3 to be 9.3/100 women-years for cystocele, 5.7/100 women-years for rectocele, and 1.5/100 women-years for uterine prolapse. This study also reported that the remission rate from grade 2 to 3 prolapse to grade 0 was 9% for cystocele and 3% for rectocele. There were no observed remissions for women with grade 2 to 3 uterine prolapse. Prolapse progression rates during this time period from grade 1 to grades 2 to 3 was 9.5% for cystocele, 14% for rectocele, and 1.9% for uterine prolapse.

Another study by Bradley and colleagues[38] used data from a 4-year period from a different WHI site. Defining prolapse based on POPQ examination at or beyond the hymen, the 1-year incidence rate was 26% and 3-year incidence was 40%. The 1-year and 3-year regression rates were 21% and 19%, respectively. Older parous women were more likely to develop new or progressive prolapse than to regress. In general, mild prolapse appeared to be a fluid state, but progression and resolution were dependent on the baseline severity of prolapse.

Costs

Data regarding the economic impact of pelvic organ prolapse are limited. One study by Subak and colleagues[42] estimated the direct costs of pelvic organ prolapse surgery based on 1997 national average Medicare reimbursement to be $1012 million, including $494 million for vaginal hysterectomy, $279 million for cystocele and rectocele repair, and $135 million for abdominal hysterectomy. Physician services accounted for 29% and hospitalization accounted for 71% of total costs. There is little information regarding costs of ambulatory care, or indirect costs associated with pelvic organ prolapse.

Anal Incontinence

Prevalence, incidence, and remission

Anal incontinence includes involuntary passage of gas, mucus, liquid, or solid stool. Similar to other pelvic floor disorders, prevalence rates are highly dependent on definitions. Most epidemiologic studies include incontinence of stool only, or fecal incontinence, and do not include flatal incontinence.

Depending on the definition used, the prevalence of fecal incontinence ranges from 2.2% to 24% in women in the United States[5,43–48] (**Table 4**). Results from the RRISK cohort reported the overall prevalence of fecal incontinence to be 24%, including 19% with less than monthly accidents, 3% with monthly, 2% with at least weekly, and less than 1% with daily fecal incontinence.[47] In this study, the overall prevalence of flatal incontinence was 71%, and 40% of women reported fecal and flatal incontinence. Whitehead and colleagues[48] reported that in the United States, 6.4% of women reported leakage of liquid stool, 2% solid stool, and 3% mucus at least once in the past month.

Table 4			
Prevalence of anal incontinence			
Study	**Definition**	**Population Age**	**Prevalence**
Nelson et al[46]	Affirmative to "... unwanted or unexpected or embarrassing loss of control of bowels or gas" past year	N/A	2.2% (men and women)
Goode et al[44]	Affirmative to "... loss of control of your bowels, even a small amount that stained the underwear?" past year	65–106 years	11.6%
Melville et al[45]	At least monthly loss of liquid or solid stool	30–90 years	7.2%
Bharucha et al[43]	Affirmative to "... accidental leakage of liquid or solid stool?" past year	20–80+ years	12.1 per 100 women (age-adjusted)
Varma et al[47]	Affirmative to "...leakage of stool, accidents or soiling because of inability to control passage of stool until you reach the toilet?" past year	40–69 years	24%
Nygaard et al[5]	At least monthly leakage of solid, liquid or mucous stool	≥20 years	9%
Whitehead et al[48]	Accidental leakage of solid, liquid or mucus at least once in past month	≥20 years	8.9%

Most studies report a significant effect of age on increasing risk of fecal inconti-nence.[45,47–49] Whitehead and colleagues[48] reported that for each 10-year increase in age, the adjusted odds of prevalent fecal incontinence increased by 1.20 (95% CI 1.10–1.31). The impact of race is inconsistent in the literature, with some studies re-porting that race and ethnicity play a significant role,[47] but other studies do not support this.[5,44,45,48] Other studies have reported that medical comorbidities (including diabetes, irritable bowel syndrome, and chronic lung disease),[47] increasing parity, and operative vaginal delivery are significant risk factors.[45,47–49] At least half of women who have fecal incontinence report that there is a significant quality-of-life impact.[45,49] Despite the significant impact on a woman's life, it is estimated that only 10% of affected women will seek care for fecal incontinence.[43] Data regarding the incidence, regression, and progression of anal incontinence are limited.

Costs

There has been limited information about the economic burden of anal incontinence. Mellgren and colleagues[50] followed 63 women in the United States with obstetric injuries and subsequent fecal incontinence and estimated the cost associated with treatment and follow-up, including physician evaluation and follow-up, treatment charges, and costs for protective materials. They estimated the average lifetime cost to be $17,166 per patient, and the average hospital costs associated with surgical treatment were $8555 per procedure (1996 dollars). A study by Deutekom and colleagues[51] estimated that total outpatient cost (outpatient health care resources, out-of-pocket expenses, and costs associated with production loss) was €2169, or approximately $3000 per anal incontinent patient per year in 2005. Sung and colleagues[52] estimated that the hospital cost of inpatient surgery for female fecal incontinence was $6000 per surgical admission in 2003, for a total of $24.5 million spent on hospital costs alone for fecal incontinence in the United States that year. This estimate did not include direct costs of physician services for the surgery, eval-uation, diagnostic tests, or indirect costs.

Painful Bladder Syndrome

Prevalence, incidence, cost

The strict criteria for interstitial cystitis, based on the National Institute of Diabetes and Digestive and Kidney Diseases, includes irritative voiding symptoms combined with cystoscopic findings after other specific bladder diseases have been excluded.[53] In 2002, the ICS defined painful bladder syndrome as "suprapubic pain related to bladder filling, accompanied by other symptoms such as increased daytime and night-time frequency, in the absence of proven urinary infection or other obvious pathology."[2] As expected, prevalence rates in the literature vary depending on how restrictive the definition is. A study by Warren and colleagues[54] reported that, in women with previ-ously diagnosed interstitial cystitis or painful bladder syndrome, only 66% met the ICS definition, suggesting that even this definition may not be sensitive.

Prevalence estimates for interstitial cystitis/painful bladder syndrome in women range from 114/100,000 women to 300/100,000 women,[55–57] and as low as 2.3% to 22%,[58–61] depending on disease definition. The incidence was estimated in one study using International Classification of Diseases, ninth revision codes to be 15/100,000 women per year.[62] These are summarized in **Table 5**.

As part of the Urologic Diseases in America Project, Payne and colleagues[63] quan-tified the burden of interstitial cystitis/painful bladder syndrome on the health care system in the United States. The annual office visit rate was 102 visits per 100,000 people, and there was a threefold increase in physician visits between 1992 and

Table 5
Prevalence of painful bladder syndrome/interstitial cystitis

Study	Definition	Prevalence
Leppilahti et al[56]	O'Leary-Sant score and clinically confirmed by cystoscopy	Probable IC: 300/100,000 Possible/probable: 680/100,000
Parsons et al[60]	Pelvic Pain and Urgency/ Frequency questionnaire	22%
Roberts et al[57]	Physician-assigned diagnosis	114/100,000
Clemens et al[55]	Physician-assigned diagnosis	197/100,000
Rosenberg et al[61]	Pelvic Pain and Urgency/ Frequency questionnaire and potassium sensitivity test or anesthetic bladder challenge	17.5% based on questionnaire 4.3% diagnosed
Link et al[59]	Symptoms suggestive of painful bladder syndrome	2.6%
Lifford et al[58]	Affirmative to "In the past 10 years, have you experienced bladder or pelvic pain associated with urinary symptoms for more than 3 consecutive months?"	2.3%

2001. In 2000, the inpatient hospitalization rate in women was 1.3/100,000 women. Between 1994 and 1996, the rate of outpatient hospital surgery in women was 22/100,000. The estimated mean annual cost per individual with interstitial cystitis was $8420 versus $4169 for those without the disorder in 2002.

Ambulatory Care and Surgical Epidemiology of Pelvic Floor Disorders

Establishing ambulatory rates for patient care associated with pelvic floor disorders is difficult and commonly relies on large, national databases. Luber and colleagues[64] estimated that projected future demands for incontinence and prolapse care will increase significantly in the future based on ambulatory care projections. Sung and colleagues[65] evaluated ambulatory care related to pelvic floor disorders in the United States from 1995 to 2006 using the National Ambulatory Medical Care Survey and the National Hospital Ambulatory Medical Care Survey. In this study, the average annual number of ambulatory visits between 2003 and 2006 was 3.9 million visits per year, representing 0.9% of all ambulatory care visits for adult women in the Unites States. This translates into an average annual visit rate of 36.3 per 1000 women. In 2006, the rate of urinary incontinence ambulatory visits was 21.7 per 1000 women, and the rate of pelvic prolapse visits was 13.5 per 1000 women.

In 1995, Olsen and colleagues[66] reported that the lifetime risk of undergoing a single operation by age 80 was 11.1%. In addition, reoperation was performed in 29.2% of cases, and the time intervals between repeat procedures decreased with each successive repair. Based on an analysis of the National Hospital Discharge Survey, the number of women who underwent inpatient surgery for stress incontinence increased from 48,345 in 1979 to 103,467 in 2004.[67] In this study, age-adjusted rates of inpatient stress incontinence procedures per 1000 women increased from 0.59 in 1979 to 0.85 in 2004, with the most remarkable increase in women 52 years of age or older. This study estimated that 34% of women having surgery for stress inconti-nence underwent prolapse surgery at the same time. This study only included inpa-tient surgical procedures. In 1996, the number of ambulatory surgeries for stress incontinence in the United States was estimated to be 15,900.[68]

A study by Waetjen and colleagues[69] in 1998 found the highest rate of surgery for incontinence was in 60- to 69-year-old women, and that the South had the highest overall rate of incontinence surgeries in the country. This study also reported large racial differences in stress incontinence surgery rates, with white women having nearly a fivefold greater rate (11.6 per 10,000 women) compared with black women (2.6 per 10,000 women). Anger and colleagues[70] reported that, among Medicare beneficiaries, white women were more likely than black women to be diagnosed and surgically treated for stress incontinence.

For pelvic organ prolapse, studies from the National Hospital Discharge Survey from 1997 estimate that 225,964 women underwent surgery for prolapse, or a rate of 22.7 per 10,000 women.[71,72] Similar to incontinence, the South had the highest rate of surgery compared with other regions, and white women had a threefold higher rate of surgery compared with African Americans (19.6 vs 6.4 per 10,000 women, respectively).

Surgical epidemiologic data for anal incontinence are limited. Using the Nationwide Inpatient Sample from 1998 to 2003, Sung and colleagues[52] estimated that 3509 inpa-tient procedures were performed for anal incontinence in 2003. Outpatient surgical data for anal incontinence is lacking.

Coexisting Pelvic Floor Disorders

It is now well recognized that pelvic floor disorders often coexist in the same woman. Nygaard and colleagues[5] estimated that in community-dwelling women in the United States, 23.7% of women had 1 or more pelvic floor disorder. Markland and colleagues[73] reported that in community-dwelling women aged 65 years and older, the prevalence of urinary incontinence was 27%, fecal incontinence 6%, and dual incontinence was 6%. Lawrence and colleagues[74] reported that the co-occurrence of pelvic floor disorders was high, with 80% of women with stress incontinence or overactive bladder, 69% with pelvic prolapse, and 48% with anal incontinence report-ing at least 1 other disorder. In this study, 56% of women reported stress incontinence and overactive bladder, 58% stress incontinence and anal incontinence, 56% overac-tive bladder and anal incontinence, and 29% pelvic organ prolapse and any incontinence.

In women enrolled in a surgical trial for treatment of stress urinary incontinence, the prevalence of coexisting monthly fecal incontinence was 16%, with 10% for liquid, and 6% for solid stool.[75] In another trial evaluating nonsurgical therapy for pure or predominant urge incontinence, the prevalence of monthly fecal incontinence was 18%, 12% for liquid stool, and 6% for solid stool.[76] In both studies, dual incontinence was associated with worse quality of life scores than isolated urinary incontinence.

A study by Bradley and colleagues[77] evaluated bowel symptoms in women enrolled in a surgical trial for pelvic organ prolapse and found that 19% of women reported anal incontinence with loose stool, 4% with formed stool, and 37% with gas. Because co-existing pelvic floor disorders are common, evaluation of all disorders at the time of evaluation and before surgical intervention could improve overall outcomes for women.

Causes and Prevention of Pelvic Floor Disorders

Prevention of pelvic floor disorders, like any disease, requires an understanding of causative factors. One model that is useful in considering the pathophysiology of pelvic floor disorders was presented by Bump and Norton[1] and is shown in **Fig. 3**. Risk factors in this model can be categorized as predisposing, inciting, promoting, or decompensating. This model is helpful in understanding the impact of various risk factors, and to potentially aid in disease prevention; however, it is often difficult to understand the significance of each factor for a specific individual or population. In addition, many risk factors may be classified into more than 1 category and the exact role, and to what degree a particular risk factor may contribute to the development of these disorders, is often unclear and difficult to quantify.

Predisposing factors
Predisposing factors can sometimes be altered or changed, but are more often those that are uncontrollable by the individual, such as gender, race, genetic collagen makeup, pelvic structure, and neurologic and muscular abnormalities.

It has been suggested that inherent physiologic makeup predisposes some racial and ethnic groups to pelvic floor dysfunction. In a study by Baragi and colleagues,[78] African American women were found to have a smaller posterior pelvic floor area compared with European American women, resulting in a 5.1% smaller total pelvic floor area. In another study using magnetic resonance imaging (MRI), white women were found to have a wider pelvic inlet, wider outlet, and shallower anteroposterior outlet compared with African American women.[79] Another study evaluating the structure and function of the continence mechanism reported that African American women had a 29% higher average urethral closure pressure during a maximum pelvic muscle contraction compared with white women.[80] However, the clinical significance of these differences and their role in the development of pelvic floor disorders remains unclear.

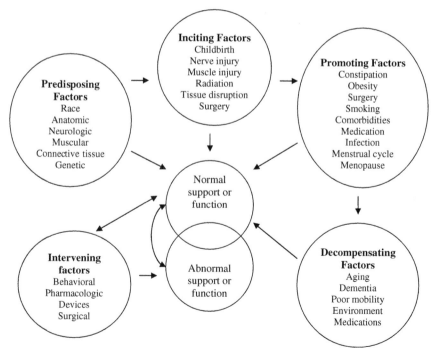

Fig. 3. Model for the development of pelvic floor dysfunction in women (*Adapted from* Bump RC, Norton PA. Epidemiology and natural history of pelvic floor dysfunction. Obstet Gynecol Clin North Am 1998;24(4):723–46; with permission.)

Quantitative and qualitative differences in collagen may contribute to pelvic floor dysfunction. Connective tissue disorders such as Marfan syndrome and Ehlers Danlos syndrome have been linked to increased prevalence of incontinence and prolapse.[81] In histologic studies, women with pelvic organ prolapse have been shown to have more type III collagen in pelvic floor connective tissues relative to other collagen subtypes[82] and differences in the regeneration of elastin fibers.[83] Other studies have shown that women with pelvic organ prolapse and stress urinary incontinence have levator ani and periurethral muscle denervation and decreased neuropeptide activity.[84] Because these are mostly cross sectional studies, it is unclear whether these histologic differences represent causes of prolapse and incontinence or subsequent effects of the disorder.

Gene expression has been found to be different in the levator ani muscles of women with prolapse, compared with controls.[85] In addition, a significant family history of hernias in men and women seems to be associated with symptoms of pelvic organ prolapse.[86] However, in a twin study by Altman and colleagues,[87] genetic effects seemed to contribute to stress incontinence and pelvic organ prolapse, but the influence of environmental factors was also substantial.

Inciting factors

Inciting factors are those that likely could be modified, but often cannot be avoided.

Although most parous women do not have pelvic floor dysfunction, one major inciting factor for pelvic floor dysfunction is childbirth. Nygaard and colleagues[5] found that the proportion of women reporting at least 1 pelvic floor disorder increased incrementally with parity, with more than 30% of women with 3 or more deliveries reporting a pelvic floor disorder. Similarly, in the RRISK cohort, Rortveit and colleagues[41] found that the risk of prolapse was significantly increased in women with 1 (odds ratio [OR] 2.8, 95% confidence interval [CI] 1.1–7.2), 2 (OR 4.1, 95% CI 1.8–9.5), and 3 or more (OR 5.3, 95% CI 2.3–12.3) vaginal deliveries compared with nulliparous women.

In the Childbirth and Pelvic Symptoms (CAPS) study, Borello-France[88] reported that women with anal sphincter injuries were twice as likely to report postpartum fecal incontinence compared with women without sphincter tears. In addition, cesarean delivery was not completely protective against anal or urinary incontinence. A second study using the CAPS data reported that the presence of antenatal urinary incontinence and increased BMI were potential modifiable risk factors that increased the risk of postpartum fecal and urinary incontinence.[89] Other studies have shown that pregnancy itself before childbirth may be a risk factor for pelvic floor dysfunction.[90–92]

Inciting factors such as radiation, pelvic surgery, and childbirth may cause injury to pelvic muscles and nerves. Delancey and colleagues[93] reported defects in the levator ani muscles of women with prolapse and a lower vaginal closure pressure during maximal contraction compared with controls. Weidner and colleagues[94] found that compared with nulliparous subjects, patients with stress urinary incontinence and pelvic prolapse had changes in the levator ani and external anal sphincter consistent with motor unit loss or failure of central activation, or both, when undergoing electromyographic examination. Other reports have described histologic differences in morphology and innervation of the pelvic floor in women with and without prolapse.[95]

Promoting factors

Promoting factors are likely the easiest factors to modify; however, the actual impact of modifying these variables on the natural history of pelvic floor dysfunction remains unclear.

Data on constipation are inconsistent regarding the relationship between constipation and pelvic organ prolapse. Some studies support that chronic constipation is more common in women with prolapse and may lead to puborectalis and external anal sphincter nerve injury.[96,97] Other studies report no, or weak, association between constipation and prolapse.[36,98–100] Bradley and colleagues[101] reported that, in women with defecatory symptoms and prolapse, 80% reported improvement in defecatory symptoms 12 months after surgical treatment of pelvic prolapse, highlighting some uncertainty on whether constipation is a cause or effect of prolapse.

In addition to chronically increased intra-abdominal pressure, neurogenic disease caused by obesity may place obese women at greater risk for prolapse and incontinence.[102] Obesity has been shown to be a risk factor for urinary incontinence.[103] Subak and colleagues[104] conducted a randomized clinical trial, the Program to Reduce Incontinence by Diet and Exercise (PRIDE), and found that a 6-month behavioral intervention targeting weight loss reduced the frequency of self-reported episodes of urinary incontinence among overweight and obese women compared with a control group. Burgio and colleagues[105] reported that, in incontinent women losing 18 or more BMI points after bariatric surgery, 71% regained urinary continence at 12 months.

Higher BMI has also been associated with pelvic organ prolapse. Hendrix and colleagues[36] reported the risk of prolapse to be 30% to 50% higher in women with a BMI of 25 or higher compared with women with lower BMI in the WHI trial. Kudish and colleagues[106] also used data from the WHI during a 5-year period to evaluate the relationship between change in weight and prolapse progression/regression in postmenopausal women. They found that overweight or obese women had an increased risk of prolapse progression compared with women of normal weight. However, prolapse regression was not associated with weight loss.

There are limited data on the effect of obesity and weight loss on anal incontinence. Richter and colleagues[107] found that the prevalence of anal incontinence was higher in morbidly obese women compared with the general population. Erekson and colleagues[108] reported that increasing BMI was significantly associated with anal incontinence. Burgio and colleagues[105] reported that following bariatric surgery, the prevalence of fecal incontinence (solid or liquid stool) decreased from 19.4% to 9.1% at 6 months and 8.6% at 12 months.

Diabetes mellitus is increasingly being recognized as a risk factor for urologic complications. In one study, women with type 1 diabetes had a nearly twofold greater prevalence of weekly urge incontinence compared with women without diabetes (8.8% vs 4.5%).[109] Danforth and colleagues[110] used data from the Nurse's Health Study I and II, and reported that the incidence of at least weekly urinary incontinence was 8.7% in women with type 2 diabetes, compared with 5.3% in women without type 2 diabetes, with an increased risk of 20% for women with diabetes. The pathways linking these conditions remain unclear, but may be a result of microvascular damage. Using data from the Action for Health in Diabetes (Look AHEAD) study evaluating overweight and obese women with type 2 diabetes, Phelan and colleagues[111] reported that weekly incontinence (27%) was reported more often than other diabetes-associated complications including retinopathy (7.5%), microalbuminuria (2.2%), and neuropathy (1.5%). The effect of strict glucose control, weight loss, or physical activity on incontinence in women with diabetes is unclear.

Daily recreational or occupational activities may have a promoting effect. The prevalence of urge and stress incontinence symptoms among nulliparous and parous elite athletes is higher than among the general population.[112] Kruger and colleagues[113] used three-dimensional ultrasound and MRI to evaluate the pelvic floor of nulliparous, high impact, frequent intensity athletes, and found an increased diameter of levator ani muscles, greater bladder neck descent, and a larger hiatal area on Valsalva maneuver compared with controls. For pelvic organ prolapse, studies have shown that women who are laborers/factory workers and homemakers were at increased risk for prolapse compared with other job categories.[114,115]

The large EPICONT study reported that former and current smoking was associated with incontinence, limited to those women who smoked 20 cigarettes a day or who had a 15 year pack history.[12,116] It may be postulated that increased prevalence of incontinence among smokers is secondary to strong and frequent coughing, and therefore increased intra-abdominal pressure. Other theories regarding smoking and its effect on incontinence include the negative effect of smoking on estrogen, and possible interference with collagen synthesis.

Smoking and chronic obstructive pulmonary disease (COPD) have also been associated with the development of pelvic organ prolapse, however no clear mechanism has been elucidated. Blandon and colleagues[117] performed a matched case-control study and found that chronic pulmonary disease was associated with an increased risk for future pelvic floor repair after hysterectomy, even after adjusting for BMI. The prevalence of urinary incontinence in older, postmenopausal women was also found to increase almost twofold with COPD.[118]

The effect of urinary tract infections on bladder function was investigated by Bergman and colleagues[119] via urodynamic evaluation. They found that, in women with significant urinary tract infection ($\geq 10^5$ CFU/mL), 45% had an unstable bladder before treatment of the infection, and 60% of those regained bladder stability after appropriate treatment. In addition, 30% of stress incontinent patients became continent after treatment of urinary infection. Brown and colleagues[120] used data from the Heart and Estrogen/progestin Replacement Study and found that the prevalence of weekly urge incontinence was twofold higher in women who reported 2 or more urinary tract infections in the prior year. In contrast, Ouslander and colleagues[121] found that eradicating bacteriuria in nursing home residents had no short-term effects on the severity of chronic urinary incontinence.

Certain medications may predispose women to pelvic floor disorders secondary to their mechanism of action (eg, by lowering bladder outlet resistance). Other drugs may predispose women secondary to side effects (eg, constipating medications or cough-inducing medications). Drugs that may predispose women to incontinence include α-adrenergics, angiotensin-converting enzyme (ACE) inhibitors, antipsychotics, benzodiazepines, and antidepressants.

The role of hormone therapy on incontinence symptoms has been evaluated.[36,122] Using data from the WHI, Hendrix and colleagues[36] reported that menopausal hormone therapy increased the incidence of all types of urinary incontinence at 1 year among women who were continent at baseline. The risk for stress incontinence was 1.87 and 2.15 fold higher for women on estrogen and progesterone therapy or estrogen therapy alone, respectively, compared with controls. The risk for mixed incontinence was 1.49- and 1.79-fold higher for women on estrogen and progesterone therapy or estrogen therapy alone, respectively, compared with controls. Townsend and colleagues[123] investigated the association of oral contraceptive use and self-reported incident urinary incontinence in premenopausal women aged 37 to 54 years enrolled in the Nurses' Health Study II. They found that ever users of oral contraception had an increased risk of incident incontinence, mainly worsening urge incontinence. In addition, the odds of incontinence increased significantly with increasing duration of oral contraceptive pill (OCP) use.

Caffeine intake is often reported to exacerbate urinary incontinence. In a case-control study, Arya and colleagues[124] found a 2.5-fold higher risk of detrusor overactivity in women with high caffeine intake and after controlling for age and smoking. In contrast, the EPINCONT study found that tea, but not coffee, was associated with incontinence.[116] The investigators theorize that tea might contain components other than caffeine that might aggravate incontinence.

The changes in circulating sex steroids that occur during the normal menstrual cycle may lead to functional changes in the lower urinary tract; however, this remains unclear. Hextell and colleagues[125] reported that the proportion of women with abnormal detrusor activity diagnosed on videocystourethrography increased significantly with time from the last menstrual period, possibly reflecting changes in the circulating level of progesterone following ovulation. However, abnormal detrusor activity was not diagnosed more frequently in women who complained of cyclical symptoms (39%) compared with women without cyclical symptoms (32%).

Transition to a hypoestrogenic state during menopause may lead to changes in the vaginal and urethral mucosa. Sherbrun and colleagues[126] reported on a population-based cohort of women in menopausal transition and found no association between the development of urinary incontinence and the transition to postmenopause. However, it is unclear when the potential effects of hypoestrogenism would manifest clinically. Furthermore, it is difficult to assess the independent effects of menopause and aging on the development or worsening of pelvic floor disorders. The effect of age on incontinence has been discussed earlier in this article.

Decompensating factors

Decompensating factors are those that are extrinsic to the pelvic floor, but can create decompensation and dysfunction of an otherwise compensated pelvic floor. Similar to its relationship to promoting factors, age is a factor that may lead to some decompensating factors, but it is difficult to say whether aging itself is a decompensating factor when considered alone. For example, mental status changes such as delirium, confusion and dementia, sometimes linked to aging, can precipitate functional decompensation of an individual, resulting in functional incontinence. Limited physical mobility, or an environment that allows for limited access to toileting, may also create a situation for functional incontinence. The same is true for conditions and medications that increase urine output and the need for toileting, or otherwise debilitating conditions such as urinary tract infections. Such decompensating factors can sometimes be remedied with interventions such as timed voids, bedside commodes, or medication alterations, but others can be more difficult to address.

SUMMARY

Pelvic floor disorders are common and have a negative impact on a woman's quality of life. Most women with these conditions will never seek care for these debilitating symptoms. Improving our understanding of risk factors, particularly modifiable factors, is critical for developing future prevention guidelines and improving the specificity of treatments.

REFERENCES

1. Bump RC, Norton PA. Epidemiology and natural history of pelvic floor dysfunction. Obstet Gynecol Clin North Am 1998;25(4):723–46.
2. Abrams P, Cardozo L, Fall M, et al. The standardisation of terminology in lower urinary tract function: report from the standardisation sub-committee of the International Continence Society. Urology 2003;61(1):37–49.
3. Milsom I. Lower urinary tract symptoms in women. Curr Opin Urol 2009;19(4): 337–41.

4. Thom D. Variation in estimates of urinary incontinence prevalence in the community: effects of differences in definition, population characteristics, and study type. J Am Geriatr Soc 1998;46(4):473–80.
5. Nygaard I, Barber MD, Burgio KL, et al. Prevalence of symptomatic pelvic floor disorders in US women. J Am Med Assoc 2008;300(11):1311–6.
6. Dooley Y, Kenton K, Cao G, et al. Urinary incontinence prevalence: results from the National Health and Nutrition Examination Survey. J Urol 2008;179(2): 656–61.
7. Waetjen LE, Liao S, Johnson WO, et al. Factors associated with prevalent and incident urinary incontinence in a cohort of midlife women: a longitudinal analysis of data: study of women's health across the nation. Am J Epidemiol 2007;165(3): 309–18.
8. Sandvik H, Seim A, Vanvik A, et al. A severity index for epidemiological surveys of female urinary incontinence: comparison with 48-hour pad-weighing tests. Neurourol Urodyn 2000;19(2):137–45.
9. Melville JL, Katon W, Delaney K, et al. Urinary incontinence in US women: a population-based study. Arch Intern Med 2005;165(5):537–42.
10. Peyrat L, Haillot O, Bruyere F, et al. Prevalence and risk factors of urinary incontinence in young and middle-aged women. BJU Int 2002;89(1):61–6.
11. Minassian VA, Stewart WF, Wood GC. Urinary incontinence in women: variation in prevalence estimates and risk factors. Obstet Gynecol 2008;111(2 Pt 1): 324–31.
12. Hannestad YS, Rortveit G, Sandvik H, et al. A community-based epidemiological survey of female urinary incontinence: the Norwegian EPINCONT study. Epidemiology of Incontinence in the County of Nord-Trondelag. J Clin Epidemiol 2000; 53(11):1150–7.
13. Coyne KS, Sexton CC, Thompson CL, et al. The prevalence of lower urinary tract symptoms (LUTS) in the USA, the UK and Sweden: results from the Epidemiology of LUTS (EpiLUTS) study. BJU Int 2009;104(3):352–60.
14. Irwin DE, Milsom I, Hunskaar S, et al. Population-based survey of urinary incontinence, overactive bladder, and other lower urinary tract symptoms in five countries: results of the EPIC study. Eur Urol 2006;50(6):1306–14 discussion 1314–5.
15. Milsom I, Abrams P, Cardozo L, et al. How widespread are the symptoms of an overactive bladder and how are they managed? A population-based prevalence study. BJU Int 2001;87(9):760–6.
16. Lukacz ES, Whitcomb EL, Lawrence JM, et al. Urinary frequency in community-dwelling women: what is normal? Am J Obstet Gynecol 2009;200(5)(552):e1–7.
17. Thom DH, van den Eeden SK, Ragins AI, et al. Differences in prevalence of urinary incontinence by race/ethnicity. J Urol 2006;175(1):259–64.
18. Ragins AI, Shan J, Thom DH, et al. Effects of urinary incontinence, comorbidity and race on quality of life outcomes in women. J Urol 2008;179(2):651–5 discussion 655.
19. Fenner DE, Trowbridge ER, Patel DA, et al. Establishing the prevalence of incontinence study: racial differences in women's patterns of urinary incontinence. J Urol 2008;179(4):1455–60.
20. Bump RC. Racial comparisons and contrasts in urinary incontinence and pelvic organ prolapse. Obstet Gynecol 1993;81(3):421–5.
21. Komesu YM, Rogers RG, Schrader RM, et al. Incidence and remission of urinary incontinence in a community-based population of women ≥50 years. Int Urogynecol J Pelvic Floor Dysfunct 2009;PMID:19229462. Epub ahead of print.

22. Brown JS, Wessells H, Chancellor MB, et al. Urologic complications of diabetes. Diabetes Care 2005;28(1):177–85.

23. Jackson RA, Vittinghoff E, Kanaya AM, et al. Urinary incontinence in elderly women: findings from the Health, Aging, and Body Composition Study. Obstet Gynecol 2004;104(2):301–7.

24. Shamliyan T, Wyman J, Bliss DZ, et al. Prevention of urinary and fecal incontinence in adults. Evid Rep Technol Assess (Full Rep) 2007;161:1–379.

25. Townsend MK, Danforth KN, Lifford KL, et al. Incidence and remission of urinary incontinence in middle-aged women. Am J Obstet Gynecol 2007;197(2)(167):e1–5.

26. Lifford KL, Townsend MK, Curhan GC, et al. The epidemiology of urinary incontinence in older women: incidence, progression, and remission. J Am Geriatr Soc 2008;56(7):1191–8.

27. Heidler S, Deveza C, Temml C, et al. The natural history of lower urinary tract symptoms in females: analysis of a health screening project. Eur Urol 2007;52(6):1744–50.

28. Wilson L, Brown JS, Shin GP, et al. Annual direct cost of urinary incontinence. Obstet Gynecol 2001;98(3):398–406.

29. Thom DH, Nygaard IE, Calhoun EA. Urologic diseases in America project: urinary incontinence in women-national trends in hospitalizations, office visits, treatment and economic impact. J Urol 2005;173(4):1295–301.

30. Kinchen KS, Long S, Orsini L, et al. A retrospective claims analysis of the direct costs of stress urinary incontinence. Int Urogynecol J Pelvic Floor Dysfunct 2003;14(6):403–11.

31. Hu TW, Wagner TH, Bentkover JD, et al. Estimated economic costs of overactive bladder in the United States. Urology 2003;61(6):1123–8.

32. Subak L, Van Den Eeden S, Thom D, et al. Urinary incontinence in women: direct costs of routine care. Am J Obstet Gynecol 2007;197(6):596 e1–e9.

33. Subak LL, Brown JS, Kraus SR, et al. The "costs" of urinary incontinence for women. Obstet Gynecol 2006;107(4):908–16.

34. Subak LL, Brubaker L, Chai TC, et al. High costs of urinary incontinence among women electing surgery to treat stress incontinence. Obstet Gynecol 2008;111(4):899–907.

35. Handa VL, Garrett E, Hendrix S, et al. Progression and remission of pelvic organ prolapse: a longitudinal study of menopausal women. Am J Obstet Gynecol 2004;190(1):27–32.

36. Hendrix SL, Clark A, Nygaard I, et al. Pelvic organ prolapse in the Women's Health Initiative: gravity and gravidity. Am J Obstet Gynecol 2002;186(6):1160–6.

37. Bump RC, Mattiasson A, Bo K, et al. The standardization of terminology of female pelvic organ prolapse and pelvic floor dysfunction. Am J Obstet Gynecol 1996;175(1):10–7.

38. Bradley CS, Zimmerman MB, Qi Y, et al. Natural history of pelvic organ prolapse in postmenopausal women. Obstet Gynecol 2007;109(4):848–54.

39. Nygaard I, Bradley C, Brandt D. Pelvic organ prolapse in older women: prevalence and risk factors. Obstet Gynecol 2004;104(3):489–97.

40. Bradley CS, Nygaard IE. Vaginal wall descensus and pelvic floor symptoms in older women. Obstet Gynecol 2005;106(4):759–66.

41. Rortveit G, Brown JS, Thom DH, et al. Symptomatic pelvic organ prolapse: prevalence and risk factors in a population-based, racially diverse cohort. Obstet Gynecol 2007;109(6):1396–403.

42. Subak LL, Waetjen LE, van den Eeden S, et al. Cost of pelvic organ prolapse surgery in the United States. Obstet Gynecol 2001;98(4):646–51.
43. Bharucha AE, Zinsmeister AR, Locke GR, et al. Prevalence and burden of fecal incontinence: a population-based study in women. Gastroenterology 2005; 129(1):42–9.
44. Goode PS, Burgio KL, Halli AD, et al. Prevalence and correlates of fecal incontinence in community-dwelling older adults. J Am Geriatr Soc 2005;53(4): 629–35.
45. Melville JL, Fan MY, Newton K, et al. Fecal incontinence in US women: a population-based study. Am J Obstet Gynecol 2005;193(6):2071–6.
46. Nelson R, Norton N, Cautley E, et al. Community-based prevalence of anal incontinence. J Am Med Assoc 1995;274(7):559–61.
47. Varma MG, Brown JS, Creasman JM, et al. Fecal incontinence in females older than aged 40 years: who is at risk? Dis Colon Rectum 2006;49(6):841–51.
48. Whitehead WE, Borrud L, Goode PS, et al. Fecal incontinence in US adults: epidemiology and risk factors. Gastroenterology 2009;137(2):512–7.
49. Boreham MK, Richter HE, Kenton KS, et al. Anal incontinence in women presenting for gynecologic care: prevalence, risk factors, and impact upon quality of life. Am J Obstet Gynecol 2005;192(5):1637–42.
50. Mellgren A, Jensen LL, Zetterstrom JP, et al. Long-term cost of fecal incontinence secondary to obstetric injuries. Dis Colon Rectum 1999;42(7):857–65 discussion 865–7.
51. Deutekom M, Dobben AC, Dijkgraaf MG, et al. Costs of outpatients with fecal incontinence. Scand J Gastroenterol 2005;40(5):552–8.
52. Sung VW, Rogers ML, Myers DL, et al. National trends and costs of surgical treatment for female fecal incontinence. Am J Obstet Gynecol 2007;197(6): 625, e1-5.
53. Gillenwater JY, Wein AJ. Summary of the National Institute of Arthritis, Diabetes, Digestive and Kidney Diseases Workshop on Interstitial Cystitis, National Institutes of Health, Bethesda, Maryland, August 28–29, 1987. J Urol 1988;140(1): 203–6.
54. Warren JW, Meyer WA, Greenberg P, et al. Using the International Continence Society's definition of painful bladder syndrome. Urology 2006;67(6):1138–42 discussion 1142–3.
55. Clemens JQ, Meenan RT, Rosetti MC, et al. Prevalence and incidence of interstitial cystitis in a managed care population. J Urol 2005;173(1):98–102 discussion 102.
56. Leppilahti M, Sairanen J, Tammela TL, et al. Prevalence of clinically confirmed interstitial cystitis in women: a population based study in Finland. J Urol 2005; 174(2):581–3.
57. Roberts RO, Bergstralh EJ, Bass SE, et al. Incidence of physician-diagnosed interstitial cystitis in Olmsted County: a community-based study. BJU Int 2003; 91(3):181–5.
58. Lifford KL, Curhan GC. Prevalence of painful bladder syndrome in older women. Urology 2009;73(3):494–8.
59. Link CL, Pulliam SJ, Hanno PM, et al. Prevalence and psychosocial correlates of symptoms suggestive of painful bladder syndrome: results from the Boston area community health survey. J Urol 2008;180(2):599–606.
60. Parsons CL, Dell J, Stanford EJ, et al. Increased prevalence of interstitial cystitis: previously unrecognized urologic and gynecologic cases identified using a new symptom questionnaire and intravesical potassium sensitivity. Urology 2002; 60(4):573–8.

61. Rosenberg MT, Page S, Hazzard MA. Prevalence of interstitial cystitis in a primary care setting. Urology 2007;69(4 Suppl):48–52.
62. Patel R, Calhoun EA, Meenan RT, et al. Incidence and clinical characteristics of interstitial cystitis in the community. Int Urogynecol J Pelvic Floor Dysfunct 2008; 19(8):1093–6.
63. Payne CK, Joyce GF, Wise M, et al. Interstitial cystitis and painful bladder syndrome. J Urol 2007;177(6):2042–9.
64. Luber KM, Boero S, Choe JY. The demographics of pelvic floor disorders: current observations and future projections. Am J Obstet Gynecol 2001; 184(7):1496–501 discussion 1501–3.
65. Sung VW, Raker C.A, Myers D.L, et al. Ambulatory care related to female pelvic floor disorders in the United States, 1995–2006. Am J Obstet Gynecol 2009;PMID:19683690. Aug 14, 2009. Epub ahead of print.
66. Olsen AL, Smith VJ, Bergstrom JO, et al. Epidemiology of surgically managed pelvic organ prolapse and urinary incontinence. Obstet Gynecol 1997;89(4): 501–6.
67. Oliphant SS, Wang L, Bunker CH, et al. Trends in stress urinary incontinence inpatient procedures in the United States, 1979–2004. Am J Obstet Gynecol 2009;200(5):521, e1-6.
68. Boyles SH, Weber AM, Meyn L. Ambulatory procedures for urinary incontinence in the United States, 1994–1996. Am J Obstet Gynecol 2004;190(1):33–6.
69. Waetjen LE, Subak LL, Shen H, et al. Stress urinary incontinence surgery in the United States. Obstet Gynecol 2003;101(4):671–6.
70. Anger JT, Rodriguez LV, Wang Q, et al. Racial disparities in the surgical management of stress incontinence among female Medicare beneficiaries. J Urol 2007; 177(5):1846–50.
71. Boyles SH, Weber AM, Meyn L. Procedures for pelvic organ prolapse in the United States, 1979–1997. Am J Obstet Gynecol 2003;188(1):108–15.
72. Brown JS, Waetjen LE, Subak LL, et al. Pelvic organ prolapse surgery in the United States, 1997. Am J Obstet Gynecol 2002;186(4):712–6.
73. Markland AD, Goode PS, Burgio KL, et al. Correlates of urinary, fecal, and dual incontinence in older African-American and white men and women. J Am Geriatr Soc 2008;56(2):285–90.
74. Lawrence JM, Lukacz ES, Nager CW, et al. Prevalence and co-occurrence of pelvic floor disorders in community-dwelling women. Obstet Gynecol 2008; 111(3):678–85.
75. Markland AD, Kraus SR, Richter HE, et al. Prevalence and risk factors of fecal incontinence in women undergoing stress incontinence surgery. Am J Obstet Gynecol 2007;197(6):662 e1–7.
76. Markland AD, Richter HE, Kenton KS, et al. Associated factors and the impact of fecal incontinence in women with urge urinary incontinence: from the Urinary Incontinence Treatment Network's Behavior Enhances Drug Reduction of Incontinence study. Am J Obstet Gynecol 2009;200(4)(424): e1–8.
77. Bradley CS, Brown MB, Cundiff GW, et al. Bowel symptoms in women planning surgery for pelvic organ prolapse. Am J Obstet Gynecol 2006;195(6):1814–9.
78. Baragi RV, Delancey JO, Caspari R, et al. Differences in pelvic floor area between African American and European American women. Am J Obstet Gynecol 2002;187(1):111–5.
79. Handa VL, Lockhart ME, Fielding JR, et al. Racial differences in pelvic anatomy by magnetic resonance imaging. Obstet Gynecol 2008;111(4):914–20.

80. Howard D, Delancey JO, Tunn R, et al. Racial differences in the structure and function of the stress urinary continence mechanism. Obstet Gynecol 2000; 95(5):713–7.
81. Carley ME, Schaffer J. Urinary incontinence and pelvic organ prolapse in women with Marfan or Ehlers Danlos syndrome. Am J Obstet Gynecol 2000;182(5): 1021–3.
82. Moalli PA, Shand SH, Zyczynski HM, et al. Remodeling of vaginal connective tissue in patients with prolapse. Obstet Gynecol 2005;106(5 Pt 1):953–63.
83. Chen B, Wen Y, Polan ML. Elastolytic activity in women with stress urinary incontinence and pelvic organ prolapse. Neurourol Urodyn 2004;23(2): 119–26.
84. Busacchi P, Perri T, Paradisi R, et al. Abnormalities of somatic peptide-containing nerves supplying the pelvic floor of women with genitourinary prolapse and stress urinary incontinence. Urology 2004;63(3):591–5.
85. Visco AG, Yuan L. Differential gene expression in pubococcygeus muscle from patients with pelvic organ prolapse. Am J Obstet Gynecol 2003;189(1):102–12.
86. McLennan MT, Harris JK, Kariuki B, et al. Family history as a risk factor for pelvic organ prolapse. Int Urogynecol J Pelvic Floor Dysfunct 2008;19(8): 1063–9.
87. Altman D, Forsman M, Falconer C, et al. Genetic influence on stress urinary incontinence and pelvic organ prolapse. Eur Urol 2008;54(4):918–22.
88. Borello-France D, Burgio KL, Richter HE, et al. Fecal and urinary incontinence in primiparous women. Obstet Gynecol 2006;108(4):863–72.
89. Burgio KL, Borello-France D, Richter HE, et al. Risk factors for fecal and urinary incontinence after childbirth: the childbirth and pelvic symptoms study. Am J Gastroenterol 2007;102(9):1998–2004.
90. Altman D, Ekstrom A, Forsgren C, et al. Symptoms of anal and urinary incontinence following cesarean section or spontaneous vaginal delivery. Am J Obstet Gynecol 2007;197(5):512 e1–7.
91. Rortveit G, Daltveit AK, Hannestad YS, et al. Urinary incontinence after vaginal delivery or cesarean section. N Engl J Med 2003;348(10):900–7.
92. O'Boyle AL, O'Boyle JD, Ricks RE, et al. The natural history of pelvic organ support in pregnancy. Int Urogynecol J Pelvic Floor Dysfunct 2003;14(1):46–9, discussion 49.
93. DeLancey JO, Morgan DM, Fenner DE, et al. Comparison of levator ani muscle defects and function in women with and without pelvic organ prolapse. Obstet Gynecol 2007;109(2 Pt 1):295–302.
94. Weidner AC, Barber MD, Visco AG, et al. Pelvic muscle electromyography of levator ani and external anal sphincter in nulliparous women and women with pelvic floor dysfunction. Am J Obstet Gynecol 2000;183(6):1390–9 discussion 1399–401.
95. Boreham MK, Wai CY, Miller RT, et al. Morphometric properties of the posterior vaginal wall in women with pelvic organ prolapse. Am J Obstet Gynecol 2002; 187(6):1501–8, discussion 1508–9.
96. Snooks SJ, Barnes PR, Swash M, et al. Damage to the innervation of the pelvic floor musculature in chronic constipation. Gastroenterology 1985;89(5):977–81.
97. Spence-Jones C, Kamm MA, Henry MM, et al. Bowel dysfunction: a pathogenic factor in uterovaginal prolapse and urinary stress incontinence. Br J Obstet Gynaecol 1994;101(2):147–52.
98. Kahn MA, Breitkopf CR, Valley MT, et al. Pelvic Organ Support Study (POSST) and bowel symptoms: straining at stool is associated with perineal and anterior

vaginal descent in a general gynecologic population. Am J Obstet Gynecol 2005;192(5):1516–22.

99. Samuelsson E, Victor A, Svardsudd K. Determinants of urinary incontinence in a population of young and middle-aged women. Acta Obstet Gynecol Scand 2000;79(3):208–15.

100. Weber AM, Walters MD, Ballard LA, et al. Posterior vaginal prolapse and bowel function. Am J Obstet Gynecol 1998;179(6 Pt 1):1446–9, discussion 1449–50.

101. Bradley CS, Nygaard IE, Brown MB, et al. Bowel symptoms in women 1 year after sacrocolpopexy. Am J Obstet Gynecol 2007;197(6)(642):e1–8.

102. Greer WJ, Richter HE, Bartolucci AA, et al. Obesity and pelvic floor disorders: a systematic review. Obstet Gynecol 2008;112(2 Pt 1):341–9.

103. Hunskaar S. A systematic review of overweight and obesity as risk factors and targets for clinical intervention for urinary incontinence in women. Neurourol Urodyn 2008;27(8):749–57.

104. Subak LL, Wing R, West DS, et al. Weight loss to treat urinary incontinence in overweight and obese women. N Engl J Med 2009;360(5):481–90.

105. Burgio KL, Richter HE, Clements RH, et al. Changes in urinary and fecal incontinence symptoms with weight loss surgery in morbidly obese women. Obstet Gynecol 2007;110(5):1034–40.

106. Kudish BI, Iglesia CB, Sokol RJ, et al. Effect of weight change on natural history of pelvic organ prolapse. Obstet Gynecol 2009;113(1):81–8.

107. Richter HE, Burgio KL, Clements RH, et al. Urinary and anal incontinence in morbidly obese women considering weight loss surgery. Obstet Gynecol 2005;106(6):1272–7.

108. Erekson EA, Sung VW, Myers DL. Effect of body mass index on the risk of anal incontinence and defecatory dysfunction in women. Am J Obstet Gynecol 2008; 198(5)(596):e1–4.

109. Sarma AV, Kanaya AM, Nyberg LM, et al. Urinary incontinence among women with type 1 diabetes–how common is it? J Urol 2009;181(3):1224–30, discussion 1230.

110. Danforth KN, Townsend MK, Curhan GC, et al. Type 2 diabetes mellitus and risk of stress, urge and mixed urinary incontinence. J Urol 2009;181(1):193–7.

111. Phelan S, Kanaya AM, Subak LL, et al. Prevalence and risk factors for urinary incontinence in overweight and obese diabetic women: the Look AHEAD study. Diabetes Care 2009;32(8):1391–7.

112. Nygaard IE, Thompson FL, Svengalis SL, et al. Urinary incontinence in elite nulliparous athletes. Obstet Gynecol 1994;84(2):183–7.

113. Kruger JA, Dietz HP, Murphy BA. Pelvic floor function in elite nulliparous athletes. Ultrasound Obstet Gynecol 2007;30(1):81–5.

114. Woodman PJ, Swift SE, O'Boyle AL, et al. Prevalence of severe pelvic organ prolapse in relation to job description and socioeconomic status: a multicenter cross-sectional study. Int Urogynecol J Pelvic Floor Dysfunct 2006;17(4):340–5.

115. Chiaffarino F, Chatenoud L, Dindelli M, et al. Reproductive factors, family history, occupation and risk of urogenital prolapse. Eur J Obstet Gynecol Reprod Biol 1999;82(1):63–7.

116. Hannestad YS, Rortveit G, Daltveit AK, et al. Are smoking and other lifestyle factors associated with female urinary incontinence? The Norwegian EPINCONT Study. BJOG 2003;110(3):247–54.

117. Blandon RE, Bharucha AE, Melton LJ 3rd, et al. Risk factors for pelvic floor repair after hysterectomy. Obstet Gynecol 2009;113(3):601–8.

118. Brown JS, Seeley DG, Fong J, et al. Urinary incontinence in older women: who is at risk? Study of Osteoporotic Fractures Research Group. Obstet Gynecol 1996; 87(5 Pt 1):715–21.

119. Bergman A, Bhatia NN. Urodynamics: effect of urinary tract infection on urethral and bladder function. Obstet Gynecol 1985;66(3):366–71.

120. Brown JS, Grady D, Ouslander JG, et al. Prevalence of urinary incontinence and associated risk factors in postmenopausal women. Heart & Estrogen/Progestin Replacement Study (HERS) Research Group. Obstet Gynecol 1999;94(1): 66–70.

121. Ouslander JG, Schapira M, Schnelle JF, et al. Does eradicating bacteriuria affect the severity of chronic urinary incontinence in nursing home residents? Ann Intern Med 1995;122(10):749–54.

122. Townsend MK, Curhan GC, Resnick NM, et al. Postmenopausal hormone therapy and incident urinary incontinence in middle-aged women. Am J Obstet Gynecol 2009;200(1)(86):e1–5.

123. Townsend MK, Curhan GC, Resnick NM, et al. Oral contraceptive use and incident urinary incontinence in premenopausal women. J Urol 2009;181(5):2170–5.

124. Arya LA, Myers DL, Jackson ND. Dietary caffeine intake and the risk for detrusor instability: a case-control study. Obstet Gynecol 2000;96(1):85–9.

125. Hextall A, Bidmead J, Cardozo L, et al. The impact of the menstrual cycle on urinary symptoms and the results of urodynamic investigation. Bjog 2001; 108(11):1193–6.

126. Sherburn M, Guthrie JR, Dudley EC, et al. Is incontinence associated with menopause? Obstet Gynecol 2001;98(4):628–33.

127. Swift SE, Tate SB, Nicholas J. Correlation of symptoms with degree of pelvic organ support in a general population of women: what is pelvic organ prolapse? Am J Obstet Gynecol 2003;189(2):372–7, discussion 377–9.

Clinical Approach and Office Evaluation of the Patient with Pelvic Floor Dysfunction

Cecilia K. Wieslander, MD*

KEYWORDS

- Pelvic floor disorders • Pelvic organ prolapse
- Urinary incontinence • Anal incontinence
- Pelvic organ quantification system

PATIENT HISTORY

Pelvic floor disorders are common and have been estimated to affect 24% to 37% of community-dwelling women in the United States.[1,2] Pelvic floor disorders are generally not life-threatening, but they can greatly impair physical functioning, emotional well-being, and quality of life. In addition, women with advanced pelvic organ prolapse (POP) have been shown to have decreased body image.[3] Pelvic floor dysfunction is a major health issue for women, as shown by the 11% lifetime risk of undergoing surgery for prolapse or urinary incontinence.[4]

Traditionally, the goal of treatment has been to restore normal pelvic anatomy. However, restoration of normal anatomy does not necessarily result in return to normal function of the pelvic organs. This problem has led to a symptom-based approach for the evaluation and treatment of pelvic floor dysfunction. During the office evaluation, it is therefore important to focus the history on the patient's specific symptoms and to what degree these symptoms affect quality of life. In addition to clinical history taking, the presence, severity, and impact of pelvic floor disorders and symptoms can be assessed via validated questionnaires. Standardized questionnaires are useful when reproducible assessment is needed at baseline and after treatment. For certain conditions, such as anal incontinence and sexual function, questionnaires may be especially helpful to clinically evaluate symptoms.[5] Several validated questionnaires are

Division of Female Pelvic Medicine and Reconstructive Surgery, Department of Obstetrics and Gynecology, David Geffen School of Medicine at UCLA, 27-139 Center for Health Sciences, Los Angeles, CA 90095-1740, USA
* Department of Obstetrics and Gynecology, Olive View-UCLA Medical Center, 14445 Olive View Drive, Room 2B-163, Sylmar, CA 91342.
E-mail address: cwieslander@dhs.lacounty.gov

Obstet Gynecol Clin N Am 36 (2009) 445–462
doi:10.1016/j.ogc.2009.09.003
0889-8545/09/$ – see front matter © 2009 Elsevier Inc. All rights reserved.

obgyn.theclinics.com

available for women with pelvic floor disorders, and a limited number have been translated to, and validated in, Spanish. Short forms have also been created and validated.

Although this article artificially divides symptoms of pelvic floor disorders into areas of POP, urinary dysfunction, anal incontinence, sexual dysfunction, and pelvic pain, many of these disorders are often present simultaneously in the same person.

Symptoms of POP

Symptomatic POP is the least common of the pelvic floor disorders, with an estimated prevalence of 2.9% to 6.0%.[1,2] However, patients with POP can be symptomatic or asymptomatic. Two of the most common symptoms associated with prolapse are seeing or feeling a vaginal bulge, or the sensation of vaginal bulging or protrusion.[6,7] Other symptoms that patients with POP may report include the inability to wear a tampon, feelings of sitting on a weight, or a bulge rubbing on their underwear.

Patients with POP often have concurrent urinary symptoms, including stress urinary incontinence, urge urinary incontinence, frequency, urgency, urinary retention, or voiding dysfunction. Although these conditions may be caused or exacerbated by prolapse, this cannot be assumed. Urodynamic testing should be performed if surgical correction is planned. In women with advanced prolapse, stress urinary incontinence can be masked by kinking an incompetent urethra, called latent, potential, or occult stress incontinence. Urethral kinking can also progress to urethral obstruction manifested by symptoms of urinary hesitancy, incomplete bladder emptying, or inability to void. The patient may have to push on the lower abdomen (Crede maneuver) to empty her bladder, or may need to manually reduce the vaginal bulge to void (splinting).

Defecatory dysfunction is often present in women with POP, and can manifest itself as straining at stool, incomplete evacuation, splinting of the posterior vaginal wall, digitation of the rectum during bowel movement, or fecal incontinence.[8,9] Although these symptoms can occur in association with posterior vaginal wall prolapse, replacement of the prolapse by surgical correction or with a pessary does not consistently cure the symptoms, and may worsen them.[10–13] For example, constipation has multiple causes besides POP. Therefore, a complete evaluation of other causes in addition to prolapse should be performed if the patient's primary symptom is defecatory dysfunction.

Anecdotal evidence suggests that many patients with POP have pelvic and low back pain. However, a cross-sectional study of 152 consecutive patients with POP did not find an association with pelvic and low back pain after controlling for age and prior surgery.[14] It is possible that the pelvic and low back pain is not due to the bulge itself, but due to altered body mechanics that result from the prolapse. Temporary pessary placement can be beneficial to determine whether certain symptoms can be attributed to the prolapse.

Urinary Dysfunction

Urinary incontinence is a common symptom of pelvic floor dysfunction and has a considerable negative impact on the health-related quality of life of women.[15] Depending on the definitions used, the prevalence of urinary incontinence, based on population studies, ranges from 15% to 28%.[1,2,16] Approximately half of patients have symptoms of mixed incontinence, 15% to 33% have symptoms of stress incontinence, and 13% have symptoms of urge incontinence.[2,16] Although history alone is a poor predictor of the type of urinary incontinence,[17–19] it is important to elicit the duration, frequency, severity, and aggravating factors. Urine loss due to elevated intra-abdominal pressure (cough, sneeze, laugh, exercise) is suggestive of stress incontinence, whereas urine leakage preceded by a strong urge to urinate (and leaking before reaching the toilet) suggests urge incontinence. Urinary frequency during the day and at night (nocturia), bed-wetting (nocturnal enuresis), and leakage associated with orgasm are associated with detrusor overactivity. To screen for urinary tract infections and cancer, one should also ask the patient about symptoms of dysuria, hematuria, and a history of previous bladder and kidney infections. Symptoms of urinary hesitancy, straining, slow urinary stream, postvoid dribble, and incomplete bladder emptying suggest voiding dysfunction. In a retrospective case-control study of 1399 women, the absence of stress incontinence symptoms, symptoms of a vaginal bulge, pelvic pressure, urinary splinting, and the presence of prolapse at or beyond the hymen were shown to be associated with elevated postvoid residual (PVR) urine (PVR $\geq$ 100 mL).[20]

Questions regarding the frequency and amount of urine loss, and the need to change underwear or use pads, suggest increased urinary severity. However, a more reliable method to determine incontinence severity is with a urinary voiding diary. The patient is given a urinary collection bowl or hat and a diary, and is asked to record the volume and frequency of all fluid intake and urine output during the day and night for 1 to 7 days. A 3-day diary has been shown to be equivalent to a 7-day diary for documenting frequency and nocturia.[21] Any episodes of urinary incontinence, and associated events and symptoms (urgency, coughing, sleeping, exercise, and so forth), are recorded. The maximum voided volume can be used to estimate the bladder capacity. The diary is then reviewed by the physician and patient, and changes in the amount or type of fluid intake, or voiding frequency, can be made to improve symptoms. The voiding diary can also be used to monitor the success of treatment, and it can be used as an educational tool to modify patient behavior.

Anal Incontinence

Anal incontinence, or the leakage of gas, liquid, or solid stool, is common in women, with a reported prevalence of 25%.[2] If leakage of flatus is excluded, the prevalence of fecal incontinence in population-based studies ranges from 7.2% to 9.0%.[1,22] The cause of fecal incontinence is multifactorial, and includes injury to the anal sphincter complex or its innervation. Other causes include diarrhea, fecal impaction, rectal prolapse, and perineal descent. To evaluate the severity of symptoms, the patient should be asked about the frequency and amount of fecal soilage (fecal staining vs larger amounts), stool consistency, and whether the incontinence occurs with liquid or solid stool. The patient should be questioned about obstetric trauma and difficult delivery, which could suggest anal sphincter injury or pudendal neuropathy. Prior anorectal surgery and chronic constipation may also be contributory factors.

Sexual Dysfunction

Female sexual dysfunction is a condition that describes patients with low libido, problems with sexual arousal, inability to achieve orgasm, and dyspareunia. Although not consistent, studies have found that sexual complaints are common in women with pelvic floor disorders.[23–25] In a community-based study of 4106 women, 86% of women with a partner were sexually active. Women with pelvic floor disorders were less likely to be sexually active, and had lower mean satisfaction scores, than unaffected women. However, after regression analysis, sexual activity and satisfaction were independent of pelvic floor disorders.[25] In contrast, in a cross-sectional study of 301 women seeking outpatient gynecologic and urogynecologic care, pelvic floor symptoms were significantly associated with reduced sexual arousal, infrequent orgasm, and dyspareunia.[26] In this study, sexual dysfunction was worse in women with symptomatic prolapse than in those with asymptomatic prolapse. Women with advanced POP have also been shown to have decreased body image, which may have an effect on sexual function. Because some prolapse procedures, such as posterior repair with levator plication, are believed to contribute to postoperative dyspareunia, care should be taken in planning appropriate surgical procedures for patients with concomitant sexual dysfunction.

Pelvic Pain

Historically, POP has been believed to cause pelvic and low back pain; however, this has not been confirmed in research studies.[14] A careful history and physical examination should be performed to evaluate the patient for gynecologic and nongynecologic causes of pelvic pain. Pelvic floor spasm (levator ani spasm, pelvic floor tension myalgia, pelvic floor hypertonia) is a chronic pain condition due to increased tone and tenderness of 1 or several muscles of the pelvic floor (see other articles in this issue). Common symptoms of women with pelvic floor spasm includes low back pain, a heavy feeling in the pelvis, leg pain, pain with defecation, constipation, coccyx pain, and dyspareunia.[27] The pain is generally worsened with activity, prolonged standing and sitting, and stress, and is improved with heat, relaxation, sedatives, and muscle relaxants.[28]

PHYSICAL EXAMINATION
General Examination

All women should have an annual well-woman examination including cancer screening. Important components of the general examination include an assessment of mental and functional status; body mass index and nutritional status; mobility and manual dexterity; abdominal and pelvic masses; and abdominal, inguinal, and femoral hernias. A urine dip or urinalysis is recommended to exclude urinary tract infection, hematuria, or glucosuria.

Neurologic Evaluation

Although the prevalence of neurologic disease causing urinary and fecal incontinence is low, not identifying these conditions can have considerable consequences to patients. Therefore, a screening neurologic examination should be performed on all patients. This examination should include an evaluation of mental status, sensory and motor function, and reflexes of the lower extremities and lumbosacral spinal cord.

Mental status is evaluated by determining the patient's level of consciousness, orientation, memory, speech, and understanding. A Mini Mental State Examination (MMSE) can be performed in 5 to 10 minutes to screen for cognitive impairment.[29] The MMSE consists of 11 questions that test 5 areas of function: orientation, registration, attention and calculation, recall, and language. The maximum score is 30, and a score of 23 or lower indicates cognitive impairment. Delirium, dementia, brain tumors, and strokes are disorders that may present with altered mental status and changes in bladder or bowel functions.

Sensory function is evaluated by testing the integrity of the lumbosacral dermatomes for the ability to discriminate between light touch, pin prick, and cold sensation. A Q-tip can be broken in half and the soft end used to assess light touch the sharp end is used to assess pin prick. Cold sensation can be assessed by using an alcohol swab. The sensory dermatomes should include the perineal and perianal skin (S2–S4). Other dermatomes of interest include mons pubis and upper labia majora (L1–L2), front of the knees (L3–L4) and the lateral part of the foot (S1).[30] A sensory deficit in a specific dermatome distribution is consistent with peripheral neuropathy. Numbness and paresthesias in a dermatome distribution can distinguish between central and peripheral neuropathies. However, there can be significant overlap between dermatomes.

Motor function of the lumbosacral cord is assessed by evaluating the strength of the lower extremities. The patient is asked to perform flexion (L2–L3) and extension (L5–S1) of the hip, flexion (L5–S1) and extension (L3–L4) of the knee, dorsiflexion (L4–L5) and plantar flexion (S1–S2) of the ankle, and inversion (L4–L5) and eversion (L5–S1) of the ankle. Motor function is graded from 0 to 5, as noted in **Table 1**.[30] The strength and tone of the levator ani muscles are assessed by palpating the vaginal wall at 5 and 7 o'clock, approximately 2 to 4 cm cephalad to the hymen. The patient is asked to squeezed her vaginal muscles as though she were holding gas or stopping urine flow. The strength of the levator ani muscles can be graded using the Modified Oxford Scale, as noted in **Table 2**.[31] The levator ani muscles should also be assessed for tenderness to palpation or spasm. If tenderness is assessed during palpation, the patient should be asked whether palpation reproduces any pain that the patient experiences in real life. Sensation of the bladder and rectum can be evaluated with cystometry and anal manometry.

The integrity of the pudendal nerve can be evaluated with the anal reflex (anal wink) and the bulbocavernosus reflex. The anal reflex is performed by gently stroking the perianal skin, which causes a reflex contraction of the external anal sphincter. In the bulbocavernosus reflex, the bulbocavernosus and ischiocavernosis muscles contract in response to tapping or squeezing the clitoris. Although absence of these reflexes can result from damage to the sacral cord or pudendal nerve, in 10% of neurologically intact patients, the response is too weak to visualize.[32] Deep tendon reflexes (L2–L4) can be helpful in distinguishing lesions above or below T12. Hyperreflexia of the deep tendon reflexes indicate an upper motor lesion, whereas diminished or absent reflexes indicate a lower motor lesion. Clinically, patients with cauda equina lesions or peripheral neuropathy demonstrate decreased bladder contractility with urinary retention and voiding difficulty.

Pelvic Examination

The goal of the pelvic examination is to objectively assess the anatomy of the pelvic floor and pelvic organs, and to attempt to correlate symptoms with anatomic findings. The severity of prolapse, the degree of pelvic floor support, and the integrity of the connective tissue of the vaginal wall is determined. The examination is performed in the dorsal lithotomy position, with the patient in stirrups. If physical findings do not

Table 1 Grading of muscle strength (Oxford scale)	
Grade	Description
0/5	No muscle movement
1/5	Muscle movement without joint motion
2/5	Movement with gravity eliminated
3/5	Movement against gravity but not against resistance
4/5	Movement against gravity and light resistance
5/5	Normal strength

Modified from LeBlond, RF, Brown D, DeGowin R. et al. DeGowin's diagnostic examination. 9th edition. USA: McGraw-Hill Co., Inc.; 2009; with permission.

Table 2
Grading of pelvic floor muscle strength (Modified Oxford Scale)

Grade	Description
0/5	No discernible pelvic floor muscle contraction
1/5	A flicker or pulsing under the examining finger; a weak contraction
2/5	A weak contraction; an increase in tension in the muscle without any discernible lift or squeeze
3/5	A moderate contraction; characterized by a degree of lifting of the posterior vaginal wall and squeezing on the base of the finger with in-drawing of the perineum. A grade 3 or higher contraction is generally discernible on visual perineal inspection
4/5	A good pelvic floor muscle contraction producing elevation of the posterior vaginal wall against resistance and in-drawing of the perineum. If 2 fingers (index and middle) are placed laterally or vertically in the vagina and separated, a grade 4 contraction can squeeze them together against resistance
5/5	A strong contraction of the pelvic floor muscle; strong resistance can be given against elevation of the posterior vaginal wall and approximation of the index and middle fingers as for grade 4/5

Modified from Haslam J, Laycock J. Therapeutic management of incontinence and pelvic pain. 2nd edition. London: Springer-Verlag; 2008; with permission.

correlate with symptoms while the patient is performing maximal valsalva, the patient can be examined in the standing position. However, studies have shown there is no difference in severity of prolapse in the lithotomy or standing position,[33] or if the patient is examined in the morning or afternoon.[34] First, the external genitalia are inspected for lesions or rashes. Pads and urine can cause a contact dermatitis or maceration of the skin of the labia majora and vulva. The labia are separated to expose the vestibule and hymen. The anterior vaginal wall and urethra are inspected and palpated. Urethral discharge, tenderness, or masses may indicate a urethral diverticulum, vaginal cyst, carcinoma, or inflammatory condition of the urethra. The patient is asked to cough or valsalva to evaluate for stress urinary incontinence. A Q-tip test (see section on Urethral Mobility) may be performed if the patient has symptoms of stress urinary incontinence. The vaginal epithelium is inspected for atrophy, and the integrity of the perineal body is assessed.

To perform the prolapse evaluation, the patient is asked to valsalva, and the maximal extent of the prolapse is noted (**Fig. 1**). The support of the apex can be evaluated by using a bivalve speculum. The movement of the cervix or vaginal cuff is noted while gradually removing an open bivalve speculum. The support of the anterior and posterior vaginal wall is assessed with a Sim speculum or the posterior blade of a bivalve speculum. The speculum is used to support the apex and posterior vaginal wall while the maximum descent and support defects of the anterior vaginal wall are assessed (**Fig. 2**). Similarly the posterior vaginal wall is evaluated while the apex and anterior vaginal wall is supported (**Fig. 3**).

Staging of POP

Two main classification systems are used to quantify the severity of prolapse. The Halfway System for Grading Pelvic Relaxations was developed by Baden and Walker in the late 1960s and modified in 1992.[35] This system is simple to use and was widely used for years by gynecologic surgeons. The most dependent portion of the pelvic organs (urethra, bladder, uterus, cul-de-sac, and rectum) during maximum straining

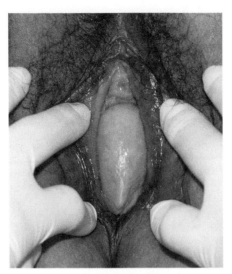

Fig. 1. Maximum extent of vaginal prolapse is seen without the use of a speculum.

or standing is graded as normal, first, second, or third degree (**Table 3**). Although the Halfway System for Grading Pelvic Relaxations quantifies specific sites of prolapse, it is only an estimation of descent relative to the hymen.

The Pelvic Organ Prolapse Quantification System (POPQ) was drafted by a subcommittee of the International Continence Society (ICS) in 1993 to more accurately quantify pelvic support findings. The POPQ was approved by the ICS in 1995, and by the American Urogynecologic Society (AUGS) and the Society of Gynecologic Surgeons (SGS) in 1996.[36] It has been shown to be a highly reproducible examination with

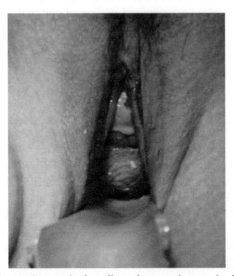

Fig. 2. Evaluation of anterior vaginal wall prolapse using a single-blade speculum to support the posterior vaginal wall and apex.

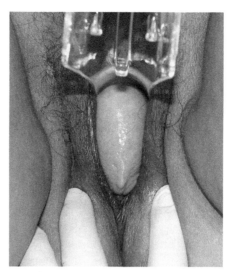

Fig. 3. Evaluation of posterior vaginal wall prolapse using a single-blade speculum to support the anterior vaginal wall and apex.

good intra- and interrater reliability.[37] The POPQ system measures 6 sites (2 on the anterior vaginal wall, 2 on the superior vaginal wall, and 2 on the posterior vaginal wall) in relation to a fixed anatomic landmark, the hymen (**Fig. 4**). The position of the 6 sites is measured in centimeters proximal (negative number) or distal (positive number) to the hymen (defined as zero).

The 2 anterior vaginal wall points are point Aa and point Ba (see **Fig. 4**). Point Aa is a fixed point located in the midline of the anterior vaginal wall 3 cm proximal to the external urethral meatus corresponding to the urethrovesical crease. By definition, the range of position of point Aa relative to the hymen is −3 to +3 cm. Point Ba represents the most distal or dependent portion of any part of the anterior vaginal wall from the vaginal cuff or anterior vaginal fornix to point Aa. By definition, point Ba is at −3 cm in the absence of prolapse, and would have a positive value equal to the position of the cuff in women with total posthysterectomy vaginal eversion. The term "anterior vaginal wall prolapse" is preferred to "cystocele" or "anterior

Table 3	
Baden Walker Halfway System for grading pelvic relaxations	
Grade	**Description. Urethrocele, Cystocele, Uterine Prolapse, Culdocele, or Rectocele: Patient Strains Firmly. Grade Posterior Urethral Descent, lowest Part other Sites**
0	Normal position for each respective site
1	Descent halfway to the hymen
2	Descent to the hymen
3	Descent halfway past the hymen
4	Maximum possible descent for each site

Modified from Baden W, Walker T. Surgical repair of vaginal defects. Philadelphia: JB Lippincott; 1992. p. 14; with permission.

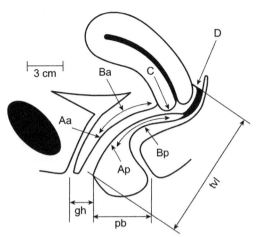

Fig. 4. Six sites (Aa, Ba, C, D, Bp, Ap), genital hiatus (gh), perineal body (pb), and total vaginal length (tvl) used for pelvic organ support quantification. (*From* Bump RC, Mattiasson A, Bo K, et al. The standardization of terminology of female pelvic organ prolapse and pelvic floor dysfunction. Am J Obstet Gynecol 1996;175:10–17; redrawn with permission.)

enterocele" because the only structure directly visible to the examiner is the surface of the vagina. Likewise, "posterior vaginal wall prolapse" is preferred to "rectocele" or "enterocele" unless the organs involved are identified by ancillary test.[36]

The 2 superior vaginal points are points C and D (see **Fig. 4**). These points represent the most proximal locations of the normally positioned lower reproductive genital tract. Point C represents the most distal or dependent edge of the cervix or the leading edge of the vaginal cuff (hysterectomy scar) after total hysterectomy. Point D represents the location of the posterior fornix or pouch of Douglas in a woman who still has a cervix. Point D represents the level of the uterosacral ligament attachment to the proximal posterior cervix. It is included as a point of measurement to differentiate suspensory failure of the uterosacral ligament complex from cervical elongation. When the location of point C is significantly more positive than the location of point D, it suggests cervical elongation. Point D is omitted in the absence of a cervix.[36]

Two points are located on the posterior vaginal wall: point Ap and Bp (see **Fig. 4**). Point Ap is a fixed point located in the midline of the posterior vaginal wall 3 cm proximal to the hymen. By definition, the range of position of point Ap relative to the hymen is −3 to +3 cm. Point Bp represents the most distal or dependent portion of any part of the upper posterior vaginal wall from the vaginal cuff or posterior vaginal fornix to point Ap. By definition, point Bp is at −3 cm in the absence of prolapse, and would have a positive value equal to the position of the cuff in a woman with total posthysterectomy vaginal eversion.[36]

Other landmarks and measurements of the POPQ include the genital hiatus (gh), perineal body (pb) and total vaginal length (tvl) (see **Fig. 4**). The genital hiatus is measured from the middle of the external urethral meatus to the posterior midline of the hymen. The perineal body is measured from the posterior midline of the hymen to the midanal opening. The total vaginal length is the greatest depth of the vagina in centimeters when points C and D are reduced to normal position. In general, all measurements except for total vaginal length are obtained with the patient performing a maximal valsalva. Measurements can be recorded as a simple line of numbers (eg, −3, −3, −7, −9, −3. −3, 9, 2, 2 for points As, Ba, C, D, Bp, Ap, tvl, gh, and pb respectively). As an alternative, a 3-by-3 grid can be used to concisely organize the measurements (**Fig. 5**), or a line diagram can be drawn of the configuration (**Figs. 6 and 7**). Stages are assigned according to the most severe position of the prolapse when the full extent of the protrusion has been demonstrated. The 5 stages of the POPQ examination are described in **Table 4**.[36]

Site-Specific Defect Analysis of the Vagina

Although the POPQ quantifies the degree of vaginal support, it does not identify specific anatomic defects that can be addressed with surgical intervention. Anterior vaginal wall defects include midline, paravaginal, and transverse defects. These defects can be assessed using ringed forceps to support aspects of the anterior vaginal wall while the posterior wall is retracted with a single-blade speculum. A midline defect is caused by a midline tear or attenuation of the anterior vaginal wall fibromuscular layer (pubocervical fascia). This defect is suspected if a midline vaginal bulge is noted when the lateral sulci and apex of the vagina are supported with ringed forceps. A midline defect can also be assessed by closing the blades of the forceps and elevating the midline of the vagina with straining. A transverse defect results from a separation of the anterior vaginal wall fibromuscular layer of the vaginal wall from its attachment to the anterior margin of the pericervical ring, or from a separation of the pericervical ring from its attachment to the uterosacral ligaments.[38] In the first case, a distinct bulging out of the anterior vaginal fornix is seen with the patient straining. The bulge may appear smooth and without rugations owing to the loss of the underlying anterior vaginal wall fibromuscular layer. In the second case, a detachment of each uterosacral ligament to the pericervical ring results in a significant cervical descensus, with no thickness of uterosacral ligaments being palpated near the pericervical ring.[39] A paravaginal defect results from a partial or complete detachment of the lateral vaginal wall from the arcus tendineus fascia pelvis or white line. These defects appear as blunting or descent of the lateral sulcus on either side with straining. Unilateral paravaginal defects can be assessed by supporting each sulcus to the

anterior wall	anterior wall	cervix or cuff
Aa	**Ba**	**C**
genital hiatus	perineal body	total vaginal length
gh	**pb**	**tvl**
posterior wall	posterior wall	posterior fornix
Ap	**Bp**	**D**

Fig. 5. Grid for recording quantitative description of pelvic organ support. (*From* Bump RC, Mattiasson A, Bo K, et al. The standardization of terminology of female pelvic organ prolapse and pelvic floor dysfunction. Am J Obstet Gynecol 1996;175:10–17; redrawn with permission.)

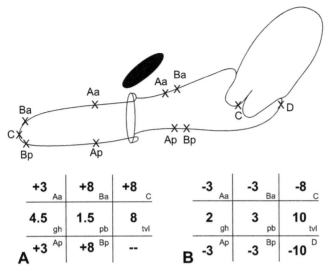

+3	+8	+8		-3	-3	-8
Aa	Ba	C		Aa	Ba	C
4.5	1.5	8		2	3	10
gh	pb	tvl		gh	pb	tvl
+3 Ap	+8 Bp	--		-3 Ap	-3 Bp	-10 D

A   **B**

Fig. 6. (A) Complete eversion of vagina. Most distal point of anterior wall (Ba), vaginal cuff scar (C), and most distal point of the posterior wall (Bp) are all at the same position (+8) and points Aa and Ap are maximally distal (+3). Because total vaginal length equals maximum protrusion, this is stage IV prolapse. (B) Normal support. Points Aa and Ba and points Ap and Bp are all −3 because there is no anterior or posterior wall descent. Lowest point of the cervix is 8 cm above the hymen (−8) and posterior fornix is 2 cm above this (−10). Vaginal length is 10 cm and genital hiatus and perineal body measure 2 and 3 cm, respectively. This condition represents stage 0 support. (*From* Bump RC, Mattiasson A, Bo K, et al. The standardization of terminology of female pelvic organ prolapse and pelvic floor dysfunction. Am J Obstet Gynecol 1996;175:10–17; redrawn with permission.)

sidewall separately with closed ring forceps. If this maneuver eliminates the bulge of the anterior vaginal wall with the patient straining, it suggests that this is the site of the support defect. Bilateral paravaginal defects are assessed by opening the blades of the ring forceps and supporting both lateral sulci along the arcus tendineus fascia pelvis. Several studies have shown that the correlation between the clinical examination and intraoperative findings may not be reliable. A retrospective study by Barber and colleagues[40] showed that of 117 women undergoing surgery for anterior vaginal wall prolapse, less than two-thirds of women believed to have paravaginal defects preoperatively had these defects confirmed intraoperatively. The sensitivity of the clinical assessment for paravaginal defects was good (92%) but the sensitivity was poor (52%).[40] A prospective study by Whiteside and colleagues[41] similarly showed poor reproducibility of the clinical examination of anterior vaginal wall defects within the same examiner and between different examiners. Because of these findings, and because, in real practice, most women have a mixture of defects, the clinical value of determining the location of midline, transverse, and paravaginal is questioned.

Apical defects can be seen in patients with uterine or vaginal cuff prolapse. In uterine prolapse, the cervix has become detached from the cardinal-uterosacral ligament complex and the anterior and posterior vaginal wall fibromuscular layers. This defect can be evaluated by using an open bivalve speculum that is slowly retracted while the patient is bearing down. The posterior and lateral fornices are seen bulging, and there is wide lateral and downward mobility of the cervix. It is important to estimate the length of the cervix, because cervical elongation can be seen with

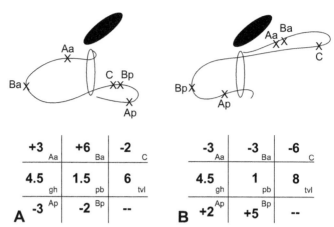

+3	+6	-2		-3	-3	-6
Aa	Ba	C		Aa	Ba	C
4.5	1.5	6		4.5	1	8
gh	pb	tvl		gh	pb	tvl
A -3 Ap	-2 Bp	--		B +2 Ap	+5 Bp	--

Fig. 7. (*A*) Predominantly anterior support defect. Leading point of prolapse is the upper anterior vaginal wall (Ba; +6). There is significant elongation of bulging at the anterior wall. Point Aa is maximally distal (+3) and vaginal cuff scar is 2 cm above hymen (C = −2). Cuff scar has undergone 4 cm of descent, because it would be at −6 (total vaginal length) if it were perfectly supported. In this example, total vaginal length is not maximum depth of vagina with elongated anterior vaginal wall maximally reduced, but depth of vagina at cuff with point C reduced to its normal full extent, as specified in the text. This condition represents stage III Ba prolapse. (*B*) Predominant posterior support defect. Leading point of prolapse is upper posterior vaginal wall, point Bp (+5). Point Ap is 2 cm distal to hymen (=2) and vaginal cuff scar is 6 cm above hymen (−6). Cuff has undergone only 2 cm of descent, because it would be at −8 (total vaginal length) if it were perfectly supported. This condition represents stage III Bp prolapse. (*From* Bump RC, Mattiasson A, Bo K, et al. The standardization of terminology of female pelvic organ prolapse and pelvic floor dysfunction. Am J Obstet Gynecol 1996;175:10–17; redrawn with permission.)

uterine prolapse. Vaginal cuff prolapse after hysterectomy results from the detachment of the cardinal and uterosacral ligaments from the vaginal apex. In addition, an apical enterocele may be present. In an apical enterocele, the anterior and posterior vaginal wall fibromuscular layers have been separated due to the disruption of the pericervical ring causing the peritoneum to be in direct contact with the vaginal epithelium. The overlying vaginal epithelium appears stretched and smooth, without rugae.[39] Occasionally, small bowel may be palpated or peristalsis may be seen though the vaginal epithelium. However, it may be difficult to discriminate between an enterocele and a high rectocele during physical examination. A rectovaginal examination may be helpful to differentiate the 2, because an enterocele may be palpated as a bulge noted to descend between the vaginal and rectal fingers while the patient is straining. Imaging techniques, such as defecography or dynamic magnetic resonance imaging (MRI) may also be helpful in discriminating between enterocele and high rectocele.

Posterior vaginal wall defects are due to breaks or global attenuation of the posterior vaginal wall fibromuscular layer (rectovaginal fascia). The defects in the posterior vaginal wall fibromuscular layer allow the rectal muscularis to bulge up against the vaginal epithelium. These defects are best evaluated via a rectovaginal examination while supporting the anterior vaginal wall and apex with a single-blade speculum. This method allows the examiner to evaluate breaks or defects and thickness of the posterior vaginal wall fibromuscular layer. Breaks in the distal third of the posterior vaginal wall are called distal posterior vaginal wall prolapse (distal rectocele), and breaks in the upper third of the vagina are called upper posterior vaginal wall

Table 4 Staging of the POPQ	
Stage	**Description**
0	No prolapse is demonstrated. Points Aa, Ap, Ba, and Bp are all at −3 cm, and point C or D is between −TVL (total vaginal length) cm and −(TVL-2) cm (ie, the quantification value for point C or D is ≤− [TVL-2] cm). **Fig. 6**B, represents stage 0
I	The criteria for stage 0 are not met, but the most distal portion of the prolapse is >1 cm above the level of the hymen (ie, its quantification value is <−1 cm)
II	The most distal portion of the prolapse is ≤1 cm proximal to or distal to the plane of the hymen (ie, its quantification value is ≥−1 cm but ≤+1 cm)
III	The most distal portion of the prolapse is >1 cm below the plane of the hymen but protrudes no further than 2 cm less than the total vaginal length in centimeters (ie, its quantification value is >+1 cm but <+[TVL-2] cm). **Fig. 7**A, represents stage II Ba, and **Fig. 7**B, represents stage III Bp prolapse
IV	Complete eversion of the total length of the lower genital tract. The distal portion of the prolapse protrudes to at least (TVL-2) cm (ie, its quantification value is ≥ +[TVL-2] cm). The leading edge of stage IV prolapse will usually be the cervix or vaginal cuff scar. **Fig. 6**A, represents stage IV C prolapse.

Modified from Bump RC, Mattiasson A, Bo K, et al. The standardization of terminology of female pelvic organ prolapse and pelvic floor dysfunction. Am J Obstet Gynecol 1996;175:10–17; with permission.

prolapse (high rectocele). Upper posterior vaginal wall prolapse appears as a bulging down of the posterior lateral walls of the vagina and cul-de-sac toward the middle third of the vagina. These high defects are associated with posterior and apical enteroceles. Richardson and colleagues[42] described site-specific defects located in the superior, inferior, right, left, and midline of the rectovaginal septum. However, the accuracy of detecting these specific defects on clinical examination is limited. In a retrospective comparison of clinical examination and intraoperative findings in 106 patients, Burrows and colleagues[43] found the sensitivity and positive predictive value for all defects to be less than 40%. Not detecting these specific defects preoperatively might be of no clinical consequence.

Evaluation of Perineum and Anal Sphincter

The perineum and anal sphincter are evaluated via inspection and rectovaginal examination. The perineal body consists of dense connective tissue and muscle fibers, and measures 3 to 4 cm in the anterior posterior direction, and 2 to 3 cm in the craniocaudal direction. It is attached anteriorly to the perineal membrane, and cranially to the posterior vaginal wall. These attachments stabilize the perineal body from downward and lateral movement. There are 5 muscles that attach to the perineal body: 2 paired bulbocavernosus muscles, 2 paired transverse perineal muscles, and the external anal sphincter. Separation of the bulbocavernosus or transverse perineal muscles causes a widened genital hiatus and a short perineal body, which can be seen during the POPQ examination with the patient at rest. A complete separation of the perineal body and external anal sphincter would be the result of a congenital cloaca or a chronic fourth degree laceration. In this situation, the perineal body would be absent.

The perineal body is attached to the sacrum indirectly via its attachment to the posterior vaginal wall fibromuscular layer, which is attached to the uterosacral ligaments. This attachment causes the perineum to be concave in shape, and limits its downward mobility to about 1 cm. Movement of the perineal body greater than

2 cm past the level of the ischial tuberosities suggests perineal descent. Perineal descent is also characterized by bulging and widening of the perineum with valsalva. On POPQ examination of a patient with perineal descent, the genital hiatus and perineal body widen as the patient strains. A perineal rectocele is caused by a complete disruption of the perineal body itself, causing the rectal muscularis to be in direct contact with the perineal skin. On physical examination, the perineal body is elongated and demonstrates ballooning as the patient strains.

To evaluate the anus, the skin of the perineum and anus should be inspected for deformity, scarring, and flattening of the gluteal creases. The presence of a "dovetail sign" suggests anterior separation of the anal sphincter. This appears as loss of the skin creases around the anterior aspect of the external anal sphincter. The patient is asked to squeeze the anal sphincter to look for uniform circular contraction of the muscle. Next, the patient is asked to strain to show perineal descent, and rectal prolapse. A digital rectal examination is performed to assess the internal and external sphincter. The initial resting tone reflects the integrity and strength of the internal anal sphincter. To assess the external anal sphincter, the patient is asked to squeeze the anus as if to hold a bowel movement. Strength, muscle defects, and early "fatigability" are assessed. The patient should also be asked to bear down with a finger still within the anus. Paradoxic contraction of the puborectalis and external anal sphincter during valsalva may indicate anismus. The presence of large amounts of fecal material in the rectum may suggest fecal impaction or neuromuscular weakness. The anus and rectum should also be assessed for masses and hemorrhoids. Ancillary tests such as endoanal ultrasound, defecography, pudendal nerve terminal motor latency, and anorectal manometry can also be ordered to evaluate the anatomy, function, and innervation of the anal sphincter and rectum.

Urethral Mobility

The support of the bladder neck is assessed by evaluating the mobility of the urethrovesical junction (UVJ). Direct visualization of the anterior vaginal wall for urethral hypermobility is generally considered inaccurate[44] unless the patient has significant anterior vaginal wall prolapse (POPQ stage II–IV).[45] Urethral hypermobility can be assessed with the Q-tip test or by imaging techniques such as lateral cystourethrogram or ultrasonography.[46] The Q-tip test is performed with the patient in the supine position. First, the external urethral meatus is cleaned with an antibacterial solution. Next, a sterile cotton-tipped applicator that has been lubricated with an anesthetic ointment is inserted transurethrally into the bladder, and then withdrawn slowly until definite resistance is felt, indicating that the cotton tip is at the bladder neck (**Fig. 8**A). The resting angle is measure with a goniometer, with the reference being parallel to the floor. The patient is then asked to valsalva or cough, and the excursion angle is measured (see **Fig. 8**B). Urethral hypermobility is generally defined as a movement with straining of more than 30° from the horizontal.[46] Although the Q-tip test reliably predicts urethral hypermobility,[47,48] it has never been demonstrated to be able to diagnose the type of incontinence,[49,50] and there is a wide overlap between continent and incontinent women.[51] Because the main goal of determining urethral hypermobility is to determine which patients benefit from surgical stabilization of the bladder neck, the Q-tip test can be omitted from the basic evaluation if a patient does not desire surgical management.

Evaluation of Urethral Sphincter and Bladder Function

The physical examination of the patient with symptoms of urinary incontinence should try to reproduce the patient's symptoms. The patient is asked to cough with the bladder comfortably full. With the patient in the supine position, the external urethral

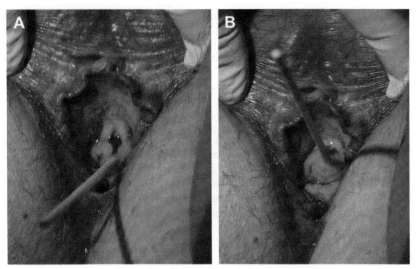

Fig. 8. (A) The Q-tip test demonstrates a normal resting angle of approximately 0°. (B) With patient straining, the Q-tip test demonstrates an angle of approximately 45°.

meatus is observed for urine loss. Small spurts of urine leakage concurrent with cough suggests stress urinary incontinence, whereas prolonged loss of urine ,or leaking after the cough has concluded, suggests detrusor overactivity. If no urine loss is noted and the patient has anterior vaginal wall prolapse, the anterior vaginal wall should be elevated with an instrument to unmask potential or occult urinary incontinence. If urine loss is not seen in the supine position, the patient should be asked to cough in the standing position.

The patient is then asked to void in private, and the voided volume is recorded. The time to void can also be recorded with a stopwatch in lieu of a formal uroflowmetry study. At this time, a clean catch urine sample can be obtained. The PVR urine is then determined via bladder ultrasound or catheterization. Normal values for PVR have not been established, and are based on expert opinion. Volumes less than 50 mL indicate adequate bladder emptying, and volumes greater than 200 mL can be considered inadequate emptying.[52] Clinical judgment must be used when interpreting PVR in the range of 50 to 200 mL, and the test should be repeated if abnormally high values are obtained.

Evaluation of bladder filling and storage can be performed in the office setting via simple cystometry (eyeball cystometry) or via multichannel cystometry. Simple cystometry is performed by placing a transurethral catheter and emptying the bladder. A 60-mL catheter-tip syringe without its piston is then attached to the catheter and held 10 to 15 cm above the pubic symphysis. With the patient in the sitting or standing position, the bladder is filled with sterile saline or water in 50-mL increments. The meniscus of the fluid in the syringe is noted throughout the procedure, because any increase in the meniscus can be due to a detrusor contraction. The patient's first bladder sensation, first desire to void, strong desire to void, and bladder capacity are also noted.[53] The definition of normal bladder capacity lacks consensus, with values ranging from 300 mL to 750 mL.[52] If the patient did not leak with coughing during the initial evaluation, a repeat cough stress test can be performed at bladder capacity after the catheter has been removed. The results of simple cystometry have been shown to be comparable with multichannel cystometry in diagnosing urodynamic stress urinary incontinence and detrusor overactivity, if these are demonstrated during simple cystometric testing.[54,55] However, a negative cystometry does not rule out the presence of urge urinary incontinence.[55] If the patient has symptoms of urge urinary incontinence and a negative cystometry, multichannel urodynamic testing can be useful.

SUMMARY

Pelvic floor disorders are common health issues for women and have a great impact on quality of life. Because these disorders can present with a wide spectrum of symptoms and anatomic defects, each patient should be evaluated based on her unique symptoms and physical findings. The goal of treatment is to provide as much symptom relief as possible. After education and counseling, patients may be candidates for nonsurgical or surgical treatment, and expectant management.

REFERENCES

1. Nygaard I, Barber M, Burgio K, et al. Prevalence of symptomatic pelvic floor disorders in US women. JAMA 2008;300(11):1311–6.
2. Lawrence J, Lukacz E, Nager C, et al. Prevalence and co-occurrence of pelvic floor disorders in community-dwelling women. Obstet Gynecol 2008;111(3): 678–85.
3. Jelovsek J, Barber M. Women seeking treatment for advanced pelvic organ prolapse have decreased body image and quality of life. Am J Obstet Gynecol 2006;194:1455–61.
4. Olsen A, Smith V, Bergstrom J, et al. Epidemiology of surgically managed pelvic organ prolapse and urinary incontinence. Obstet Gynecol 1997;89(4):501–6.
5. Barber M. Questionnaires for women with pelvic floor disorders. Int Urogynecol J Pelvic Floor Dysfunct 2007;18(4):461–5.
6. Ellerkmann R, Cundiff G, Melick C, et al. Correlation of symptoms with location and severity of pelvic organ prolapse. Am J Obstet Gynecol 2001;185:1332–8.
7. Bradley C, Zimmerman M, Wang Q, et al. Vaginal descent and pelvic floor symptoms in postmenopausal women. A longitudinal study. Obstet Gynecol 2008; 111(5):1148–53.
8. Kahn M, Breitkopf C, Valley M, et al. Pelvic organ support study (POSST) and bowel symptoms: straining at stool is associated with perineal and anterior vaginal descent in a general gynecology population. Am J Obstet Gynecol 2005;192:1516–22.
9. Weber A, Walters M, Ballard L, et al. Posterior vaginal prolapse and bowel function. Obstet Gynecol 1998;179(6):1446–9.
10. Cundiff G, Weidner A, Visco A, et al. An anatomic and functional assessment of the discrete defect rectocele repair. Am J Obstet Gynecol 1998;179(6):1451–7.
11. Kenton K, Shott S, Brubaker L. The anatomic and functional variability of rectoceles in women. Int Urogynecol J Pelvic Floor Dysfunct 1999;10(2):96–9.
12. Mellgren A, Anzén B, Nilsson B, et al. Results of rectocele repair. A prospective study. Dis Colon Rectum 1995;38(1):7–13.
13. Kahn M, Stanton S. Posterior colporrhaphy: its effects on bowel and sexual function. Br J Obstet Gynaecol 1997;104(1):82–6.
14. Heit M, Culligan P, Rosenquist C, et al. Is pelvic organ prolapse a cause of pelvic or low back pain? Obstet Gynecol 2002;99(1):23–8.

15. Monz B, Pons M, Hampel C, et al. Patient-reported impact of urinary incontinence – results from treatment seeking women in 14 European countries. Maturitas 2005;52S:S24–34.
16. Melville J, Katon W, Delaney K, et al. Urinary incontinence in US women: a population-based study. Arch Intern Med 2005;165:537–42.
17. Harvey M, Versi E. Predicting value of clinical evaluation of stress urinary incontinence: a summary of the published literature. Int Urogynecol J Pelvic Floor Dysfunct 2001;12:31–7.
18. Sand P, Hill R, Ostergard D. Incontinence history as a predictor of detrusor stability. Obstet Gynecol 1988;71:257–60.
19. Jensen J, Nielsen F, Ostergard D. The role of patient history in the diagnosis of urinary incontinence. Obstet Gynecol 1994;83:904–10.
20. Lukacz E, DuHamel E, Menefee S, et al. Elevated postvoid residual in women with pelvic floor disorders: Prevalence and associated risk factors. Int Urogynecol J Pelvic Floor Dysfunct 2007;18:397–400.
21. Brown J, McNaughton K, Wyman J, et al. Measurement characteristics of a voiding diary for use by men and women with overactive bladder. Urology 2003;61(4):802–9.
22. Melville J, Fan M, Newton K, et al. Fecal incontinence in US women: a population-based study. Am J Obstet Gynecol 2005;193:2071–6.
23. Barber M, Visco A, Wyman J, et al. Sexual function in women with urinary incontinence and pelvic organ prolapse. Obstet Gynecol 2002;99:281–9.
24. Handa V, Harvey L, Cundiff G, et al. Sexual function among women with urinary incontinence and pelvic organ prolapse. Am J Obstet Gynecol 2004;191:751–6.
25. Lukacz E, Whitcomb E, Lawrence L, et al. Are sexual activity and satisfaction affected by pelvic floor disorders? Analysis of a community-based survey. Am J Obstet Gynecol 2007;197(88):e1–6.
26. Handa V, Cundiff G, Chang H, et al. Female sexual function and pelvic floor disorders. Obstet Gynecol 2008;111:1045–52.
27. Sinaki M, Meritt J, Stillwell G. Tension myalgia of pelvic floor. Mayo Clin Proc 1977;52(11):717–22.
28. Marvel R. Pelvic floor tension myalgia. In: Bent AE, Cundiff GW, Swift SW, editors. Ostergard's urogynecology and pelvic floor dysfunction. 6th edition. Philadelphia: Lippincott Williams & Wilkins; 2008. p. 133–47.
29. Folstein M, Folstein S, McHugh P. "Mini-mental state" a practical method for grading the cognitive state of patients for the clinician. J Psychiatr Res 1975;12(3):189–98.
30. LeBlond R, Brown D, DeGowin R. The neurologic examination. Chapter 14. In: Shanahan J, Edmonson KG, editors. DeGowin's diagnostic examination, 9th edition. USA: McGraw-Hill Medical; 2009. p. 683–763.
31. Laycock J, Whelan M, Dumoulin C. Patient assessment. Chapter 7. In: Haslam J, Laycock J, editors. Therapeutic management of incontinence and pelvic pain, 2nd edition. London: Springer-Verlag; 2008. p. 62.
32. Blavias JG, Zayed AAH, Kamal BC. The bulbocavenosus reflex in urology; a prospective study of 299 patients. J Urol 1981;126(2):197–9.
33. Swift S, Herring M. Comparison of pelvic organ prolapse in the dorsal lithotomy compared with the standing position. Obstet Gynecol 1998;91:961–4.
34. Pearce M, Swift S, Goodnight W. Pelvic organ prolapse: is there a difference in POPQ exam results based on time of day, morning or afternoon? Am J Obstet Gynecol 2008;199(200):e1–5.
35. Baden W, Walker T. Surgical repair of vaginal defects. Philadelphia: JB Lippincott; 1992.

36. Bump R, Mattiasson A, Bo K, et al. The standardization of terminology of female pelvic organ prolapse and pelvic floor dysfunction. Am J Obstet Gynecol 1996;175:10–7.

37. Hall A, Theofrastous J, Cundiff G, et al. Interobserver and intraobserver reliability of the proposed International Continence Society, Society of Gynecologic Surgeons, and American Urogynecologic Society pelvic organ prolapse classification system. Am J Obstet Gynecol 1996;175:1467–71.

38. Richardson A, Lyon J, Williams N. A new look at pelvic relaxation. Am J Obstet Gynecol 1976;126:569–73.

39. Cundiff G. The clinical evaluation of pelvic organ prolapse. In: Bent AE, Cundiff GW, Swift SW, editors. Ostergard's urogynecology and pelvic floor dysfunction. 6th edition. Philadelphia: Lippincott Williams & Wilkins; 2008. p. 422–39.

40. Barber M, Cundiff G, Weidner A, et al. Accuracy of clinical assessment of paravaginal defects in women with anterior vaginal wall prolapse. Am J Obstet Gynecol 1999;181(1):87–90.

41. Whiteside J, Barber M, Paraiso M, et al. Clinical evaluation of anterior vaginal support defects: interexaminer and intraexaminer reliability. Am J Obstet Gynecol 2004;191:100–4.

42. Richardson A. The rectovaginal septum revisited: its relationship to rectocele and its importance in rectocele repair. Clin Obstet Gynecol 1993;36:976–83.

43. Burrows L, Sewell C, Leffler K, et al. The accuracy of clinical evaluation of posterior vaginal wall defects. Int Urogynecol J Pelvic Floor Dysfunct 2003;14:160–3.

44. Montella JM, Ewing S, Cater J. Visual assessment of urethrovesical junction mobility. Int Urogynecol J Pelvic Floor Dysfunct 1997;8(1):13–7.

45. Noblett K, Lane F, Driskill C. Does pelvic organ prolapse quantification exam predict urethral mobility in stages 0 and I prolapse? Int Urogynecol J Pelvic Floor Dysfunct 2005;16(4):268–71.

46. Karram M, Bhatia N. The Q-tip test: standardization of the technique and its interpretations in women with urinary incontinence. Obstet Gynecol 1988;71(6):807–11.

47. Thorp J, Jones L, Wells E, et al. Assessment of pelvic floor function: a series of simple tests in nulliparous women. Int Urogynecol J Pelvic Floor Dysfunct 1996;7(2):94–7.

48. Crystle C, Charme L, Copeland W. Q-tip test in stress urinary incontinence. Obstet Gynecol 1971;38:13–7.

49. Fantl J, Hurt W, Bump R, et al. Urethral axis and sphincteric function. Am J Obstet Gynecol 1986;155(3):554–8.

50. Walters M, Shields L. The diagnostic value of history, physical examination, and the Q-tip cotton swab test in women with urinary incontinence. Am J Obstet Gynecol 1988;159(1):145–9.

51. Walters M, Diaz K. Q-tip test: a study of continent and incontinent women. Obstet Gynecol 1987;70(2):208–11.

52. Walters M. ACOG practice bulletin #63: urinary incontinence in women. Obstet Gynecol 2005;105(6):1533–45.

53. Swift S, Bent A. Basic evaluation of the incontinent female patient. In: Bent AE, Cundiff GW, Swift SW, editors. Ostergard's urogynecology and pelvic floor dysfunction. 6th edition. Philadelphia: Lippincott Williams & Wilkins; 2008. p. 65–77.

54. Ouslander J, Leach G, Abelson S, et al. Simple versus multichannel cystometry in the evaluation of bladder function in an incontinent geriatric population. J Urol 1988;140(6):1482–6.

55. Wall L, Wiskind A, Taylor P. Simple bladder filling with a cough stress test compared with subtracted cystometry for the diagnosis of urinary incontinence. Am J Obstet Gynecol 1994;171(6):1472–7.

Pathophysiology of Urinary Incontinence, Voiding Dysfunction, and Overactive Bladder

David D. Rahn, MD*, Shayzreen M. Roshanravan, MD

KEYWORDS

- Detrusor overactivity • Instability • Urinary stress incontinence
- Neuroanatomy • Neurophysiology

DEFINITIONS, TERMINOLOGY

Pelvic floor dysfunction may include problems of urine storage and evacuation, inadequate support of the pelvic viscera, colorectal/anal disorders, and acute or chronic pelvic pain. When considering just the disorders of the lower urinary tract, there is an abundance of terms describing the various symptoms and suspected etiologies of these storage and evacuation problems; miscommunication and confusion may result. The International Continence Society has attempted to standardize several definitions based on patients' symptoms to facilitate more effective communication between physicians, patients, and researchers.[1] These urinary disorders may be divided into three categories: problems with storage, voiding, and postmicturition.

Among the storage symptoms, urinary incontinence is broadly defined as "the complaint of any involuntary leakage of urine." More specifically, stress urinary incontinence is "involuntary leakage on effort or exertion, or on sneezing or coughing." Urinary urgency is "the complaint of a sudden compelling desire to pass urine which is difficult to defer" and urgency incontinence is "the complaint of involuntary leakage accompanied by or immediately preceded by urgency."[1,2] Taken together, overactive bladder syndrome is "urgency, with or without urgency incontinence usually with increased daytime frequency and nocturia."[2]

Voiding symptoms include problems with slow urinary stream, splitting or spraying, intermittency or hesitancy with the urine flow, or straining to void. Postmicturition symptoms include feelings of incomplete emptying and postmicturition dribble. Although all of these labels may help characterize patients by their predominant

Division of Female Pelvic Medicine and Reconstructive Surgery, Department of Obstetrics and Gynecology, University of Texas Southwestern Medical Center, 5323 Harry Hines Boulevard, Dallas, TX 75390-9032, USA
* Corresponding author.
E-mail address: david.rahn@utsouthwestern.edu (D.D. Rahn).

Obstet Gynecol Clin N Am 36 (2009) 463–474
doi:10.1016/j.ogc.2009.08.012
0889-8545/09/$ – see front matter © 2009 Elsevier Inc. All rights reserved.

symptoms, they do not provide insight into the degree to which symptoms bother patients nor the etiology of these symptoms. This article presents a simplified explanation of the mechanics of urine storage and emptying, establishing a framework to understand how different physiologic and pathologic states may contribute to the disorders mentioned earlier.

PHYSIOLOGIC NEUROANATOMY OF URINE STORAGE AND EVACUATION

The anatomy of the lower urinary tract is closely related to its function of storage and evacuation of urine. The bladder remains relaxed during the storage phase and contracts during the evacuation phase. The urethra acts in synchrony with the bladder but has reciprocal actions: contracting during storage and relaxing during evacuation. The coordinated function of this system depends on complex interactions between the nervous system and the lower urinary tract anatomy.

Anatomy: Bladder

The urinary bladder is a muscular organ that consists of coarse bundles of smooth muscle known as the detrusor muscle (**Fig. 1**). The bladder is lined by transitional epithelium, which merges with the squamous epithelium of the urethra. Approximately at the level of the ureteral orifices, the bladder can be divided into two parts: a body (or dome) and a base. The base of the bladder includes the vesical trigone, which is bounded by the two ureteral orifices and the internal urethral opening. An important distinction between the dome and the base is the type of neurotransmitter receptor that predominates (see **Fig. 1**). At the dome, beta-adrenergic and cholinergic receptors predominate, whereas alpha-adrenergic receptors predominate at the base and the proximal urethra. The primary cholinergic (muscarinic) receptor subtypes in the human bladder are M2 and M3. Although there are more M2 receptors, the M3

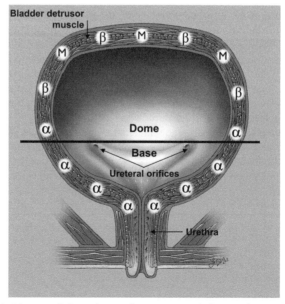

Fig. 1. Urinary bladder. α, alpha adrenergic receptors; β, beta adrenergic; M, muscarinic (cholinergic). (*Courtesy of* Lindsay Oksenberg, Dallas, TX)

receptors predominate in the mediation of detrusor contraction.[3] The vesical neck is that area of the bladder where the urethral lumen passes through the musculature of the bladder base.[4]

Anatomy: Urethra

In women, the urethra is a complex 3 to 4 cm structure that extends from the bladder to the external urethral opening (**Fig. 2**A, B). Surrounding the mucosal lining of the urethra is a submucosal layer that contains a prominent vascular plexus. This plexus is thought to contribute to the watertight closure of the urethral lumen. Adjacent to the submucosal layer lie two layers of smooth muscle: a well-developed inner longitudinal and a poorly defined outer circular layer. These smooth muscle layers are thought to assist with constriction and opening of the urethral lumen. The most external layer of the urethral wall consists of the striated urogenital sphincter muscles (see **Fig. 2B**).[5,6] This complex consists of the sphincter urethrae and two strap like bands of muscle, the urethrovaginal sphincter and compressor urethrae muscles (**Fig. 3**).[7,8] The sphincter urethrae surrounds the proximal region of the urethra. This muscle is an integral part of the urethral wall and its fibers are oriented in a circular fashion. The compressor urethrae and urethrovaginal sphincter muscles arch over the ventral surface of the urethra and are found just superior to the perineal membrane (see **Fig. 3**).

Peripheral nervous system

Understanding the normal physiologic function of the lower urinary tract requires a basic understanding of its peripheral innervation.[9] The peripheral nervous system has a somatic and an autonomic component. The somatic component innervates skeletal or striated muscle, whereas the autonomic component innervates smooth muscle, cardiac muscle, and glands. In the lower urinary tract, somatic nerves innervate the muscles that comprise the striated urogenital sphincter complex. Autonomic nerves supply the detrusor muscle of the bladder and smooth muscle of the urethra (**Fig. 4**).

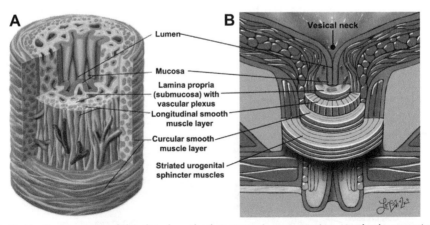

Fig. 2. Urethral anatomy. (*A*) Isolated urethral anatomy in cross section. Urethral coaptation results in part from filling of the rich subepithelial vascular plexus. (*B*) Vesical neck and urethral anatomy. (*From* Wai CY. Urinary incontinence. In: Schorge JO, Schaffer JI, Halvorson LM, et al, editors. Williams Gynecology, 1st edition. New York: McGraw Hill Medical; 2008. p. 517; *with permission.*) (*Courtesy of* Lindsay Oksenberg, Dallas, TX).

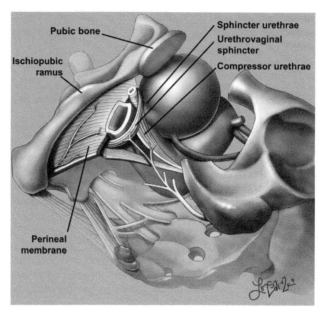

Fig. 3. Striated urogenital sphincter anatomy. With the perineal membrane removed or reflected, one encounters the three component muscles of the striated urogenital sphincter. (*Courtesy of* Lindsay Oksenberg, Dallas, Texas).

The autonomic nervous system is further divided into sympathetic and parasympathetic divisions. Fibers arising from the intermediolateral gray column of the tenth thoracic and first two lumbar spinal cord segments form the pelvic sympathetic division. The pelvic parasympathetic division consists of fibers arising from the intermediolateral cell columns of the second through fourth sacral cord segments. Autonomic fibers that supply the pelvic viscera course in the superior and inferior hypogastric plexuses (**Fig. 5**). The superior hypogastric plexus primarily contains sympathetic fibers from the T10 to L2 cord segments and terminates by dividing into right and left hypogastric nerves. The inferior hypogastric plexus, also known as the pelvic plexus, is formed by visceral efferents from S2 to S4, which provide

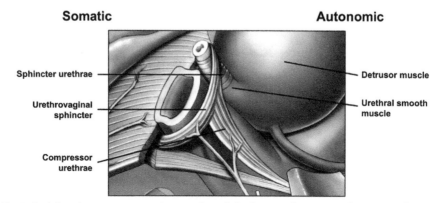

Fig. 4. Peripheral nervous system innervation of the lower urinary tract. (*Courtesy of* Lindsay Oksenberg, Dallas, TX).

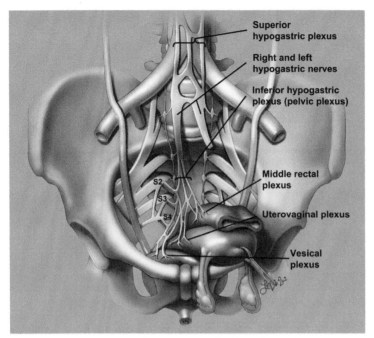

Fig. 5. The pelvic plexus. (*Courtesy of* Lindsay Oksenberg, Dallas, TX).

the parasympathetic component by way of the pelvic nerves. The lateral extensions of the superior hypogastric plexus, the hypogastric nerves and rami from the sacral portion of the sympathetic chain, contribute the sympathetic component to the pelvic plexus. The pelvic plexus divides into three portions according to the course and distribution of its fibers: the middle rectal plexus, uterovaginal plexus (or Frankenhauser's ganglion), and vesical plexus (see **Fig. 5**).[10]

The somatic component of the peripheral nervous system that is relevant to lower urinary tract function takes origin from Onuf's somatic nucleus (**Fig. 6**). Onuf's nucleus, located in the ventral horn of the gray matter of S2 through S4, contains the neuronal cell bodies of the fibers that supply the striated urogenital sphincter complex. The urethrovaginal sphincter and compressor urethrae are innervated by the perineal branch of the pudendal nerve. The sphincter urethrae are variably innervated by somatic efferents that travel in the pelvic nerves.

Neurophysiology

Normal voiding function requires higher cortical areas of the brain, which allow for voluntary control over the primitive autonomic reflex arcs found within the sacral spinal cord. This central coordination of micturition largely occurs in the pontine micturition center. The parietal lobes and thalamus receive and coordinate the bladder detrusor afferent stimuli, whereas the frontal lobes and basal ganglia modulate with inhibitory signals. There is also peripheral coordination that occurs in the sacral micturition center (S2–4). Precise knowledge of the neural pathways involved in voiding remains controversial; the concepts presented here represent a summary of the major pathways.

Urine storage depends predominantly on sympathetic neural activity. During storage, bladder distention results in afferent input from sensory neurons located in

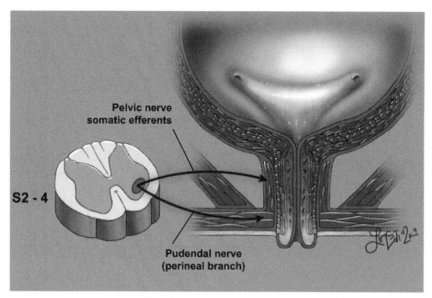

Fig. 6. Onuf's somatic nucleus. (*Courtesy of* Lindsay Oksenberg, Dallas, TX).

the bladder wall. This leads to activation of urethral motor neurons in Onuf's nucleus, which results in contraction of the striated urogenital sphincter muscles by way of the pudendal nerve. Simultaneously, activation of the spinal sympathetic reflex (T11–L2) by way of the hypogastric nerves results in alpha-adrenergic contraction of urethral smooth muscle with increased tone at the vesical neck and inhibition of parasympathetic transmission, which inhibits detrusor contraction.[11] The net effect is that urethral pressure remains greater than detrusor pressure, facilitating storage (**Fig. 7**). When there are increases in abdominal pressure, a fascial and muscular urethral support hammock compresses the urethra to help maintain continence[12]; this is also accomplished when the pelvic muscles are contracted.

Voiding is largely a parasympathetic event. This begins with efferent impulses from the pontine micturition center, which results in inhibition of somatic fibers in Onuf's nucleus and voluntary relaxation of the striated urogenital sphincter muscles. These efferent impulses also result in preganglionic sympathetic inhibition with opening of the vesical neck and parasympathetic stimulation, which results in detrusor muscarinic contraction. The net result is relaxation of the striated urogenital sphincter complex causing decreased urethral pressure, followed almost immediately by detrusor contraction and voiding (**Fig. 8**).

NEUROGENIC CAUSES OF URINE STORAGE AND EVACUATION DYSFUNCTION

Voluntary control of the micturition reflex is mediated by connections between the frontal cerebral cortex and the pons. Voluntary control of the striated urogenital sphincter muscles is through the corticospinal pathway connecting the frontal cortex with Onuf's somatic nucleus. Disruption of these neural pathways can result in dysfunctional storage and voiding patterns.

Lesions in the cortical centers of the brain can result in urge incontinence, enuresis, and urethral spasm. Patients may be unaware of their incontinence. Patients suffering from stroke, Alzheimer disease, multi-infarct dementia, other dementias, Parkinson

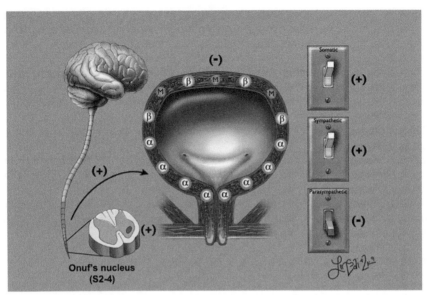

Fig. 7. Urine storage. Bladder distention from filling leads to alpha-adrenergic contraction of the urethral smooth muscle and increased tone at the vesical neck (T11-L2 spinal sympathetic reflex); activation of urethral motor neurons in Onuf's nucleus with contraction of striated urogenital sphincter muscles (by way of the pudendal nerve); and inhibited parasympathetic transmission with decreased detrusor pressure. α, alpha adrenergic receptors; β, beta adrenergic; M, muscarinic (cholinergic). (*Courtesy of* Lindsay Oksenberg, Dallas, TX).

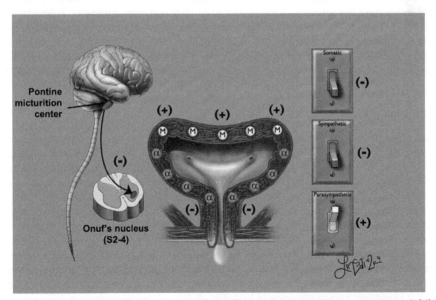

Fig. 8. Urine evacuation. Efferent impulses from the pontine micturition center cause inhibition of somatic fibers in Onuf's nucleus with voluntary relaxation of the striated urogenital sphincter muscles; preganglionic sympathetic inhibition with relaxation at the vesical neck; and parasympathetic stimulation with detrusor muscle contraction. α, alpha adrenergic receptors; M, muscarinic (cholinergic). (*Courtesy of* Lindsay Oksenberg, Dallas, Texas).

disease, or multiple sclerosis with suprapontine lesions may experience involuntary detrusor contractions, which occur in synchrony with relaxation of the urethra. These contractions can result in neurogenic detrusor overactivity with urgency/frequency and urgency incontinence.

High spinal cord or upper motor neuron lesions can also result in neurogenic detrusor overactivity. However, the detrusor contractions are not synchronized with urethral relaxation, resulting in detrusor-sphincter dyssynergia where patients can also have urinary retention. This dyssynergia can be seen with acute spinal cord trauma, cervical or lumbar stenosis, disc herniation, or chronic conditions involving the spinal cord, such as multiple sclerosis.

Lastly, lower motor neuron lesions, as seen with injury to the peripheral nervous system, may result in reduced contraction of the detrusor muscle. This may manifest as overflow incontinence. In developed countries, the most common cause of peripheral neuropathy is diabetes. Injury to the pelvic plexus can be seen with resection surgery, such as radical hysterectomy or rectal surgery. In these cases, parasympathetic innervation is mainly affected.

MUSCULAR CAUSES OF URINE STORAGE AND EVACUATION DYSFUNCTION

The detrusor muscle's functional ability to contract appropriately may be altered as a result of aging, atrophy, trauma, or decreased muscular innervation. The smooth muscle contractions of the detrusor require several interacting biochemical pathways to raise intracellular calcium levels; these include adenosine triphosphate (ATP) phosphorylation, protein kinases, and potassium and calcium channels. Alterations in any of these pathways may result in inappropriate contractions or loss in contractility.[13,14] Studies have demonstrated that women who have detrusor overactivity have structural changes in their bladder walls at the tissue and cellular levels. Electron microscopy examining the ultrastructural anatomy of detrusor cells suggests that patients who have overactivity have an abnormal number of intercellular connections used for communication between smooth muscle cells, which may facilitate the generation of inappropriate detrusor contractions.[15] At a light microscopic level, overactive bladder tissue has demonstrated increases in elastin, collagen, and segments of denervated muscle.[16]

STRESS URINARY INCONTINENCE

Theories regarding the maintenance of urinary continence during increases in intra-abdominal pressure involve concepts of pressure transmission, anatomic support, and urethral integrity. Most simply, continence during these times of physical stress requires anatomic urethral support and urethral integrity. Ideal support requires intact and healthy (1) ligaments along the lateral aspects of the urethra, termed the pubourethral ligaments; (2) anterior vaginal wall and its lateral fascial condensation; (3) arcus tendinous fascia pelvis; and (4) levator ani muscles. Collectively, this support provides a firm backboard against which the urethra is supported during increases in intra-abdominal pressure. With the loss of this support, downward forces, such as from a cough, sneeze, or laugh, are not countered as they should be; the urethra funnels at the urethrovaginal junction; the urethra becomes more patent and has a reduced closing pressure; and continence is lost (**Fig. 9**).[17]

Mechanical closure/integrity of the urethra is also necessary to prevent stress urinary incontinence. This closure/integrity requires mucosal surface coaptation and intact viscoelastic properties of the urethral epithelium, a healthy underlying urethral vascular plexus, and contraction of the surrounding musculature (see **Fig. 2**). Defects

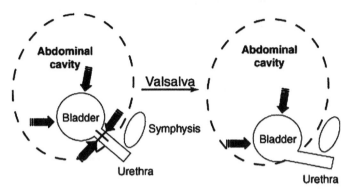

Fig. 9. Stress urinary incontinence: the pressure-transmission theory. (*From* Wai CY. Urinary incontinence. In: Schorge JO, Schaffer JI, Halvorson LM, et al, editors. Williams Gynecology. 1st edition. New York: McGraw Hill Medical; 2008. p. 518; with permission.)

in any of these components may contribute to stress incontinence by way of "intrinsic sphincter deficiency."[12] Possible etiologies of such defects include prior retropubic surgery with denervation or scarring of the urethra and supporting tissue, prior pelvic radiotherapy, hypoestrogenism, diabetic neuropathy, and other degenerative neuronal diseases. Childbirth and associated trauma can physically disrupt the musculature of the urogenital sphincter or its supportive fascia or muscles (levator ani) or may cause nerve damage with immediate or delayed stress urinary incontinence.

COMORBID CONDITIONS AND OTHER FACTORS AFFECTING URINE STORAGE AND EVACUATION

Urinary incontinence often reflects multidimensional and multiple impairments. Besides requiring intact micturition physiology (including the lower urinary tract, pelvic, and neurologic components described earlier), continence depends on an intact functional ability to toilet oneself. Several medical conditions and pharmacologic agents can negatively impact this ability. One pneumonic designed to highlight these potentially reversible or transient contributors to urinary incontinence is DIAPPERS: Dementia/delirium, Infection, Atrophic vaginitis, Psychological, Pharmacologic, Endocrine, Restricted mobility, and Stool impaction.[18]

Continence requires the cognitive ability to recognize and react appropriately to the sensation of a full bladder, motivation to maintain dryness, sufficient mobility and manual dexterity, and ready access to toilet facilities. Patients who have dementia or significant psychological impairments often do not have this necessary cognitive ability or motivation for maintenance of continence, and women who have severe physical handicaps or restricted mobility may simply not have time to reach the toilet, especially in the setting of urinary urgency/overactive bladder.

Urinary tract infections cause inflammation of the bladder mucosa. Sensory afferent activity increases with this inflammation, which contributes to an overactive bladder. Similarly, estrogen deficiency may lead to atrophic vaginitis and urethritis with increased local irritation and a greater risk of urinary tract infection and overactive bladder. Topical estrogen may ameliorate symptoms and infections should be treated before other incontinence interventions are considered.[3]

Table 1			
Medications that may contribute to voiding dysfunction			
Medication	**Examples**	**Mechanism**	**Effect**
Alcohol	Beer, wine, liquor	Diuretic effect, sedation, immobility	Polyuria, frequency
Alpha-adrenergic agonist	Decongestants, diet pills	IUS contraction	Urinary retention
Alpha-adrenergic blockers	Prazosin, terazosin, doxazosin	IUS relaxation	Urinary leakage
Anticholinergic agents		Inhibit bladder contraction, sedation, fecal impaction	Urinary retention or functional incontinence
Antihistamines	Diphenhydramine, scopolamine, dimenhydrinate		
Antipsychotics	Thioridazine, chlorpromazine, haloperidol		
Antiparkinsonians	Trihexyphenidyl, benztropine mesylate		
Skeletal muscle relaxants	Orphenadrine, cyclobenzaprine		
Tricyclic antidepressants	Amitriptyline, imipramine, nortriptyline, doxepin		
Miscellaneous	Dicyclomine, disopyramide		
Angiotensin-converting enzyme inhibitors	Enalapril, captopril, lisinopril, losartan	Chronic cough	Urinary leakage
Calcium-channel blockers	Nifedipine, nicardipine, isradipine, felodipine	Relaxes bladder, fluid retention	Urinary retention, nocturnal diuresis
Cyclooxygenase-2 selective NSAID	Celecoxib	Fluid retention	Nocturnal diuresis
Diuretics	Caffeine, HCTZ, furosemide, bumetanide, acetazolamide, spironolactone	Increases urinary frequency, urgency	Polyuria
Narcotic analgesics	Opiates	Relaxes bladder, fecal impaction, sedation	Urinary retention and/or functional incontinence
Thiazolidinediones	Rosiglitazone, pioglitazone, troglitazone	Fluid retention	Nocturnal diuresis

Abbreviations: HCTZ, hydrochlorothiazide; IUS, internal urethral sphincter; NSAID, nonsteroidal antiinflammatory drug. *From* Wai CY. Urinary incontinence. In: Schorge JO, Schaffer JI, Halvorson LM, et al, editors. Williams Gynecology. 1st edition. New York: McGraw Hill Medical; 2008. p. 521; with permission.

Although incontinence should not be viewed as a normal consequence of aging, there are several physiologic changes that occur in the lower urinary tract with aging that may predispose one to incontinence, overactive bladder, or other voiding difficulties. First, the prevalence of involuntary detrusor contractions increases with aging, with detrusor overactivity being found in 21% of healthy, continent, community-dwelling elderly.[19] Total bladder capacity may diminish and the ability to postpone voiding decreases, leading to urinary frequency. Meanwhile, urinary flow rate decreases in older men and women likely because of an age-related decrease in detrusor contractility.[20] In women, postmenopausal decrease in estrogen levels results in atrophy of the urethral mucosal seal, loss of compliance, and bladder irritation, which may predispose to stress and urgency urinary incontinence. Age-related changes in renal filtration rate and alterations in diurnal levels of antidiuretic hormone and atrial natriuretic factor shift the diurnal pattern of fluid excretion toward increased volume of urine excreted later in the day.[21] Comorbid conditions, such as congestive heart failure, hypothyroidism, venous insufficiency, and the effects of certain medications all contribute to peripheral edema leading to urinary frequency and nocturia when a patient is supine.

Diabetes mellitus can lead to osmotic diuresis and polyuria when there is poor glucose control. Polydipsia from diabetes insipidus or excessive intake of caffeine or alcohol can also lead to polyuria/urinary frequency. Similarly, abnormalities of arginine vasopressin with its impaired secretion or action may cause polyuria and nocturia; these carefully selected patients may benefit from desmopressin therapy.[3]

Finally, stool impaction resulting from poor bowel habits and constipation can contribute to overactive bladder symptoms, perhaps from local irritation or direct compression against the bladder wall.

As alluded to earlier, there are many medications that may cause or worsen urinary incontinence or other forms of voiding dysfunction. This dysfunction occurs through changes in rate of urine production, the integrity of the sympathetic and parasympathetic nervous systems, and cognition. It is important to note patients' use of diuretics, anticholinergic medications, alcohol, psychotropic medications, narcotics, alpha agonists or antagonists, beta mimetics, or calcium channel blockers (see **Table 1**).

SUMMARY

The coordinated function of the lower urinary tract system depends on the normal and complex interactions between the nervous system and the lower urinary tract anatomy. A thorough understanding of these components and their interactions is essential to properly diagnose and manage lower urinary tract dysfunction.

ACKNOWLEDGMENTS

The authors thank Ms. Lindsay Oksenberg, medical illustrator, University of Texas Southwestern Office of Medical Education, for use of the many illustrations demonstrating lower urinary tract neurophysiology.

REFERENCES

1. Abrams P, Cardozo L, Fall M, et al. The standardisation of terminology of lower urinary tract function: report from the Standardisation Sub-committee of the International Continence Society. Am J Obstet Gynecol 2002;187(1):116–26.
2. Abrams P, Artibani W, Cardozo L, et al. Reviewing the ICS 2002 terminology report: the ongoing debate. Neurourol Urodyn 2009;28(4):287.

3. Ouslander JG. Management of overactive bladder. N Engl J Med 2004;350(8): 786–99.

4. DeLancey JO. Correlative study of paraurethral anatomy. Obstet Gynecol 1986; 68(1):9–17.

5. Berkow SG. The corpus spongiosum of the urethra: its possible role in urinary control and stress incontinence in women. Am J Obstet Gynecol 1953;65(2): 346–51.

6. Rud T, Andersson KE, Asmussen M, et al. Factors maintaining the intraurethral pressure in women. Invest Urol 1980;17(4):343–7.

7. Gosling JA. Structure of the lower urinary tract and pelvic floor. Clin Obstet Gynaecol 1985;12(2):285–94.

8. Oelrich TM. The striated urogenital sphincter muscle in the female. Anat Rec 1983;205(2):223–32.

9. Benson JT, Walters MD. Neurophysiology and pharmacology of the lower urinary tract. In: Walters MD, Karram MM, editors. Urogynecology and reconstructive pelvic surgery. 3rd edition. Philadelphia: Mosby Elsevier; 2007. p. 31–43.

10. Ashley FL, Anson BJ. The pelvic autonomic nerves in the male. Surg Gynecol Obstet 1946;82:598–608.

11. Van Arsdalen K, Wein A. Physiology of micturition and continence. In: Krane RJ, Siroky MB, editors. Clinical neuro-Urology. 2nd edition. Boston: Little, Brown; 1995. p. 25.

12. DeLancey JOL. Structural aspects of the extrinsic continence mechanism. Obstet Gynecol 1988;72:296–301.

13. Blakeman P, Hilton P. Cellular and molecular biology in urogynaecology. Curr Opin Obstet Gynaecol 1996;8(5):357–60.

14. Levin RM, Levin SS, Wein AJ. Etiology of incontinence: a review and hypothesis. Scand J Urol Nephrol Suppl 1996;179:15–25.

15. Elbadawi A, Yalla SV, Resnick NM. Structural basis of geriatric voiding dysfunction. III. Detrusor overactivity. J Urol 1993;150(5 Pt 2):1668–80.

16. Brading AF. A myogenic basis for the overactive bladder. Urology 1997;50(Suppl 6A):57–67.

17. Wai CY. Urinary incontinence. In: Schorge JO, Schaffer JI, Halvorson LM, et al, editors. Williams gynecology. 1st edition. New York: McGraw Hill Medical; 2008. p. 517–8.

18. Swift SE, Bent AE. Basic evaluation of the incontinent female patient. In: Bent AE, Cundiff GW, Swift SE, editors. Ostergard's urogynecology and pelvic floor dysfunction. 6th edition. Philadelphia: Lippincott Williams and Wilkins; 2008. p. 67.

19. Resnick NM, Elbadawi A, Yalla SV. Age and the lower urinary tract: what is normal? Neurourol Urodyn 1995;14:577.

20. Resnick NM. Voiding dysfunction in the elderly. In: Yalla SV, McGuire EJ, Elbadawi A, et al, editors. Neurourology and urodynamics: principles and practice. New York: MacMillan; 1984. p. 303.

21. Kirkland JL, Lye M, Levy DW, et al. Patterns of urine flow and excretion in healthy elderly people. Br Med J 1983;287:1665–7.

Behavioral Treatment of Urinary Incontinence, Voiding Dysfunction, and Overactive Bladder

Kathryn L. Burgio, PhD

KEYWORDS

- Behavioral treatment • Urinary incontinence
- Voiding dysfunction • Overactive bladder
- Pelvic floor muscle • Physical therapy • Biofeedback

Behavioral treatments have been used for several decades to treat urinary incontinence, overactive bladder (OAB), and other lower urinary tract symptoms. They have been adopted by several disciplines and are implemented in many different ways. The spectrum of behavioral treatments includes those that target voiding habits and life style, as well as those that train pelvic floor muscles to improve strength and control. What they all have in common is that they improve symptoms by teaching skills and by changing the patient's behavior.

When used in clinical practice, behavioral programs are usually comprised of multiple components and individualized according to the needs of the patient and her unique situation. Behavioral programs are generally built around one of two approaches. One approach focuses on modifying bladder function by changing voiding habits, such as with bladder training and delayed voiding. Another approach targets the bladder *outlet*, teaching skills for improving pelvic floor muscle strength and control and behavioral training with urge suppression. Components of behavioral treatment can include self-monitoring (bladder diary), scheduled voiding, delayed voiding, pelvic floor muscle training and exercise, active use of pelvic floor muscles for urethral occlusion ("stress strategies"), urge suppression techniques (urge strategies), urge control techniques (distraction, self-assertions), biofeedback, electrical stimulation, fluid management, dietary changes, weight loss, and other life style changes.

All of these behavioral techniques require the active participation of the patient and they require time and effort from the clinician. Most patients are not cured through

University of Alabama at Birmingham, Department of Medicine and Birmingham/Atlanta Geriatric Research, Education, and Clinical Center, Department of Veterans Affairs, 700 South 19th Street (11G), Birmingham, Alabama, 35233, USA
E-mail address: kburgio@uab.edu

Obstet Gynecol Clin N Am 36 (2009) 475–491
doi:10.1016/j.ogc.2009.08.005
0889-8545/09/$ – see front matter. Published by Elsevier, Inc.

obgyn.theclinics.com

behavioral intervention, but the abundance of literature tells us that most patients experience significant reductions in symptoms and improvements in quality of life. Behavioral treatments should be a mainstay in the care of women of all ages with incontinence or other lower urinary tract symptoms.

THE BLADDER DIARY

Self-monitoring is a common first step in any behavioral program. When treating bladder symptoms, it is useful to have the patient complete a bladder diary for 5 to 7 days.[1] The diary is a valuable clinical tool for the patient, as well as the clinician. In the evaluation phase, it provides information on the type and frequency of urine loss, frequency of urination, and other symptoms, which helps the clinician plan appropriate components of behavioral intervention. Usually, patients are asked to record the time of each incontinent episode, its size, and the circumstances or reasons for the episode. In addition, it is useful to have patients record the times that they void, which provides a foundation for determining voiding intervals in bladder training programs. Voided volumes are more burdensome to document and are usually recorded for only 24 to 48 hours, but they provide a practical estimate of patients' functional bladder capacity in their daily lives.

During the course of treatment, the diary can be used to monitor symptoms and to track the efficacy of various treatment components and guide the intervention. In addition to guiding the clinician, the self-monitoring effect of completing the diary enhances patients' awareness of voiding habits and helps them recognize how their incontinence may be related to their activities. By reviewing the bladder diary with the clinician, patients can identify the times when they are at increased risk of an incontinence episode and activities that can trigger incontinence. In particular, learning about the circumstances that precipitate urine leakage prepares patients to implement the continence skills they are about to learn.

PELVIC FLOOR MUSCLE TRAINING AND EXERCISE

Pelvic floor muscle training and exercise is a cornerstone of behavioral treatment for both stress and urge urinary incontinence. It was originally designed to teach patients how to control and exercise peri-urethral muscles with the goal of strengthening the muscles and reducing stress incontinence. It was first popularized by Arnold Kegel, a gynecologist who proposed that stress incontinence was due to a lack of awareness of function and coordination of pelvic floor muscles,[2] and who also demonstrated that women could reduce their stress incontinence through pelvic floor muscle training and exercise.[2,3] Over the decades, this intervention has evolved both as a behavior therapy and as a physical therapy, combining principles from both fields into a widely accepted conservative treatment for stress, as well as urge incontinence. The literature on pelvic floor muscle training and exercise has demonstrated that it is effective for reducing stress, urge, and mixed incontinence in most outpatients who cooperate with training.[4–12]

Teaching Pelvic Floor Muscle Control

The goal of behavioral treatment for stress incontinence is to teach patients how to improve urethral closure by voluntarily contracting pelvic floor muscles during coughing, sneezing, lifting, or whatever physical activities precipitate urine leakage. The first step in training is to assist the woman to identify the pelvic floor muscles and to contract and relax them selectively (without increasing intra-abdominal pressure on the bladder or pelvic floor). Confirming that patients have identified and isolated the correct muscles is essential and often overlooked. Failure to find the pelvic floor muscles or to exercise them correctly is perhaps the most common reason for failure with this treatment modality. Although it is easy for the clinician to give patients a pamphlet or brief verbal instructions to "lift the pelvic floor" or to interrupt the urinary stream during voiding, this approach does not ensure that she understands which muscles to use before she is sent home to begin her exercises. Several techniques can be used to help patients learn to exercise correctly, including biofeedback,[11,13,14] verbal feedback based on vaginal or anal palpation,[15] or electrical stimulation.[16] Although some clinicians advocate the use of a resistive device or weighted vaginal cones to improve the effects of exercise on the pelvic floor muscles, there has been little research to support these modalities.[7]

A common problem encountered in learning to control the pelvic floor muscles is that patients tend to recruit other muscles, such as the rectus abdominis muscles or gluteal muscles. Contracting certain abdominal muscles can be counterproductive when it increases pressure on the bladder or pelvic floor. Thus, it is important to observe for this valsalva response and to help patients to exercise pelvic floor muscles selectively while relaxing these abdominal muscles.

Some clinicians advocate coordinated training of transversus abdominus muscles, because it is believed that they facilitate pelvic floor muscle contraction. However, this approach remains controversial and a recent review article indicates an absence of evidence for this type of training.[17]

Daily Pelvic Floor Muscle Exercise

Once patients demonstrate the ability to properly contract and relax the pelvic floor muscles selectively in the clinic, a regimen of daily practice and exercise is recommended. The purpose of daily exercise is not only to increase muscle strength, but also to enhance motor skills through practice. Exercise regimens vary considerably in frequency and intensity, and the optimal exercise regimen has yet to be determined. However good results are generally achieved using 45 to 50 exercises per day.[4] It is usually recommended that patients space the exercises across the day, typically in 2 to 5 sessions per day to avoid muscle fatigue. Practicing the exercises while in the lying position is often recommended at first, but it is important to progress patients to sitting or standing positions as well, so that they become comfortable and skilled using their muscles to avoid incontinence in any position.

To improve muscle strength, contractions should be sustained for 2 to 10 seconds, depending on the patient's initial ability. Exercise regimens can be individualized so that patients begin with a comfortable duration and gradually progress to 10 seconds. Each exercise consists of muscle contraction followed by a period of relaxation using a 1:1 or 1:2 ratio.[18] This allows the muscles to recover between contractions.

Using Muscles to Prevent Stress Incontinence

Although exercise alone has been known to improve urethral pressure and structural support and reduce incontinence,[19] in recent years, more emphasis has been placed on teaching patients to consciously contract the pelvic floor muscles to occlude the urethra during physical activities that cause stress incontinence.[16,20] This skill has been referred to as the "stress strategy,"[16] "counterbracing," "perineal co-contraction," "the Knack,"[20] and "the perineal blockage before stress technique."[21] Initially, this new skill requires vigilance and a conscious effort on the part of the patient, but with time and consistent practice, patients can develop the habit of using muscles to occlude the urethra and it eventually becomes automatic. Although it is ideal for a woman to have strong pelvic floor muscles, even those with weak muscles can benefit from simply learning how to control their pelvic floor muscles and use them to prevent incontinence.[20] Others will need a more comprehensive program of pelvic floor muscle rehabilitation to increase strength in addition to skill.

BEHAVIORAL TRAINING AND URGE SUPPRESSION STRATEGIES

Historically, pelvic floor muscle training and exercise was used almost exclusively for the treatment of stress incontinence. In the 1980s, it became evident that voluntary pelvic floor muscle contraction can also be used to suppress detrusor contraction.[13] The technique can be learned by most patients and is used increasingly as a central element in the treatment of urge incontinence and overactive bladder.[13,22] Generally, patients with urge incontinence are taught pelvic floor muscle control and exercise in the same manner as those with stress incontinence. What differs is how they use their muscles to prevent urine loss. In addition to using active muscle contraction to occlude the urethra to prevent urine loss during detrusor contraction, patients learn to use volitional pelvic floor muscle contractions to inhibit or suppress bladder contraction.

Urge suppression skills are an essential component in teaching patients a new way of responding to the sensation of urgency. Ordinarily, women with OAB or urge incontinence feel compelled to rush to the nearest bathroom when they feel the urge to void. In behavioral training, they learn how this natural response is actually counterproductive, because it increases physical pressure on the bladder, enhances the feeling of fullness, exacerbates urgency, exposes them to visual cues that can trigger incontinence, and increases the risk of an incontinent episode. Although counterintuitive at first, patients are taught not to rush to the bathroom when they feel the urge to void. Instead, they are advised to stay away from the bathroom. They are encouraged to pause, sit down if possible, relax the entire body, and contract pelvic floor muscles repeatedly to diminish urgency, inhibit detrusor contraction, and prevent urine loss. They concentrate on voluntarily inhibiting the urge sensation and wait for the urge to subside before they walk at a normal pace to the toilet.

In addition to the normal daily exercises to increase strength and control, one exercise found to be helpful for patients with urge incontinence is to interrupt or slow the urinary stream during voiding once per day. Not only does this provide practice in occluding the urethra and interrupting detrusor contraction, it does so in the presence of the urge sensation, when patients with urge incontinence or OAB need the skill most. Some clinicians have expressed concerns that repeated interruption of the urinary stream may lead to incomplete bladder emptying in certain groups of patients. Therefore, caution should be used when recommending this technique for patients who may be susceptible to voiding dysfunction.

The effectiveness of behavioral training for urge incontinence has been established in several clinical series studies[13,23,24] and in controlled trials using intention-to-treat models, in which mean reductions of incontinence range from 60% to 80%.[15,22] In the first randomized controlled trial, behavioral training reduced incontinence episodes significantly more than drug treatment and patient perceptions of improvement and satisfaction with their progress were higher.[22]

NOCTURIA

Nocturia is a multifactorial condition that requires differential diagnosis. When it is truly related to fluid intake or overactive bladder, behavioral interventions can be helpful. Although getting up once per night to void is widely regarded as normal, getting up 2 or more times can be very bothersome when it results in sleep disruption or daytime fatigue, or increases the risk of falls. One simple method to overcoming nocturia is to restrict fluid intake for 3 to 4 hours before bedtime. Although there is little scientific evidence for the efficacy of fluid restriction, it has been known to help in many individual cases. In patients who retain fluid during the day and have nocturia due to mobilization of fluid at night, interventions focus on managing daytime accumulation of fluid. Patients are advised to wear support stockings, elevate the lower extremities in the late afternoon, or use a diuretic. For patients who are already taking a diuretic, nocturia can often be improved by altering the timing of the diuretic (so that most of the effect has occurred before bed time) or by using a long-acting diuretic.

In addition to the medical management of nocturia, behavioral training for urge incontinence has also been shown to reduce nocturia.[25] Patients are instructed to use the urge suppression strategy when they wake up at night. If the urge subsides, they are encouraged to go back to sleep. If after a minute or two the urge to void has not remitted, they should get up and void so as not to interfere unnecessarily with their sleep. In one trial, both behavioral training and drug therapy reduced nocturia more than placebo, and behavioral training was significantly more effective than drug therapy (median reduction = 0.50 versus 0.30 episodes per night; $P = .02$).[25]

VOIDING DYSFUNCTION

With most pelvic floor muscle training programs, the focus of treatment is on active contraction of the muscles, because the goal is to occlude the urethra. For patients who have voiding dysfunction owing to pelvic floor tension, the focus of behavioral treatment is on teaching volitional relaxation of pelvic floor muscles in the context of voiding. Normal voiding is a coordinated response in which detrusor contraction is accompanied by pelvic floor relaxation, which lowers intraurethral pressure and facilitates urine flow. In fact, pelvic floor relaxation is regarded as the initiating event in voiding, and inability to relax these muscles is one cause of voiding dysfunction in women.

Treatment begins with educating the patient regarding bladder and pelvic floor anatomy and function, in particular the coordinated responses that comprise normal voiding. Some women habitually void by valsalva in the belief that they need to bear down to empty the bladder. These patients in particular need to understand that the normal bladder empties itself by means of detrusor contraction, which they can facilitate through pelvic floor muscle relaxation.

Initially, the pelvic floor muscles are evaluated by digital palpation to assess contraction strength, resting tone, and the ability to relax. Some women present with an "overactive pelvic floor" characterized by high resting tone. Others may have increased muscle tension only in the context of voiding. Pelvic floor muscle training focuses first on developing an awareness of muscle tension versus relaxation. Active muscle contraction is used to demonstrate the sensations associated with muscle tension to assist patients to discriminate and contrast it with the sensations of relaxation. The active contraction also effects a more complete subsequent relaxation. Perineal or vaginal biofeedback can be especially useful for bringing muscle tension to a conscious level.[26]

As described above, daily pelvic floor muscle exercise involves not only contracting, but also relaxing muscles fully between contractions, so that these muscles can recover. This is particularly important practice for patients with voiding dysfunction. To facilitate relaxation, these patients can focus more on the relaxation phase, which can be extended with a 1:2 ratio or longer as appropriate.

Once the patient has learned good pelvic floor relaxation in the clinic, it is important to address voiding habits at home and elsewhere, so that the relaxation skills can be generalized. For many women, voiding is an activity that is rushed due to a busy life-style, and they do not take the time they need to void normally. Rushing can inhibit pelvic floor relaxation, and valsalva voiding can increase pelvic floor tension resulting in incomplete emptying. Behavioral treatment begins by encouraging the patient to create a relaxing environment and taking adequate time for voiding. They are in-structed to slow down, take a deep breath, relax their body, relax their pelvic floor muscles, and wait for the urine to flow. Good voiding technique involves relaxation as the initiating event. Anecdotally, some women have benefitted from double voiding, or lingering until another detrusor contraction brings about more complete emptying.

BIOFEEDBACK

Biofeedback is a teaching technique that helps patients learn by giving them precise, instantaneous feedback of their pelvic floor muscle activity. In his original work, Kegel used a biofeedback device he designed and named the perineometer.[3] It consisted of a pneumatic chamber (placed in the vagina) and a hand-held pressure gauge, which displayed the pressure generated by circumvaginal muscle contraction. This device provided immediate visual feedback of pelvic floor muscle contraction to the woman learning to identify her muscles and monitor her practice.

Most biofeedback instruments in current use are computerized and display feedback visually on a monitor. Pelvic floor muscle activity can be measured by manometry or electromyography, using vaginal or anal probes or surface electrodes. Signals are augmented through the computer, and immediate feedback is provided on a monitor for visual feedback or via speakers for auditory feedback. When patients observe the results of their attempts to control bladder pressure and pelvic floor muscle activity, learning occurs by means of operant conditioning (trial and error learning). Biofeed-back-assisted behavioral training has been tested in several studies, producing mean reductions of incontinence ranging from 60% to 85%.[11,13–16,22,24]

Biofeedback technology is an excellent method to help patients identify the pelvic floor muscles and exercise them properly, but it requires special equipment and expertise, increasing the time and cost of treatment. There is a small body of literature examining the therapeutic role of biofeedback and whether it is improves outcomes over other forms of teaching. The earliest studies investigating the role of biofeedback were conducted in the treatment of stress incontinence. These studies were small and provided evidence that biofeedback does improve the patient's ability to learn a correct pelvic floor muscle contraction and increase the probability of a successful outcome.[14,27]

However, two randomized controlled trials did not replicate these findings. In the first, older women with stress-predominant incontinence received pelvic floor muscle training with or without biofeedback. Pelvic floor muscle exercise yielded a mean 61% reduction of incontinence when taught with biofeedback versus a mean 54% reduc-tion when taught without biofeedback. Both approaches were significantly more effec-tive than the no-treatment control condition, but they were not significantly different from each other.[11]

In a later study, women with stress incontinence received 6 months of pelvic floor muscle training supervised by a physical therapist, with or without home-based biofeedback. In this study, biofeedback was used to reinforce the learning at home, but not to teach proper pelvic floor muscle control in the clinic. Training enhanced with home biofeedback resulted in higher rates of objective cure, but the difference between groups was not statistically significant.[28] The authors noted that the value of the home biofeedback may have been that it motivated many women to adhere to the program and should be an option in clinical practice.

The role of biofeedback for treatment of urge incontinence has been examined in two randomized trials. The first was a small trial in 20 elderly, nondemented patients with persistent urge-predominant incontinence.[29] Those trained without biofeedback responded as well to treatment as those trained with bladder-sphincter biofeedback. In a larger trial in 222 older women with urge-predominant incontinence, patients were randomly assigned to behavioral training with biofeedback, behavioral training without biofeedback (verbal feedback based on vaginal palpation), or behavioral training with a self-help booklet. Patients in the biofeedback group showed a 63% reduction of incontinence, which was not significantly different from the 69% reduction in the verbal feedback group.[15] This study indicates that careful training with verbal feedback can be at least as effective as biofeedback in the first line treatment of urge incontinence. This means that behavioral training, because it does not require biofeedback in most patients, can be used more widely and particularly in settings where biofeedback is not available. Thus, biofeedback can be used as a first-line approach to teaching or it can be reserved for those patients who cannot successfully identify their muscles by other methods.

VOIDING HABITS AND SCHEDULES
Bladder Training

Bladder training is a behavioral intervention developed originally for the treatment of urge incontinence. The premise of bladder training is that habitual frequent urination can reduce bladder capacity and lead to bladder overactivity, which in turn causes urge incontinence.[30] The goal of the training is to break this cycle using consistent incremental voiding schedules to reduce voiding frequency, increase bladder capacity, and restore normal bladder function.

Its precursor, first described in the 1970s, was the bladder drill, an intensive intervention that was usually conducted in a hospital setting. Bladder drill procedures imposed an immediate lengthened interval between voids, usually 4 hours, to force a normal frequency of urination and were reported to result in normalization of bladder function. Women with urge incontinence were treated in the hospital for a period of 7 to 10 days, where they were placed on the strict voiding schedule and monitored by nurses. Bladder drills were often combined with anticholinergic medications and sedatives to help cope with severe urgency. Cure rates of 82% to 86% were reported in women 15 to 77 years of age.[30,31]

Bladder training is a modification of bladder drill that is conducted in a more gradual fashion on an outpatient basis. Similar results have been demonstrated using this less intensive approach or a combination of inpatient and outpatient intervention. As with bladder drill, the woman voids at predetermined intervals, rather than in response to urgency. She first completes a voiding diary, which shows the clinician when and how often she voids. After reviewing the diary with the patient, a voiding interval is selected based on the longest time interval between voids that is comfortable for the patient. She is then given instructions to void first thing in the morning, every time the interval passes, and before going to bed at night. Over time, the voiding interval is increased at comfortable intervals to a maximum of every 3 to 4 hours.

To comply with the voiding schedule, patients must resist the sensation of urgency and postpone urination. Although the hallmark of bladder training is the expanded voiding interval, more attention is now focused on helping patients to control the urge to urinate while they wait for their voiding interval to pass. The traditional approach to helping patients cope with urgency in bladder training has been to suggest various techniques for relaxation or distraction to another activity.[32,33] Patients are encouraged to get their minds off the bladder by engaging in a task that requires mental but not physical effort. Examples include reading, calling a friend, or making a to-do list. Also used are affirming self-statements such as "I am in control of my bladder," or "I can wait." More recently, traditional bladder training has been enhanced by incorporating the urge suppression techniques from behavioral training. Repeated contractions of the pelvic floor muscles are used to control urgency and detrusor contractions while the patient postpones urination.

Several studies have demonstrated the efficacy of bladder training.[32–41] The most definitive study is a randomized clinical trial that showed a mean 57% reduction in frequency of incontinence in older women.[32] In this trial, bladder training not only reduced incontinence associated with detrusor overactivity, but also incontinence associated with sphincter insufficiency, possibly because patients acquired a greater awareness of bladder function or that having to postpone urination increased pelvic floor muscle activity. In another trial that compared bladder training to oxybutynin, 73% of women in bladder training were reported to be "clinically cured."[41]

Delayed Voiding

Delayed voiding is another approach to helping patients to expand the interval between voids, but without placing them on a predetermined voiding schedule. As in behavioral training with urge suppression, patients are encouraged not to run to the bathroom whenever they have an urge to void, but to use their urge suppression techniques and wait for the urge to subside. Instead of going to the bathroom immediately after this, they expand their ability to postpone urination by waiting 5 minutes before voiding.

In patients who have experienced incontinence, even a small sensation of urge can trigger a degree of anxiety, which they tend to avoid by going to the bathroom as soon as possible, rather than exercising any control they may have. However, even the most urgent patient can usually be convinced to try a 5-minute delay, and are often surprised to find that after a brief wait, the urge subsides or disappears altogether. This enhances their sense of control, and once confidence has been restored, the delay interval can be gradually increased to achieve a normal frequency.

Increasing Voiding Frequency

Many health care providers advise their female patients to increase frequency of urination as a way to prevent urgency and incontinence by avoiding a full bladder. This approach can provide immediate relief in the short-term. However, the long-term result is most likely counterproductive, because the patient can lose the ability to accommodate a full bladder and may reduce functional bladder capacity. In addition, it feeds the cycle of urgency and frequency that is thought to perpetuate overactive bladder and urge incontinence over time. Increasing the frequency of urination is generally reserved for women who void less often than normal (eg, fewer than five times per day) or in patients with dementia or other cognitive impairment, who are thus incapable of learning new skills for bladder control. Women who have reduced bladder sensation may also benefit.

BEHAVIORAL LIFE STYLE CHANGES

Life style changes are generally used as adjuncts to a primary behavioral intervention such as pelvic floor muscle training or behavioral training with urge suppression strategies. Life style changes include fluid management, reducing caffeine and other bladder irritants, weight control, and bowel management.

Fluid Management

Changes in the volume of fluid intake are recommended by many behavioral clinicians either as a primary or as an adjunctive strategy to optimize outcomes. Many women attempt to control their incontinence by restricting their overall fluid intake or by not drinking at particular times of day when they do not have access to a toilet. In some cases, particularly in older women, the resulting fluid intake may be inadequate and places them at risk of dehydration. Although it may seem counterintuitive, it is usually good advice to encourage the patient to consume at least 6 glasses of fluid each day.[42] Some believe that this will also dilute the urine making it less irritating to the bladder.

It is also common to encounter patients who increase their fluid intake deliberately in an effort to "flush" their kidneys, lose weight, or avoid dehydration. In others it is simply an unconscious habit. For patients who consume an unnecessarily high volume of fluid (eg, > 2100 mL of output per 24 hours), reducing excess fluids can relieve problems with sudden bladder fullness and resulting urgency or incontinence.[43] Avoiding excessive fluid intake in the evening hours may also be helpful for reducing nocturia.

Caffeine Reduction

Caffeine, in addition to being a diuretic, has also been reported to be a bladder irritant for many women. Urodynamic studies have shown that caffeine increases detrusor pressure[44] and is a risk factor for detrusor instability.[45,46] There is also evidence that reducing caffeine intake can help to reduce episodes of both stress and urge incontinence.[47–49] It can be difficult for coffee drinkers to eliminate their morning coffee and patients are often reluctant at first to forgo their caffeinated beverages. However, if it is presented as a trial period, they may be convinced to try it for 3 to 5 days. If they experience relief from their symptoms, they are often more willing to reduce or eliminate caffeinated beverages from their diet altogether. To avoid problems with caffeine withdrawal, it is recommended that caffeine reduction be approached gradually and may include mixing caffeinated and decaffeinated beverages incrementally.

Bladder Irritants

Although data are scarce, there are a number of other substances that have been implicated as bladder irritants, including sugar substitutes, citrus fruits, and tomato products. There are innumerable clinical cases in which these substances appear to be aggravating incontinence, and reducing them has provided clinical improvement. However, this should not be interpreted to mean that all patients need to eliminate these foods from their diets. A diary of food and beverage intake is useful for identifying which substances are irritants for individual patients, and a trial period of eliminating these substances can be used to confirm the relationship.

Prescription diuretics are also known to aggravate incontinence by increasing the rate of bladder filling and producing sudden urges. Such effects can sometimes be avoided by altering the type, dose, or timing of diuretic medication.

Weight Loss

Obesity is a prevalent health problem that is now recognized as an established risk factor for urinary incontinence in women. Women with high body mass index are not only more likely to develop incontinence, they also tend to have more severe incontinence than women with lower body mass index.[50] Research on the relationship between body mass index and incontinence reports that each 5-unit increase in body mass index increases the risk of daily incontinence by approximately 60%.[50,51] Intervention studies of morbidly obese women report significant improvement in symptoms of incontinence with weight loss of 45 to 50 kg following bariatric surgery.[52–54] Similarly, significant improvements in continence status have been demonstrated with as little as 5% weight reduction in more traditional weight loss programs.[55]

In a recent randomized controlled trial, 338 overweight and obese women were assigned to an intensive 6-month group-administered, weight loss program (including diet, exercise, and behavior modification) or to a structured education control program. Both groups received a booklet describing a step-by-step self-administered behavioral program to reduce incontinence. After a mean weight loss of 8.0%, the intervention group reported a greater reduction in incontinence episodes compared with the control group (mean = 47% versus 28%; P = .01).[56] Because this degree of weight loss is an achievable goal for many overweight women, it is reasonable to recommend weight loss as a component in an individualized behavioral program for incontinence in overweight women.

Bowel Management

Fecal impaction and constipation have been cited as factors contributing to urinary incontinence in women, particularly in nursing home populations.[57] In severe cases, fecal impaction can be an irritating factor in overactive bladder or obstruct normal voiding, causing incomplete bladder emptying and overflow incontinence. Some patients experience immediate relief with disimpaction, but a bowel management program is often needed to maintain regularity and avoid recurrence. Bowel management may consist of recommendations for normal fluid intake and dietary fiber (or supplements) to maintain normal stool consistency and regular bowel movements. When hydration and fiber are not enough, enemas may be used to stimulate a regular daily bowel movement, preferably after a regular meal such as breakfast to take advantage of postprandial motility.

COMBINING BEHAVIORAL TREATMENT WITH OTHER MODALITIES

Despite the good evidence for the effectiveness of behavioral treatments, most patients do not achieve complete control with this modality. One way to potentially improve the efficacy of behavioral treatments is to combine them with other conservative treatments that may have additive effects.

Combining Behavioral and Drug Therapy

Some clinicians combine behavioral and drug treatments based on the premise that relaxing the bladder with a medication makes it easier for the patient to gain volitional control over detrusor contraction. Others believe that drugs are helpful, but patients do not fully regain continence without using their own efforts to control the bladder. Although the therapeutic mechanisms of behavioral and drug therapies have not been established completely, there is evidence that they work by different mechanisms, suggesting that they may have additive effects.[58] The issue of combining behavioral treatment with drug therapy has been addressed in a small number of studies.

One controlled study examined the effects of bladder drill with and without anticholinergic medication.[59] Combined therapy did not significantly improve the cure rate (83%) over that achieved with bladder drill alone (79%). In a second study, prompted voiding was combined with oxybutynin or a placebo in functionally impaired nursing home patients with detrusor instability. Although patients in both groups improved significantly, adding oxybutynin did not enhance the outcomes of prompted voiding in the nursing home setting.[60] Although the results of these early studies were not encouraging, a larger study has demonstrated that adding simple written instructions for bladder training to tolterodine led to greater changes in voiding frequency and voided volumes than were achieved with tolterodine alone.[61] However, combined therapy did not produce greater improvements in incontinence (Median reduction of incontinence = 87% versus 81% with drug alone).

Biofeedback-assisted behavioral training has also been combined with an anticholinergic drug to test whether combined therapy may be more effective than either treatment alone.[62] Patients who were not completely satisfied with 8 weeks of behavioral treatment or drug treatment (oxybutynin) alone were offered combined therapy for an additional 8 weeks. Subjects who initially received behavioral treatment showed further improvement with the addition of oxybutynin ($P = .034$). Subjects who were initially assigned to drug therapy also showed further improvement with the addition of behavioral treatment ($P = .001$).[62] Thus the data indicate that for patients who achieve a less than satisfactory result with drug or behavioral training alone, adding another therapy in a stepped program can produce better outcomes.

A more recent study examined whether combining behavioral and drug therapy from the beginning of treatment would enable women with urge-predominant incontinence to discontinue their drug therapy and maintain a clinically significant reduction in incontinence episodes.[63] It also investigated the short-term (10-week) impact of combined therapy compared with drug therapy alone. The BE-DRI study (Behavior Enhances Drug Reduction of Incontinence) was a multicenter, randomized, controlled trial conducted by the National Institute of Diabetes and Digestive and Kidney Diseases (NIDDK) Urinary Incontinence Treatment Network. Results indicated that women who underwent behavioral training in addition to drug therapy were no more likely to discontinue drug therapy and sustain improvements in continence status than women treated with drug alone. However, women who received combined therapy reported greater improvements on several secondary outcome measures, including patient perception of improvement, patient satisfaction, and validated measures of symptom distress and bother (Urogenital Distress Inventory and Overactive Bladder Questionnaire) while on active therapy and after 6 months from the time drug therapy was discontinued.

Another large multicenter trial examined the effects of tolterodine extended release plus a self-administered behavioral intervention (educational pamphlet with verbal reinforcement) in patients who were previously treated and dissatisfied with tolterodine or other antimuscarinics.[64] This was not a controlled trial, but it demonstrated that 91% of subjects were least "a little satisfied" after 8 weeks of treatment, including 53% who reported being "very satisfied." Further, all bladder diary variables were significantly improved by week 4 ($P < .0001$). Thus, combined therapy resulted in high treatment satisfaction and improved bladder diary variables in patients who were previously treated and dissatisfied with antimuscarinic therapy.

Less is known about combining behavioral and drug treatments for stress incontinence. A single study has compared the effects of pelvic floor muscle training combined with duloxetine to duloxetine alone, pelvic floor muscle training alone, and placebo. The results indicated that combined therapy was superior to either treatment alone. As in the case of urge incontinence, combining treatments for stress incontinence is thought to improve outcomes owing to the different modes of action of behavioral and drug therapies.[65] Taken together, the research on combining behavioral and drug therapies indicates that for many patients, combined therapy will be the best way to optimize therapeutic outcomes.

Combining Behavioral Treatment with Electrical Stimulation

Patients with very weak pelvic floor muscles often have difficulty identifying and using their muscles to prevent stress incontinence. Some clinicians have advocated using electrical stimulation to facilitate training by helping patients better identify and strengthen their muscles. Two studies have examined whether adding electrical stimulation might lead to better outcomes of pelvic floor muscle training. One study explored whether combining training with home-based, low intensity electrical stimulation or clinic-based maximal intensity electrical stimulation would yield better results than pelvic floor muscle training alone.[66] All three groups demonstrated significant improvement in muscle strength and pad test results, but electrical stimulation did not produce better outcomes than pelvic floor muscle exercise alone.

Another trial examined whether adding daily home electrical stimulation would enhance the effectiveness of biofeedback-assisted behavioral training for stress incontinence.[16] Patients in the biofeedback group had a mean 68% reduction in the frequency of urine loss. Outcomes for patients who received biofeedback plus electrical stimulation were not significantly better than those who received training without electrical stimulation. Thus, whereas pelvic floor muscle electrical stimulation is an effective treatment for urge or stress incontinence in women,[67,68] the research does not show that it improves outcomes over that achieved through pelvic floor muscle training alone.

WHO IS A CANDIDATE FOR BEHAVIORAL TREATMENT?

Although there are many studies that report the effects of behavioral treatment for urinary incontinence in a variety of populations, relatively few report on variables that might influence or predict the outcome of treatment. Most patients who are motivated and cooperative with behavioral treatment experience some degree of improvement, but there is wide variation in outcome and little is known of the characteristics of patients who respond best to behavioral therapy. Most studies have found that outcomes are not related to the type of incontinence or urodynamic diagnosis.[8,32,33,69,70] There is some evidence that patients with more severe incontinence have greater improvements following behavioral treatment.[32,71] In contrast, other studies have shown that patients with more severe incontinence have poorer outcomes,[23,70,71] or no relationship between severity and outcome.[24,33,69,72] Studies are also inconsistent with regard to the effect of age.[23,24,32,72] Thus, the literature on predictors of outcomes is inconsistent and many studies have inadequate sample sizes.

The existing literature suggests that treatment outcome is unaffected by race, 2° or 3° cystocele, diuretic use, parity, history of hysterectomy, uterine prolapse, hormone therapy, body mass index, or urodynamic parameters. At this time, response to treatment cannot be predicted from the type of incontinence, the patient's medical or obstetric history, the results of her pelvic or rectal examination, nor the findings on her urodynamic testing. Aside from the baseline frequency of incontinence and history of previous treatment, there is little information in the usual clinical evaluation of a patient with stress or urge incontinence that would indicate the likelihood of her success with behavioral treatment. Thus, given that most motivated patients receive some benefit from behavioral treatment and it involves minimal risk or discomfort, there is no reason to discourage any woman with stress or urge incontinence who is willing and motivated to exert the effort necessary to participate in behavioral treatment.

ADHERENCE

It is widely acknowledged that the effectiveness of behavioral interventions depend on the active participation of an involved and motivated patient. However, most studies provide little information about how compliant patients are with pelvic floor muscle exercise, behavioral strategies, voiding schedules, or other components of behavioral treatment.[7,28,73] Measurement of adherence to behavioral protocols is often neglected in research, and the literature is sparse on methods to identify barriers and improve adherence.

One of the greatest challenges lies in how to motivate patients not only to be actively involved, but to persist in their efforts for a long enough time that they will experience noticeable change in bladder control. The fact that progress is usually gradual and progressive makes compliance even more difficult for patients who expect immediate results. Clinically, we can optimize adherence by making it clear to the patient that her progress will be gradual and will depend on her consistent practice and use of her new skills. Clinicians can provide support by scheduling follow-up appointments to create accountability, track and reinforce progress, identify and address barriers, adjust the daily regimen, and encourage persistence.

Most clinicians agree that adherence to a maintenance protocol is also necessary for long-term effectiveness. Yet, little work has been completed on the durability of behavioral treatments. The few studies of long-term outcomes are inconsistent, but promising in that many patients are able to sustain improvements in bladder control over time.[71,73,74] There is clearly a need for more studies of long-term outcomes to understand the reasons for regression and to learn how the effects of treatment can be maintained over a lifetime.

SUMMARY

Behavioral interventions are a diverse group of treatments that improve symptoms by altering bladder habits and teaching new skills. They have been used for decades to improve incontinence and other lower urinary tract symptoms in women of all ages. The collective literature on outpatient behavioral treatments has demonstrated that they are effective for reducing stress, urge, and mixed incontinence in most women who cooperate with training. Although they are not curative in the majority of women, most can achieve significant improvements in symptoms. Behavioral interventions are safe and reversible, and can be implemented by advanced practice nurses, physical therapists, physicians, or other providers in outpatient practice. They do not require special equipment, but they do require the time of a knowledgeable clinician and the active participation of a motivated patient. This makes them very reasonable first-line approaches to the treatment of urinary incontinence and other lower urinary tract symptoms in women.

REFERENCES

1. Locher JL, Roth DL, Goode PS, et al. Reliability assessment of the bladder diary for urinary incontinence in older women. J Gerontol A Biol Sci Med Sci 2001;56: M32–5.
2. Kegel AH. Progressive resistance exercise in the functional restoration of the perineal muscles. Am J Obstet Gynecol 1948;56:238–48.

3. Kegel AH. Stress incontinence of urine in women: physiologic treatment. J Int Coll Surg 1956;25:487–99.
4. Hay Smith J, Berghmans B, Burgio K, et al. Adult conservative management. In: Abrams P, Cardozo L, Khoury S, et al, editors. Incontinence, 4th international consultation on incontinence. Paris, France: Health Publications Ltd; 2009. p. 1025–120.
5. Hay-Smith EJC, Dumoulin C. Pelvic floor muscle training versus no treatment, or inactive control treatments, for urinary incontinence in women. Cochrane Database Syst Rev 2006;1:CD005654.
6. Shamliyan TA, Kane RL, Wyman J, et al. Systematic review: randomized, controlled trials of nonsurgical treatments for urinary incontinence in women. Ann Intern Med 2008;148:1–15.
7. Bo K, Talseth T. Single blind randomized controlled trial of pelvic floor exercises, electrical stimulation, vaginal cones, and no treatment in management of genuine stress incontinence in women. Br Med J 1999;318:487–93.
8. Nygaard IE, Kreder KJ, Lepic MM, et al. Efficacy of pelvic floor muscle exercises in women with stress, urge, and mixed urinary incontinence. Am J Obstet Gynecol 1996;174:120–5.
9. Wells TJ, Brink CA, Diokno AD, et al. Pelvic muscle exercise for stress urinary incontinence in elderly women. J Am Geriatr Soc 1991;39:785–91.
10. Dougherty M, Bishop K, Mooney R, et al. Graded pelvic muscle exercise. Effect on stress urinary incontinence. J Reprod Med 1993;39:684–91.
11. Burns PA, Pranikoff K, Nochajski TH, et al. A comparison of effectiveness of biofeedback and pelvic muscle exercise treatment of stress incontinence in older community-dwelling women. J Gerontol 1993;48:167–74.
12. Wilson PD, Herbison GP. A randomized controlled trial of pelvic floor muscle exercises to treat postnatal urinary incontinence. Int Urogynecol J Pelvic Floor Dysfunct 1998;9:257–64.
13. Burgio KL, Whitehead WE, Engel BT. Urinary incontinence in the elderly: bladder-sphincter biofeedback and toileting skills training. Ann Intern Med 1985;104:507–15.
14. Burgio KL, Robinson JC, Engel BT. The role of biofeedback in Kegel exercise training for stress urinary incontinence. Am J Obstet Gynecol 1986;157:58–64.
15. Burgio KL, Goode PS, Locher JL, et al. Behavioral training with and without biofeedback in the treatment of urge incontinence in older women: a randomized controlled trial. JAMA 2002;288:2293–9.
16. Goode PS, Burgio KL, Locher JL, et al. Effect of behavioral training with or without pelvic floor electrical stimulation on stress incontinence in women: a randomized controlled trial. JAMA 2003;290:345–52.
17. Bo K, Morkved S, Frawley H, et al. Evidence for benefit of transversus abdominus training alone or in combination with pelvic floor muscle training to treat female urinary incontinence: a systematic review. Neurourol Urodyn 2009;28:368–73.
18. Kisner C, Colby LA. Therapeutic exercise. Foundations and techniques. 4th edition. Philadelphia: FA Davis; 2003.
19. Bo K. Pelvic floor muscle exercise for the treatment of stress urinary incontinence: an exercise physiology perspective. Int Urogynecol J 1995;6:282–91.
20. Miller JM, Ashton-Miller JA, DeLancey JOL. A pelvic muscle precontraction can reduce cough-related urine loss in selected women with mild SUI. J Am Geriatr Soc 1998;46:870–4.

21. Bourcier AP, Juras JC, Jacquetin B. Urinary incontinence in physically active and sportswomen. In: Appell RA, Bourcier AP, La Torre F, editors. Pelvic floor dysfunction: investigations and conservative treatment. Rome (Italy): C.E.S.I; 1999. p. 9–17.
22. Burgio KL, Locher JL, Goode PS, et al. Behavioral versus drug treatment for urge incontinence in older women: a randomized clinical trial. JAMA 1998;23: 1995–2000.
23. Baigis-Smith J, Smith DAJ, Rose M, et al. Managing urinary incontinence in community-residing elderly persons. Gerontologist 1989;229:33.
24. McDowell BJ, Burgio KL, Dombrowski M, et al. Interdisciplinary approach to the assessment and behavioral treatment of urinary incontinence in geriatric outpatients. J Am Geriatr Soc 1992;40:370–4.
25. Johnson TM, Burgio KL, Goode PS, et al. Effects of behavioral and drug therapy on nocturia in older incontinent women. J Am Geriatr Soc 2005;53:846–50.
26. Shelly B, Knight S, King P, et al. Treatment of pelvic pain. In: Laycock J, Haslem J, editors. Therapeutic management of incontinence and pelvic pain. London: Springer; 2002. p. 177–89, Chapter 27.
27. Shepherd AM, Montgomery E, Anderson RS. Treatment of genuine stress incontinence with a new perineometer. Physiotherapy 1983;69:113.
28. Morkved S, Bo K, Fjortoft T. Effect of adding biofeedback to pelvic floor muscle training to treat urodynamic stress incontinence. Obstet Gynecol 2002;100: 730–9.
29. Burton JR, Pearce KL, Burgio KL, et al. Behavioral training for urinary incontinence in elderly ambulatory patients. J Am Geriatr Soc 1988;36:693–8.
30. Frewen WK. Role of bladder training in the treatment of the unstable bladder in the female. Urol Clin North Am 1979;6:273–7.
31. Frewen WK. A reassessment of bladder training in detrusor dysfunction in the female. Br J Urol 1982;54:372–3 Gynaecol 1989;96:607–12.
32. Fantl JA, Wyman JF, McClish DK, et al. Efficacy of bladder training in older women with urinary incontinence. JAMA 1991;265:609–13.
33. Wyman JF, Fantl JA, McClish DK, et al. Comparative efficacy of behavioral interventions in the management of female urinary incontinence. Am J Obstet Gynecol 1998;179:999–1007.
34. Elder DD, Stephenson TP. An assessment of the Frewen regime in the treatment of detrusor dysfunction in females. Br J Urol 1980;52:467–71.
35. Jarvis GJ, Millar DR. Controlled trial of bladder drill for detrusor instability. Br Med J 1980;281:1322–3.
36. Jarvis GJ. A controlled trial of bladder drill and drug therapy in the management of detrusor instability. J Urol 1981;53:565–6.
37. Jarvis GJ. The management of urinary incontinence due to primary vesical sensory urgency by bladder drill. Br J Urol 1982;54:374–6.
38. Pengelly AW, Booth CM. A prospective trial of bladder training as treatment for detrusor instability. Br J Urol 1980;52:463–6.
39. Svigos JM, Matthews CD. Assessment and treatment of female urinary incontinence by cystometrogram and bladder retraining programs. Obstet Gynecol 1977;50:9–12.
40. Jeffcoate TNA, Francis WJ. Urgency incontinence in the female. Am J Obstet Gynecol 1966;94:604–18.
41. Colombo M, Zanetta G, Scalambrino S, et al. Oxybutynin and bladder training in the management of female urinary urge incontinence: a randomized study. Int Urogynecol J 1995;6:63–7.

42. Dowd TT, Campbell JM, Jones JA. Fluid intake and urinary incontinence in older community-dwelling women. J Community Health Nurs 1996;13:179–86.

43. Swithinbank L, Hashim H, Abrams P. The effect of fluid intake on urinary symptoms in women. J Urol 2005;174:187–9.

44. Creighton SM, Stanton SL. Caffeine: does it affect your bladder? Br J Urol 1990; 66:613–4.

45. Arya LA, Myers DL, Jackson ND. Dietary caffeine intake and the risk for detrusor instability: a case-control study. Obstet Gynecol 2000;96:85–9.

46. Holroyd-Leduc JM, Straus SE. Management of urinary incontinence in women: scientific review. JAMA 2004;291:986–95.

47. Tomlinson BU, Dougherty MC, Pendergast JF, et al. Dietary caffeine, fluid intake and urinary incontinence in older rural women. Int Urogynecol J Pelvic Floor Dysfunct 1999;10:22–8.

48. Bryant CM, Dowell CJ, Fairbrother G. Caffeine reduction education to improve urinary symptoms. Br J Nurs 2002;11:560–5.

49. Gray M. Caffeine and urinary continence. J Wound Ostomy Continence Nurs 2001;28:66–9.

50. Brown J, Grady D, Ouslander J, et al. Prevalence of urinary incontinence and associated risk factors in postmenopausal women. Heart & Estrogen/Progestin Replacement Study (HERS) Research Group. Obstet Gynecol 1999;94:66.

51. Brown J, Seeley D, Feng J, et al. Urinary incontinence in older women: who is at risk? Study of Osteoparotic Fractures Research Group. Obstet Gynecol 1996;87: 715.

52. Bump R, Sugerman H, Fantl J, et al. Obesity and lower urinary tract function in women: effect of surgically induced weight loss. Am J Obstet Gynecol 1992; 166:392.

53. Deitel M, Stone E, Kassam HA, et al. Gynecologic-obstetric changes after loss of massive excess weight following bariatric surgery. J Am Coll Nutr 1988;7:147.

54. Burgio KL, Richter HE, Clements RH, et al. Changes in urinary and fecal incontinence symptoms with weight loss surgery in morbidly obese women. Obstet Gynecol 2007;110:1034–40.

55. Subak LL, Johnson CEW, Boban D, et al. Does weight loss improve incontinence in moderately obese women? Int Urogynecol J Pelvic Floor Dysfunct 2002;13:40.

56. Subak LL, Wing R, West DS, et al. Weight loss to treat urinary incontinence in overweight and obese women. N Engl J Med 2009;360:481–90.

57. Ouslander JG, Schnelle JF. Incontinence in the nursing home. Ann Intern Med 1995;122:438–49.

58. Goode PS, Burgio KL, Locher JL, et al. Urodynamic changes associated with behavioral and drug treatment of urge incontinence in older women. J Am Geriatr Soc 2002;50:808–16.

59. Fantl JA, Hurt WG, Dunn LJ. Detrusor instability syndrome: the use of bladder retraining drills and with and without anticholinergics. Am J Obstet Gynecol 1981;140:885–90.

60. Ouslander JG, Schnelle JF, Uman G, et al. Does oxybutynin add to the effectiveness of prompted voiding for urinary incontinence among nursing home residents? A placebo-controlled trial. J Am Geriatr Soc 1995;43:610–7.

61. Mattiasson A, Blaakaer J, Hoye K, et al. Simplified bladder training augments the effectiveness of tolterodine in patients with an overactive bladder. BJU Int 2003; 91:54–60.

62. Burgio KL, Locher JL, Goode PS. Combined behavioral and drug therapy of urge incontinence in older women. J Am Geriatr Soc 2000;48:370–4.

63. Burgio KL, Kraus SR, Menefee S, et al. Behavior therapy to enable drug discontinuation in the treatment of urge incontinence: a randomized controlled trial. Ann Intern Med 2008;149:161–9.

64. Klutke CG, Burgio KL, Wyman JF, et al. Combined effects of behavioral intervention and tolterodine in subjects dissatisfied with their overactive bladder medication. J Urol 2009;181:2599–607.

65. Ghoniem GM, van Leeuwen JS, Elser DM, et al. Bump RC for the duloxetine/pelvic floor muscle training clinical trial group. A randomized controlled trial of duloxetine alone, pelvic floor muscle training alone, combined treatment, and no active treatment in women with stress urinary incontinence. J Urol 2005;173:1647–53.

66. Knight S, Laycock J, Naylor D. Evaluation of neuromuscular electrical stimulation in the treatment of genuine stress incontinence. Physiotherapy 1998;84:61–71.

67. Sand PK, Richardson DR, Staskin SE, et al. Pelvic floor stimulation in the treatment of genuine stress incontinence: a multicenter placebo-controlled trial. Am J Obstet Gynecol 1995;173:72–9.

68. Yamanishi T, Yasuda K, Sakakibara R, et al. Pelvic floor electrical stimulation in the treatment of stress incontinence: an investigational study and a placebo controlled double-blind trial. J Urol 1997;158:2127–31.

69. Subak LL, Quesenberry CP, Posner SF, et al. The effect of behavioral therapy on urinary incontinence: a randomized controlled trial. Obstet Gynecol 2002;100:72–8.

70. Burgio KL, Goode PS, Locher JL, et al. Predictors of outcome in the behavioral treatment of urinary incontinence in women. Obstet Gynecol 2003;102:940.

71. Weinberger MW, Goodman BM, Carnes M. Long-term efficacy of nonsurgical urinary incontinence treatment in elderly women. J Gerontol 1999;54:M117–21.

72. Theofrastous JP, Wyman JF, Bump RC, et al. Effects of pelvic floor muscle training on strength and predictors of response in the treatment of urinary incontinence. Neurourol Urodyn 2002;21:486–90.

73. Bo K, Talseth T. Long-term effect of pelvic floor muscle exercise 5 years after cessation of organized training. Obstet Gynecol 1996;87:261–5.

74. Cammu H, Van Nylen M. Pelvic floor muscle exercises: 5 years later. Urology 1995;45:113–8.

Pharmacologic Management of Urinary Incontinence, Voiding Dysfunction, and Overactive Bladder

Emily K. Saks, MD*, LilyA. Arya, MD, MS

KEYWORDS

- Urinary incontinence • Overactive bladder • Female
- Medication • Treatment

The bladder and urethra comprise the female lower urinary tract and function in concert to store and expel urine at the proper times. Urinary incontinence and voiding dysfunction are the result of an inability to appropriately store or empty urine. The capability of the female lower urinary tract to efficiently store urine and release it at appropriate intervals requires an intact and functioning nervous system.

The female bladder and urethra are supplied by the somatic (pudenal) and autonomic (sympathetic and parasympathetic) nerves (**Fig. 1**).[1] The pudendal nerve, originating from the anterior horn of the second, third, and fourth sacral nerve roots, supplies the external urethral sphincter and is under voluntary control. The parasympathetic nerves are derived from dorsolateral ganglion of the second, third, and fourth sacral segments of the spinal cord and have long preganglionic nerves that synapse close to the bladder. The short postganglionic nerves end primarily on muscarinic receptors of the detrusor muscle. Sympathetic nerve supply of the bladder is derived from the thoracolumbar segments (T10–L2) of the spinal cord. The short preganglionic fibers synapse in the sympathetic trunk and the long postganglionic fibers terminate in adrenergic receptors of the urethra and the bladder neck. The pharmacologic treatment of urinary incontinence and voiding dysfunction is focused on modulating sphincter function or detrusor contractility through its effect on the nerve supply of the lower urinary tract.

Division of Urogynecology and Pelvic Reconstructive Surgery, Department of Obstetrics and Gynecology, University of Pennsylvania School of Medicine, 1000 Courtyard, Philadelphia, PA 19104, USA
* Corresponding author.
E-mail address: emily.saks@uphs.upenn.edu (E.K. Saks).

Obstet Gynecol Clin N Am 36 (2009) 493–507
doi:10.1016/j.ogc.2009.08.001   obgyn.theclinics.com
0889-8545/09/$ – see front matter © 2009 Elsevier Inc. All rights reserved.

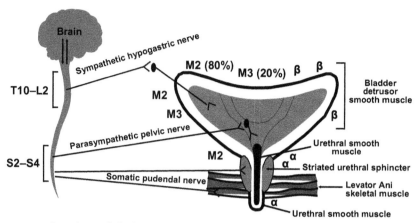

Fig. 1. Neurophysiology of the lower urinary tract. (*Adapted from* Wein AJ. Pharmacological agents for the treatment of urinary incontinence due to overactive bladder. Expert Opin Investig Drugs 2001;10(1):65–83; with permission. *Data from* Abrams P, Andersson KE, Buccafusco JJ, et al. Muscarinic receptors: their distribution and function in body systems, and the implications for treating overactive bladder. Br J Pharmacol 2006;148(5):565–78; and Benson JT, Walters MD. Neurophysiology and pharmacology of the lower urinary tract. In: Walters MD, Karram MM, editors. Urogynecology and reconstructive surgery. 3rd edition. Philadelphia: Mosby and Elsevier; 2007. p. 33.).

STRESS URINARY INCONTINENCE

Numerous drugs have been investigated as potential treatments for stress urinary incontinence, but unfortunately few have made significant impact. This is likely because the main underlying cause of stress urinary incontinence is mechanical displacement of the bladder neck and urethra.[2] Pharmacologic therapies for stress urinary incontinence are targeted toward improving urethral muscle tone by stimulation of adrenergic receptors at the urethra and bladder neck, where α-adrenoceptors predominate over β-adrenoceptors.[3]

Adrenergic agonists, such as pseudoephedrine and ephedrine, have long been used off-label for stress urinary incontinence with some beneficial results in uncontrolled studies.[4] A recent Cochrane review[5] concluded that the potential of serious side effects, such as hypertension, arrhythmias, and cardiovascular events, severely limits the use of these medications for stress urinary incontinence.

Imipramine inhibits reuptake of norepinephrine and serotonin and is thought to improve contraction of urethral smooth muscle. Imipramine may also have some benefit in the treatment of detrusor hyperactivity because it exerts weak antimuscarinic properties in the bladder. There are no well-conducted studies proving efficacy of the drug in stress or urge incontinence.[6–8] Additionally, there is concern regarding associated side effects including peripheral antimuscarinic effects, hypertension, and orthostatic hypotension, especially in older adults.

Duloxetine, an antidepressant, inhibits presynaptic reuptake of serotonin and norepinephrine in the sacral spinal cord, which leads to increased activity of the urethral striated sphincter. Duloxetine may also reduce detrusor overactivity and increase bladder capacity through a central mechanism.[9] Although randomized clinical trials have shown overall decreases in the frequency of stress and urge incontinence episodes and improvements in quality of life, it remains unclear whether these effects are sustainable.[10–12] High rates of nausea lead to significant dropout (over

50%) in the clinical trials.[13] The drug is not approved for urinary incontinence in the United States and carries a black box warning regarding suicidal tendencies during early use.

Because of the limited efficacy of medications in women with stress urinary incontinence, pharmacotherapy should be used in conjunction with behavioral therapies. Behavioral treatments and surgical procedures remain the mainstay of treatment for stress urinary incontinence.

URGE URINARY INCONTINENCE AND OVERACTIVE BLADDER

Antimuscarinic medications serve as the foundation of therapy for urge urinary incontinence and overactive bladder and have been used for several decades. Recently, with the development of slow-release and transdermal formulations, and novel antimuscarinic medications, a variety of treatment options have emerged. Multiple studies have established their safety and tolerability. Although these drugs produced significant improvements in symptoms and quality of life as compared with placebo,[14] the overall cure rate (ie, the number of patients reporting no urinary leakage) is low.

Acetylcholine, the main contractile neurotransmitter of the detrusor muscle, acts by stimulation of the muscarinic receptors.[15] Antimuscarinic agents act during the filling-storage phase of the micturition cycle by inhibiting afferent (sensory) input from the bladder, and directly inhibiting smooth muscle contractility. Clinically, antimuscarinic agents reduce urinary frequency, urgency, and the number of incontinence episodes, while increasing the warning time to get to the bathroom and the volume of each void. Antimuscarinic medications may be prescribed for overactive bladder when behavioral measures, such as caffeine restriction, fluid manipulation, bladder retraining, and pelvic physical therapy, have failed to control symptoms.

Five subtypes of muscarinic receptors are found throughout the human body including the central nervous system, salivary glands, heart, and bowel.[16] Urinary smooth muscle and urothelium contain mainly M2 and M3 receptors. Although M2 receptors account for 80% of the receptors in the urinary tract, M3 receptors are primarily responsible for bladder contraction. Unfortunately, M2 and M3 receptors are also present in other tissues of the body (eg, M3 in bowel, salivary glands, and eye; M2 in cardiac smooth muscle), making it difficult to develop purely uroselective drugs. Most of the current antimuscarinic medications used in the treatment of urge incontinence produce varying degrees of common antimuscarinic side effects, such as dry mouth, blurred vision, confusion, constipation, and rarely increased heart rate. Although these medications have varying selectivity for the different subtypes of muscarinic receptors, it is unclear whether this results in clinically significant differences in efficacy and tolerability.

Historical antimuscarinics, such as urospas, propiverine, and flavoxate, are no longer recommended because of lack of efficacy. Data on the efficacy of tricyclic antidepressants, α-adrenergic agonists, afferent nerve inhibitors, prostaglandin antagonists, β-adrenergic agonists, and calcium channel blockers for overactive bladder are lacking and are generally not used.[17] Currently, six main anticholinergic drugs are available in the United States for the treatment of urge urinary incontinence and overactive bladder. The receptor selectivity, dose, and pharmacodynamics of these drugs are listed in **Table 1**.

Oxybutynin[18] is one of the earliest medications used for the treatment of overactive bladder and has a combination of antimuscarinic, antispasmodic, and local anesthetic properties.[19] The drug seems to have the greatest affinity for M1 and M3 receptors, but may have more selectivity for salivary gland tissue than bladder smooth muscle[20]

Table 1
Dose, receptor selectivity, and pharmacodynamics of antimuscarinic medications

Generic Name	Brand Name	Subtype of Muscarinic Blockade[20]	Dose	Peak Plasma Level[a]	Elimination Half-Life[a]
Darifenacin	Enablex	Relatively selective for M3	7.5–15 mg daily	7 h	13–19 h
Fesoterodine	Toviaz	Similar block of M3 and M2	4–8 mg daily	3–8 h	45–68 h
Oxybutinin IR	Ditropan[b]	Relatively selective for M3 and M1	5 mg two to four times daily	1 h	2–3 h
Oxybutinin ER	Ditropan XL[b]	Relatively selective for M3 and M1	5–30 mg daily	4–6 h	13 h
Oxybutinin transdermal patch	Oxytrol	Relatively selective for M3 and M1	One patch every 3–4 d	10 h	7–8 h
Oxybutinin transdermal gel	Gelnique	Relatively selective for M3 and M1	1g gel daily	7–8 h	64 h
Solifenacin	Vesicare	Relatively selective for M3 and M1	5–10 mg daily	3–8 h	45–68 h
Tolterodine IR	Detrol	Similar block of M3 and M2, relatively nonselective	1–2 mg twice a day	0.5–2 h	2.4 h
Tolterodine ER	Detrol LA	Similar block of M3 and M2, relatively nonselective	2–4 mg daily	2–6 h	7–9 h
Tropsium IR	Sanctura	Similar block of M3 and M2, relatively nonselective	20 mg twice a day	5–6 h	20 h
Tropsium ER	Sanctura XR	Similar block of M3 and M2, relatively nonselective	60 mg daily	4–5 h	35 h

[a] Pharmacodynamic data obtained from drug prescribing information.
[b] Generic form also available.

as reflected in the significantly high rates of dry mouth. Most of the side-effects of oxy-butynin are caused by its active metabolite, N-desethyloxyloxybutynin, produced through the extensive first-pass metabolism in the gut.[21] Alternate formulations of oxy-butynin, such as an extended-release formulation,[22] a transdermal patch,[23] and a new transdermal gel,[24] produce lower levels of N-desethyloxyloxybutynin by reducing the first-pass effect. They have similar efficacy rates with fewer side effects than the immediate-release oral preparation. The transdermal patches have been associated with local skin irritation, such as pruritis and erythema.[23] Because of its local anes-thetic properties, oxybutynin may be of some benefit in patients with urgency, frequency, and bladder pain.[25]

Tolterodine[26] was the first drug to be developed specifically for treatment of over-active bladder. It is a relatively nonselective muscarinic receptor antagonist, but may have more affinity for the receptors of the bladder than of the salivary gland, likely contributing to the reports of significantly less dry mouth than oxybutynin.[20] The extended-release formulation was developed to reduce side effects. In clinical trials, the extended-release formulation was 18% more effective and had a 27% decrease in the rate of dry mouth than the immediate-release formulation.[22]

Trospium[27] was approved for use in the United States in 2004 but has been approved in Europe for over 25 years. In contrast to other antimuscarinics, which are negatively charged tertiary amines, tropsium is a positively charged, hydrophilic, quaternary amine.[28] This structure results in impaired absorption from the gut that is even worse if taken with food. It does not cross the blood-brain barrier and very few effects on the central nervous system have been reported in clinical trials. It is the only drug, other than fesoterodine, not metabolized by the liver and has lower potential for side effects. Because it is excreted by the kidneys, there is concern for toxicity in patients with renal impairment.[28] It does not seem, however, that the dose needs to be adjusted in elderly patients.[29] The drug binds to all muscarinic receptors with similar affinity and the extended-release formulation has fewer side effects than the immediate-release drug.

Solifenacin[30] primarily blocks M1 and M3 receptors and may be more selective for M3 receptors on bladder smooth muscle cells than for salivary gland tissue, explaining the low rate of dry mouth in clinical trials.[31] As compared with placebo, there is a reduction in the mean number of voids and daily incontinence episodes and an increase in the mean voided volume. As compared with tolterodine extended-release, slightly improved efficacy, fewer side effects, and lower drug discontinuation rates were observed with solifenacin.[32]

Darifenacin[33] is a relatively selective M3 muscarinic receptor antagonist. Consis-tent with its low relative affinity for M1 and M2 receptors, it has few effects on cogni-tive function or the cardiovascular system. Darifenacin is metabolized by the liver and is not recommended for patients with severe liver impairment.[34] It is unclear if improved M3 selectivity of darifenacin correlates with improved efficacy and tolerability.

Festoterodine,[35] the newest antimuscarinic compound for the treatment of overac-tive bladder and urge urinary incontinence, was approved by the Food and Drug Administration in October of 2008. It is a prodrug of tolterodine that is nonhepatically metabolized and has demonstrated acceptable efficacy and safety with both the 4- and 8-mg doses in two recent, placebo-controlled, phase three trials.[35,36] Fesotero-dine was found to be superior to placebo in decreasing the number of voids, number of incontinence, and urgency episodes in a 24-hour period and increasing mean voided volume. Side effects of fesoterodine are similar to that of other antimuscarinic medications.

INTERPRETATION OF CLINICAL TRIAL DATA

Most clinical trials on antimuscarinic medications assess efficacy by using objective measures, such as pad counts, pad weights, voiding diary variables, and urodynamic parameters. It is clear that improvements in some of these objective measures may not correspond to the patient's perception of improvement in symptoms or address the most disabling aspects of urinary incontinence. Currently, few clinical trials include patient-reported outcomes and there are insufficient data to compare the effects of individual antimuscarinic medications on health-related quality of life.[37] Future well-designed clinical trials should routinely include validated instruments to measure symptomatic improvements and treatment-related enhancement in quality of life.

COMPLIANCE

Although numerous well-performed studies have demonstrated the efficacy of anti-muscarinic medications, their effectiveness in real life is limited by poor adherence. Because overactive bladder is a symptom-based disease, adherence may be an over-all marker of the efficacy/side effect ratio, with women likely to continue the drug if they experience significant improvement. Studies have reported discontinuation rates of up to 80% at 1 year.[38–40] Side effects along with patient perception of inadequate relief of symptoms may be contributing factors to high discontinuation rates.[41]

WHICH ANTIMUSCARINIC?

To help guide clinicians in their choice of antimuscarinic drugs, a Cochrane review[42] analyzed 49 randomized clinical trials that compared two formulations of antimuscar-inic medications or one antimuscarinic drug with another and concluded that overall efficacies of the varied antimuscarinic drugs are similar. Chapple and coworkers[43] recommended that if one drug does not seem to provide satisfactory relief of symptoms, the clinician should choose an alternate drug. The initial choice of antimuscar-inic agent should be based on its side effect profile. Major studies comparing different antimuscarinic medications are summarized in **Table 2**.

CONSIDERATIONS IN THE ELDERLY

Although the prevalence of overactive bladder increases with age, there are relatively little data on the safety and the efficacy of antimuscarinic medications in older women. In a community-based study in women 65 years and older, side effects were similar to those observed in younger women with no increase in serious adverse events.[44] Although drug absorption is generally unchanged with aging, drug distribution may change because of decreased muscle mass with decreased water content and renal impairment. These factors become particularly important in the frail elderly, and in women with comorbidities or on multiple medications. When prescribing antimuscar-inic medications to older women, care should be taken regarding the overall antimus-carinic burden because several other medications used in older women (eg, those for Parkinson's disease or dementia) also have antimuscarinic effects. There is significant concern for cognitive side effects with antimuscarinics in older women and studies have shown impaired memory recall and immediate learning with oxybutynin.[45] Dar-fenicin, transdermal oxybutynin, tolterodine,[46] and solifenacin[47] have been shown to have relatively few cognitive side effects in clinical studies of older women. Close monitoring is required when these medications are prescribed to elderly women, especially in long-term care facilities.

Table 2
Comparative efficacy of different antimuscarinic medications

Study	Drugs Compared	Efficacy	Side Effects
Pooled data (Cochrane, 2005)[42]	Oxybutinin and tolterodine	Similar in most outcome variables	Slightly less dry mouth and withdrawals with tolterodine
Pooled data (Cochrane, 2005)[42]	Oxybutinin ER and tolterodine ER	Similar in most outcome variables	Slightly less dry mouth with tolterodine ER
OPERA (Diokno et al, 2003)[22]	Oxybutinin ER and tolterodine ER	Similar in most outcome variables	Slightly less dry mouth with tolterodine ER, overall tolerability similar
Trospium and oxybutinin (Halaska et al, 2003)[82]	Oxybutinin and trospium	Similar in most outcome variables	Slightly less dry mouth with trospium
STAR (Chapple et al, 2005)[31]	Solifenacin and tolterodine ER	Solifenacin had slightly better efficacy than tolterodine ER	Similar rates of side effects
Tolterodine and fesoterodine (Chapple et al, 2008)[83]	Tolterodine and fesoterodine	Fesoterodine had slightly better efficacy than tolterodine ER	Slightly less dry mouth with tolterodine ER

BOTULINUM-A TOXIN

Injection of botulinum toxin into the detrusor muscle for the treatment of neurogenic detrusor overactivity was first described by Schurch and coworkers.[48] Botulinum toxin, a potent neurotoxic protein produced by the bacterium *Clostridium botulinum*, binds to the presynaptic terminals of motor neurons and impedes the fusion of synaptic vesicles with the neuronal membrane.[49] This inhibits the release of neurotransmitters, including acetylcholine, causing an interruption in neuronal transmission that affects both the efferent and the afferent branches of the micturition reflex and inhibits detrusor contractions. It may also decrease sensory input to the bladder by down-regulating the neurotransmitter receptors of afferent neurons in the detrusor muscle.[50] In clinical practice, the technique for botulinum injection has not been standardized. It usually involves multiple injections of the drug into the detrusor muscle of the bladder under cystoscopic guidance using local anesthesia, with sparing of the trigone.

Botulinum toxin injections have been shown to be beneficial in several conditions associated with neurogenic detrusor overactivity, including neurogenic detrusor hyperreflexia and detrusor external sphincter dyssynergia. In a large review of patients with neurogenic detrusor overactivity, there was marked reduction in the number of incontinence episodes in between episodes of clean intermittent self-catheterization with improved quality of life.[50] The effects were noted within 1 to 2 weeks of treatment and lasted for 8 to 9 months. Urodynamics showed reduced mean detrusor pressures with increased postvoid residual volumes. There were minimal injection sites or systemic adverse effects.

The role of botulinum toxin injection has also been investigated in the treatment of refractory, idiopathic, urge incontinence in neurologically normal women.[51] In a clinical trial investigating botulinum injection in women with urge incontinence refractory to at least two other first-line treatments, significant improvement in symptoms were noted in 60% women with sustained clinical effects for almost 1 year. Unexpectedly high rates of urinary retention and urinary tract infections led to early discontinuation of the trial. The clinical significance of asymptomatic increased postvoid residual volume remains unclear.

A Cochrane review[52] evaluating botulinum toxin for both neurogenic and idiopathic overactive bladder concluded that although the drug can improve symptoms of overactive bladder, too little data exist on safety and efficacy compared with placebo and other treatments. A clear consensus on use of the drug in clinical practice including optimal dose, location, and number and timing of initial and repeat injections has not yet emerged. Experts recommend use of the drug in treatment of refractory symptoms in neurogenic and idiopathic detrusor overactivity[53] but recommend caution because the risk of voiding difficulty and duration of effect have not yet been accurately evaluated.[54]

DRUGS TO DECREASE AFFERENTS

The afferent nerve input for the voiding reflex from bladder to brain requires stimulation of the A delta fibers that detect bladder fullness and increased wall tension and C fibers that detect noxious stimuli and initiate painful sensations. Abnormal detrusor contractions may be triggered by hypersensitive C fiber afferent neurons.[55] Intravesical instillation of vanilloid neurotoxins, resiniferatoxin and capsaicin, have been investigated for the treatment of refractory neurogenic and nonneurogenic idiopathic detrusor overactivity. Intravesically administered neurotoxin, such as capsaicin and its analog resiniferatoxin, bind to vanilloid receptors in the bladder epithelium and desensitize the C fiber sensory neurons while sparing the A delta unmyelinated fibers involved in the normal micturition reflex.[15] Both drugs have similar rates of reduced urinary frequency and incontinence episodes; however, resiniferatoxin causes less side effects, such as acute pain and irritation, than capsaicin.[55] Because of the lack of well-designed randomized controlled trials, neither is approved for use in the United States. A small study showed that botulinum toxin may be better than resiniferatoxin in the treatment of refractory detrusor overacitivity.[56] The use of either resiniferatoxin or botulinum toxin for overactive bladder is off-label, should be considered experimental, and probably restricted to patients who have failed conventional therapies.[57]

Desmopressin nasal spray,[58] an oxytocin analog, is currently the only medication approved for nocturia. Nocturia is common in older women and often coexists with sleep disorders, such as insomnia and sleep apnea.[59] Because of the risk of hyponatremia, the drug should be prescribed with extreme caution in older women.

VOIDING DYSFUNCTION

Anatomic bladder outlet obstruction is rare in women and is usually iatrogenic (postsurgical). Functional causes of bladder outlet obstruction including detrusor sphincter dysynnergia, and primary bladder neck obstruction along with other causes of urinary retention, such as impaired detrusor contractility and detrusor hyperactivity with impaired contractility, are treated primarily with clean intermittent self-catheterization. Drug therapy has a small secondary role in their management.

Detrusor sphincter dyssynergia, characterized by a lack of coordination of detrusor muscle contraction with external sphincter relaxation, usually occurs as a result of a neurologic lesion caudal to the pontine micturition center. It is usually treated with clean intermittent self-catheterization to prevent increased intravesical pressures and overflow incontinence. Intraurethral injections of botulinum toxin may be beneficial in improving voiding function as suggested in several small studies of patients with spinal cord injury and detrusor sphincter dysynnergia.[60–62] Attempts have also been made to decrease outlet resistance with baclofen or diazepam.[15]

Primary bladder neck obstruction has an unclear etiology in women. Suggested underlying causes include hypertrophy of the bladder neck or increased tone of urethral smooth muscle from an increased number of α-adrenergic receptors.[63] Most treatment options for primary bladder neck obstruction in women, including pharmacologic and surgical therapies, are based on anecdotal evidence. Although some studies suggest that α-adrenergic antagonists, such as terazosin or doxazosin, may be effective, there are little available scientific data.[64,65] Postural hypotension is a significant side effect.

Impaired detrusor contractility may be a side effect of various drugs and the first-line treatment should be to stop these medications if possible. If the condition persists, the mainstay of treatment is clean intermittent self-catheterization while attempting to improve detrusor contractions with muscarinic agonists or β-adrenergic antagonists.[66] Bethanechol, a muscarinic agonist, has been used anecdotally, but does not have proved efficacy.[67]

Detrusor hyperactivity with impaired contractility is a condition characterized by urge incontinence and retention of urine with prominent detrusor trabeculations on cystoscopy and is common in older women with overactive bladder.[68] Patients with detrusor hyperactivity with impaired contractility may benefit from antimuscarinic medications or botulinum toxin,[69] recognizing that women may require intermittent catheterization even after injection.

ESTROGEN

The increased prevalence of urgency, frequency, and incontinence in postmenopausal women may at least partially be caused by the urogenital effects of estrogen loss including thinning of mucosa, loss of sphincter muscle tone, and alteration of the urethrovesical angle.[70] Although oral estrogen replacement seems to improve some urogenital symptoms, such as urgency, frequency, and recurrent urinary tract infections in menopausal women, estrogen does not improve incontinence symptoms.[71,72] In two large clinical trials, women taking oral hormone-replacement therapy reported significantly more incontinence symptoms when compared with controls.[73,74] Vaginal estrogen may be the most useful form of administration for reducing irritative voiding symptoms and recurrent infections.[71]

ROLE OF BEHAVIORAL THERAPIES WITH PHARMACOLOGIC MANAGEMENT

A recent Cochrane review reported that in women with overactive bladder, symptom improvement is greater when antimuscarinics are combined with bladder training as compared with each therapy alone.[75] Studies have also suggested additive effects of behavioral therapy when combined with pharmacologic agents in the treatment of stress urinary incontinence. A recent trial comparing antimuscarinic medication alone with combined medication and behavioral therapies in the treatment of overactive bladder found no difference in the number of women who remained off anti-muscarinics or reported a reduction in incontinence episodes among the two groups, but women who received both behavioral treatment and antimuscarinic medications reported greater satisfaction as compared with the women who received antimuscarinics alone.[76]

NEW HORIZONS

Several neurotransmitters are being recognized as having a role in urinary storage and voiding through their effect on central and peripheral pathways. These include glutamate and serotonin for central pathways and norepinephrine, nitric oxide, tachykinins, and dopamine for peripheral pathways. Several new drugs, targeted toward these neurotransmitters, are currently under investigation for the treatment of overactive bladder. Preclinical studies suggest that β_3-adrenergic receptors predominate in the detrusor muscle[77] and preliminary data evaluating solabegron, a β_3-adrenergic agonist, seem promising.[57] Two additional clinical trials assessing mirabegron[78] and solabegron[79] were completed earlier this year and results should be available shortly. Gabapentin, which binds to calcium channels, is being investigated in patients with neurogenic and idiopathic detrusor overactivity.[57] Tramadol is a weak μ-receptor agonist that also inhibits serotonin and norepinephrine reuptake. Both actions may inhibit bladder contractions and improve the symptoms of overactive bladder.[80] Tachykinins including substance P and neurokinins A and B play a role in the mincturition reflex. Neurokinin receptors are found on neurons of the dorsal horn and it is thought that upregulation of tachykinin-mediated bladder-spinal reflex signaling may lead to urge urinary incontinence. Initial clinical trials with aprepitant, a neurokinin-1 receptor antagonist, have shown promising preliminary results in the treatment of urge urinary incontinence.[81]

SUMMARY

Most pharmacologic agents used for the treatment urinary incontinence and voiding dysfunction exert their effect on the neuromuscular transmission of the central or peripheral nervous system. Surgery remains the mainstay of treatment for stress urinary incontinence. Several different antimuscarinic medications are available for the treatment of overactive bladder. Despite multiple routes of administration, most of these drugs have similar efficacy and tolerability. Overall adherence to the medications is low. Despite the high prevalence of overactive bladder in the elderly, studies regarding safety and efficacy of these drugs in this population are lacking. Several medications with different mechanisms of action are being investigated for urge urinary incontinence and overactive bladder and are still in the preclinical phase. Clean intermittent self-catheterization is the mainstay of treatment for voiding dysfunction with medications playing a small secondary role.

REFERENCES

1. de Groat WC. A neurologic basis for the overactive bladder. Urology 1997; 50(Suppl 6A):36–52.
2. DeLancey JO. Structural support of the urethra as it relates to stress urinary incontinence: the hammock hypothesis. Am J Obstet Gynecol 1994;170(6): 1713–20.
3. Fraser MO, Chancellor MB. Neural control of the urethra and development of pharmacotherapy for stress urinary incontinence. BJU Int 2003;91(8):743–8.

4. Diokno AC, Taub M. Ephedrine in treatment of urinary incontinence. Urology 1975;5(5):624–5.
5. Mariappan P, Ballantyne Z, N'Dow JM, et al. Serotonin and noradrenaline reuptake inhibitors (SNRI) for stress urinary incontinence in adults. Cochrane Database Syst Rev 2005;(3):CD004742.
6. Hunsballe JM, Djurhuus JC. Clinical options for imipramine in the management of urinary incontinence. Urol Res 2001;29(2):118–25.
7. Castleden CM, Duffin HM, Gulati RS. Double-blind study of imipramine and placebo for incontinence due to bladder instability. Age Ageing 1986;15(5):299–303.
8. Woodman PJ, Misko CA, Fischer JR. The use of short-form quality of life questionnaires to measure the impact of imipramine on women with urge incontinence. Int Urogynecol J Pelvic Floor Dysfunct 2001;12(5):312–5.
9. Thor KB, Katofiasc MA. Effects of duloxetine, a combined serotonin and norepinephrine reuptake inhibitor, on central neural control of lower urinary tract function in the chloralose-anesthetized female cat. J Pharmacol Exp Ther 1995;274(2):1014–24.
10. Bump RC, Norton PA, Zinner NR, et al. Mixed urinary incontinence symptoms: urodynamic findings, incontinence severity, and treatment response. Obstet Gynecol 2003;102(1):76–83.
11. Steers WD, Herschorn S, Kreder KJ, et al. Duloxetine compared with placebo for treating women with symptoms of overactive bladder. BJU Int 2007;100(2):337–45.
12. Norton PA, Zinner NR, Yalcin I, et al. Duloxetine versus placebo in the treatment of stress urinary incontinence. Am J Obstet Gynecol 2002;187(1):40–8.
13. Bump RC, Voss S, Beardsworth A, et al. Long-term efficacy of duloxetine in women with stress urinary incontinence. BJU Int 2008;102(2):214–8.
14. Nabi G, Cody JD, Ellis G, et al. Anticholinergic drugs versus placebo for overactive bladder syndrome in adults. Cochrane Database Syst Rev 2006;(4):CD003781.
15. Wein AJ, Rovner ES. Pharmacologic management of urinary incontinence in women. Urol Clin North Am 2002;29(3):537–50, viii.
16. Abrams P, Andersson KE, Buccafusco JJ, et al. Muscarinic receptors: their distribution and function in body systems, and the implications for treating overactive bladder. Br J Pharmacol 2006;148(5):565–78.
17. Roxburgh C, Cook J, Dublin N. Anticholinergic drugs versus other medications for overactive bladder syndrome in adults. Cochrane Database Syst Rev 2007;(4):CD003190.
18. Anderson RU, Mobley D, Blank B, et al. Once daily controlled versus immediate release oxybutynin chloride for urge urinary incontinence. OROS Oxybutynin Study Group. J Urol 1999;161(6):1809–12.
19. Andersson KE, Chapple CR. Oxybutynin and the overactive bladder. World J Urol 2001;19(5):319–23.
20. Hegde SS. Muscarinic receptors in the bladder: from basic research to therapeutics. Br J Pharmacol 2006;147(Suppl 2):S80–7.
21. Zobrist RH, Quan D, Thomas HM, et al. Pharmacokinetics and metabolism of transdermal oxybutynin: in vitro and in vivo performance of a novel delivery system. Pharm Res 2003;20(1):103–9.
22. Diokno AC, Appell RA, Sand PK, et al. Prospective, randomized, double-blind study of the efficacy and tolerability of the extended-release formulations of oxybutynin and tolterodine for overactive bladder: results of the OPERA trial. Mayo Clin Proc 2003;78(6):687–95.

23. Dmochowski RR, Sand PK, Zinner NR, et al. Comparative efficacy and safety of transdermal oxybutynin and oral tolterodine versus placebo in previously treated patients with urge and mixed urinary incontinence. Urology 2003; 62(2):237–42.

24. Staskin DR, Dmochowski RR, Sand PK, et al. Efficacy and safety of oxybutynin chloride topical gel for overactive bladder: a randomized, double-blind, placebo controlled, multicenter study. J Urol 2009;181(4):1764–72.

25. Diokno A, Ingber M. Oxybutynin in detrusor overactivity. Urol Clin North Am 2006; 33(4):439–45, vii.

26. Van Kerrebroeck P, Kreder K, Jonas U, et al. Tolterodine once-daily: superior efficacy and tolerability in the treatment of the overactive bladder. Urology 2001; 57(3):414–21.

27. Cardozo L, Chapple CR, Toozs-Hobson P, et al. Efficacy of trospium chloride in patients with detrusor instability: a placebo-controlled, randomized, double-blind, multicentre clinical trial. BJU Int 2000;85(6):659–64.

28. Staskin DR. Trospium chloride: distinct among other anticholinergic agents available for the treatment of overactive bladder. Urol Clin North Am 2006;33(4): 465–73, viii.

29. Rovner ES. Trospium chloride in the management of overactive bladder. Drugs 2004;64(21):2433–46.

30. Cardozo L, Lisec M, Millard R, et al. Randomized, double-blind placebo controlled trial of the once daily antimuscarinic agent solifenacin succinate in patients with overactive bladder. J Urol 2004;172(5 Pt 1):1919–24.

31. Simpson D, Wagstaff AJ. Solifenacin in overactive bladder syndrome. Drugs Aging 2005;22(12):1061–9.

32. Chapple CR, Martinez-Garcia R, Selvaggi L, et al. A comparison of the efficacy and tolerability of solifenacin succinate and extended release tolterodine at treating overactive bladder syndrome: results of the STAR trial. Eur Urol 2005;48(3): 464–70.

33. Haab F, Stewart L, Dwyer P. Darifenacin, an M3 selective receptor antagonist, is an effective and well-tolerated once-daily treatment for overactive bladder. Eur Urol 2004;45(4):420–9.

34. Zinner N. Darifenacin: a muscarinic M3-selective receptor antagonist for the treatment of overactive bladder. Expert Opin Pharmacother 2007;8(4):511–23.

35. Chapple C, Van KP, Tubaro A, et al. Clinical efficacy, safety, and tolerability of once-daily fesoterodine in subjects with overactive bladder. Eur Urol 2007; 52(4):1204–12.

36. Nitti VW, Dmochowski R, Sand PK, et al. Efficacy, safety and tolerability of fesoterodine for overactive bladder syndrome. J Urol 2007;178(6):2488–94.

37. Khullar V, Chapple C, Gabriel Z, et al. The effects of antimuscarinics on health-related quality of life in overactive bladder: a systematic review and meta-analysis. Urology 2006;68(Suppl 2):38–48.

38. Gopal M, Haynes K, Bellamy SL, et al. Discontinuation rates of anticholinergic medications used for the treatment of lower urinary tract symptoms. Obstet Gynecol 2008;112(6):1311–8.

39. Shaya FT, Blume S, Gu A, et al. Persistence with overactive bladder pharmacotherapy in a Medicaid population. Am J Manag Care 2005;11(Suppl 4): S121–9.

40. Yu YF, Nichol MB, Yu AP, et al. Persistence and adherence of medications for chronic overactive bladder/urinary incontinence in the California Medicaid program. Value Health 2005;8(4):495–505.

41. Kelleher CJ, Cardozo LD, Khullar V, et al. A medium-term analysis of the subjective efficacy of treatment for women with detrusor instability and low bladder compliance. Br J Obstet Gynaecol 1997;104(9):988–93.
42. Hay-Smith J, Herbison P, Ellis G, et al. Which anticholinergic drug for overactive bladder symptoms in adults. Cochrane Database Syst Rev 2005;(3):CD005429.
43. Chapple CR, Khullar V, Gabriel Z, et al. The effects of antimuscarinic treatments in overactive bladder: an update of a systematic review and meta-analysis. Eur Urol 2008;54(3):543–62.
44. Sand P, Zinner N, Newman D, et al. Oxybutynin transdermal system improves the quality of life in adults with overactive bladder: a multicentre, community-based, randomized study. BJU Int 2007;99(4):836–44.
45. Malavaud B, Bagheri H, Senard JM, et al. Visual hallucinations at the onset of tolterodine treatment in a patient with a high-level spinal cord injury. BJU Int 1999; 84(9):1109.
46. Kay G, Crook T, Rekeda L, et al. Differential effects of the antimuscarinic agents darifenacin and oxybutynin ER on memory in older subjects. Eur Urol 2006;50(2): 317–26.
47. Wagg A, Wyndaele JJ, Sieber P. Efficacy and tolerability of solifenacin in elderly subjects with overactive bladder syndrome: a pooled analysis. Am J Geriatr Pharmacother 2006;4(1):14–24.
48. Schurch B, Stohrer M, Kramer G, et al. Botulinum-A toxin for treating detrusor hyperreflexia in spinal cord injured patients: a new alternative to anticholinergic drugs? Preliminary results. J Urol 2000;164(3 Pt 1):692–7.
49. Cruz F, Dinis P. Resiniferatoxin and botulinum toxin type A for treatment of lower urinary tract symptoms. Neurourol Urodyn 2007;26(Suppl 6):920–7.
50. Karsenty G, Denys P, Amarenco G, et al. Botulinum toxin A (Botox) intradetrusor injections in adults with neurogenic detrusor overactivity/neurogenic overactive bladder: a systematic literature review. Eur Urol 2008;53(2):275–87.
51. Brubaker L, Richter HE, Visco A, et al. Refractory idiopathic urge urinary incontinence and botulinum A injection. J Urol 2008;180(1):217–22.
52. Duthie J, Wilson DI, Herbison GP, et al. Botulinum toxin injections for adults with overactive bladder syndrome. Cochrane Database Syst Rev 2007;(3):CD005493.
53. Apostolidis A, Dasgupta P, Denys P, et al. Recommendations on the use of botulinum toxin in the treatment of lower urinary tract disorders and pelvic floor dysfunctions: a European consensus report. Eur Urol 2008. September 17, 2009. Epub ahead of print.
54. Giannantoni A, Mearini E, Del ZM, et al. Six-year follow-up of botulinum toxin a intradetrusorial injections in patients with refractory neurogenic detrusor overactivity: clinical and urodynamic results. Eur Urol 2009;55(3):705–11.
55. Chancellor MB, de Groat WC. Intravesical capsaicin and resiniferatoxin therapy: spicing up the ways to treat the overactive bladder. J Urol 1999;162(1):3–11.
56. Giannantoni A, Mearini E, Di Stasi SM, et al. New therapeutic options for refractory neurogenic detrusor overactivity. Minerva Urol Nefrol 2004;56(1):79–87.
57. Andersson KE, Chapple CR, Cardozo L, et al. Pharmacological treatment of overactive bladder: report from the International Consultation on Incontinence. Curr Opin Urol 2009;19(4):380–94.
58. Hashim H, Abrams P. Novel uses for antidiuresis. Int J Clin Pract Suppl 2007;(155):32–6.
59. Gopal M, Sammel MD, Pien G, et al. Investigating the associations between nocturia and sleep disorders in perimenopausal women. J Urol 2008;180(5): 2063–7.

60. Dykstra DD, Sidi AA. Treatment of detrusor-sphincter dyssynergia with botulinum A toxin: a double-blind study. Arch Phys Med Rehabil 1990;71(1):24–6.

61. de Seze M, Petit H, Gallien P, et al. Botulinum a toxin and detrusor sphincter dyssynergia: a double-blind lidocaine-controlled study in 13 patients with spinal cord disease. Eur Urol 2002;42(1):56–62.

62. Phelan MW, Franks M, Somogyi GT, et al. Botulinum toxin urethral sphincter injection to restore bladder emptying in men and women with voiding dysfunction. J Urol 2001;165(4):1107–10.

63. Nitti VW, Tu LM, Gitlin J. Diagnosing bladder outlet obstruction in women. J Urol 1999;161(5):1535–40.

64. Kumar A, Mandhani A, Gogoi S, et al. Management of functional bladder neck obstruction in women: use of alpha-blockers and pediatric resectoscope for bladder neck incision. J Urol 1999;162(6):2061–5.

65. Low BY, Liong ML, Yuen KH, et al. Terazosin therapy for patients with female lower urinary tract symptoms: a randomized, double-blind, placebo controlled trial. J Urol 2008;179(4):1461–9.

66. Taylor JA III, Kuchel GA. Detrusor underactivity: clinical features and pathogenesis of an underdiagnosed geriatric condition. J Am Geriatr Soc 2006;54(12):1920–32.

67. Finkbeiner AE. Is bethanechol chloride clinically effective in promoting bladder emptying? A literature review. J Urol 1985;134(3):443–9.

68. Resnick NM, Yalla SV. Detrusor hyperactivity with impaired contractile function: an unrecognized but common cause of incontinence in elderly patients. JAMA 1987;257(22):3076–81.

69. Kuo HC. Effect of botulinum a toxin in the treatment of voiding dysfunction due to detrusor underactivity. Urology 2003;61(3):550–4.

70. Schaffer J, Fantl JA. Urogenital effects of the menopause. Baillieres Clin Obstet Gynaecol 1996;10(3):401–17.

71. Cardozo L, Lose G, McClish D, et al. A systematic review of the effects of estrogens for symptoms suggestive of overactive bladder. Acta Obstet Gynecol Scand 2004;83(10):892–7.

72. Cardozo L, Lose G, McClish D, et al. A systematic review of estrogens for recurrent urinary tract infections: third report of the Hormones and Urogenital Therapy (HUT) Committee. Int Urogynecol J Pelvic Floor Dysfunct 2001;12(1):15–20.

73. Hendrix SL, Cochrane BB, Nygaard IE, et al. Effects of estrogen with and without progestin on urinary incontinence. JAMA 2005;293(8):935–48.

74. Grady D, Brown JS, Vittinghoff E, et al. Postmenopausal hormones and incontinence: the Heart and Estrogen/Progestin Replacement Study. Obstet Gynecol 2001;97(1):116–20.

75. Alhasso AA, McKinlay J, Patrick K, et al. Anticholinergic drugs versus non-drug active therapies for overactive bladder syndrome in adults. Cochrane Database Syst Rev 2006;(4):CD003193.

76. Burgio KL, Kraus SR, Menefee S, et al. Behavioral therapy to enable women with urge incontinence to discontinue drug treatment: a randomized trial. Ann Intern Med 2008;149(3):161–9.

77. Drake MJ. Emerging drugs for treatment of overactive bladder and detrusor overactivity. Expert Opin Emerg Drugs 2008;13(3):431–46.

78. Available at: http://clinicaltrials.gov/ct2/show/NCT00343486?intr=%22GW427353%22&rank=1. Accessed June 6, 2009.

79. Available at: http://clinicaltrials.gov/ct2/show/NCT00527033?cond=%22Urinary+Bladder%2C+Overactive%22&rank=1. Accessed June 6, 2009.
80. Safarinejad MR, Hosseini SY. Safety and efficacy of tramadol in the treatment of idiopathic detrusor overactivity: a double-blind, placebo-controlled, randomized study. Br J Clin Pharmacol 2006;61(4):456–63.
81. Green SA, Alon A, Ianus J, et al. Efficacy and safety of a neurokinin-1 receptor antagonist in postmenopausal women with overactive bladder with urge urinary incontinence. J Urol 2006;176(6 Pt 1):2535–40.
82. Halaska M, Ralph G, Wiedemann A, et al. Controlled, double-blind, multicentre clinical trial to investigate long-term tolerability and efficacy of trospium chloride in patients with detrusor instability. World J Urol 2003;20(6):392–9.
83. Chapple CR, Van Kerrebroeck PE, Junemann KP, et al. Comparison of fesoterodine and tolterodine in patients with overactive bladder. BJU Int 2008;102(9): 1128–32.
84. Wein AJ. Pharmacological agents for the treatment of urinary incontinence due to overactive bladder. Expert Opin Investig Drugs 2001;10(1):65–83.
85. Benson JT, Walters MD. Neurophysiology and pharmacology of the lower urinary tract. In: Walters MD, Karram MM, editors. Urogynecology and reconstructive surgery. 3rd edition. Philadelphia: Mosby and Elsevier; 2007. p. 33.

Surgical Treatment for Stress and Urge Urinary Incontinence

Clifford Y. Wai, MD

KEYWORDS

- Urodynamic stress incontinence • Anti-incontinence surgery
- Bulking agents • Slings • Burch retropubic urethropexy

Urinary incontinence is defined as any involuntary leakage of urine. According to International Continence Society guidelines, urinary incontinence is a symptom and a sign, as well as a condition.[1] Urinary incontinence is a symptom when a patient complains of involuntary leakage. As a sign, urinary incontinence is the observation of involuntary leakage from the urethra. As a condition, urinary incontinence is objectively demonstrated on urodynamic evaluation. Urinary incontinence is a major health problem with social, economic, and psychological consequences affecting approximately 25% of ambulatory women in the United States.[2] In 1995, the annual direct cost of urinary incontinence for women in the United States was estimated to be $12.4 billion per year.[3] The most common type is stress urinary incontinence, with one study reporting 78% of women presenting with the symptom of stress urinary incontinence (49% with pure stress urinary incontinence and 29% with both stress and urge urinary incontinence).[4,5] According to a study using the National Hospital Discharge Survey and National Census data, approximately 129,778 women underwent surgery for stress urinary incontinence in the United States in 2003 (a rate of 12 per 10,000 women).[6] Approximately 30% of women with stress urinary incontinence in the United States opt for surgical treatment.[7]

Although conservative treatment is a reasonable initial approach for urinary incontinence, surgical management is appropriate when conservative treatment is unsuccessful or not desired. Over 200 operations have been developed for the treatment of incontinence,[8] many of which have been abandoned because of poor efficacy and durability. There is no consensus on which is the single "best" treatment for urinary incontinence and therapy should be individualized for each patient. When selecting a surgical procedure for incontinence, factors that should be considered include history of prior anti-incontinence surgery, obesity, concurrent surgery for

Division of Female Pelvic Medicine and Reconstructive Surgery, Department of Obstetrics and Gynecology, University of Texas Southwestern Medical Center, 5323 Harry Hines Boulevard, Dallas, TX 75390-9032, USA
E-mail address: clifford.wai@utsouthwestern.edu

Obstet Gynecol Clin N Am 36 (2009) 509–519
doi:10.1016/j.ogc.2009.08.009
0889-8545/09/$ – see front matter © 2009 Elsevier Inc. All rights reserved.

obgyn.theclinics.com

pelvic organ prolapse, chronic increases in intra-abdominal pressure, mixed incontinence or concurrent overactive bladder, and whether the patient has multiple medical problems or is an appropriate candidate for surgery. This review focuses mainly on the surgical treatment of stress urinary incontinence.

STRESS INCONTINENCE

Continence is maintained through the interplay of normal anatomic and physiologic properties of the bladder, urethra, sphincter, and pelvic floor and the innervation coordinating these structures. Although there is no guaranteed method of ensuring which is the best procedure for every circumstance, a brief understanding of some of the theories behind the pathophysiology of stress urinary incontinence can aid in making the decision and provide some rationale for selecting a particular procedure. Theories on continence are abundant and involve concepts relating to pressure transmission, anatomic support, and urethra integrity.[9,10] Simplistically, stress incontinence can be conceptualized in terms of loss of bladder and urethral support (anatomic stress incontinence) or loss of urethral integrity (sphincteric deficiency).

Anatomic Stress Incontinence

In an ideally supported urogenital tract, increases in intra-abdominal pressure are equally transmitted to the bladder, bladder base, and urethra. This support is derived from (1) ligaments along the lateral aspects of the urethra, termed the *pubourethral ligaments*; (2) the vagina and its lateral fascial condensation; (3) the arcus tendinous fascia pelvic; and (4) levator ani muscles. In women who are continent, increases in intra-abdominal pressure from coughing, laughing, sneezing, or performing a Valsalva maneuver, are countered by supportive tissue tone provided by the levator ani muscle and surrounding vaginal and pelvic connective tissue, thus providing a "backboard" of support. In those with inadequate support, however, these intra-abdominal forces are not countered. This leads to funneling of the urethrovesical junction or a patent urethra, an inability to resist increases in bladder pressure, and in turn, incontinence. This mechanistic theory is the basis for surgical procedures directed at reestablishing this anatomic support of the urethrovesical junction and proximal urethra and stablizing the vagina and urethra during increases in intra-abdominal pressures. An example of such a procedure is the retropubic colposuspension (eg, Burch and Marshall-Marchetti-Kranz [MMK] retropubic urethropexies).

Sphincteric Deficiency

The urethra also maintains continence through the combination of urethral mucosal coaptation, the viscoelastic properties of the urethral epithelium, the underlying urethral vascular plexus, and contraction of appropriate surrounding musculature. Defects in any of these components may lead to urine leakage. For instance, prior surgery in the retropubic space may cause denervation and scarring of the urethra and its supporting tissue. These effects may damage the urethral sphincter, subsequently impede urethral closure, and lead to incontinence. Similarly, incontinence may result from the extensive scarring that may follow local radiotherapy for gynecologic malignancy. The resulting failure of the urethral sphincteric mechanism is commonly termed *intrinsic sphincteric deficiency* and is colloquially referred to as a "lead-pipe" or "low-pressure" urethra. Commonly this condition is defined on urodynamic testing as either a leak point pressure less than 60 cm H_2O or a maximal urethral closure pressure (MUCP) less than 20 cm H_2O.[11] Although these terms and concepts provides the rationale for procedures aimed at correcting stress incontinence, the values used to define intrinsic sphincteric deficiency are not well standardized and have not been consistently found to influence surgical outcomes.[12,13] Surgical treatment directed at restoring urethral integrity includes transurethral injection of bulking agents and surgical sling procedures. Bulking agents, such as collagen, are placed below the urethral muscularis at the level of the urethrovesical junction to elevate the epithelium and promote coaptation. Alternatively, the partially obstructive nature of traditional sling procedures enhances urethral integrity.

Procedures

The three most common operations for the surgical management of stress urinary incontinence are injection of urethral bulking agents, retropubic urethropexy, and sling procedures.

Urethral bulking agents

Injection of bulking agents has been traditionally indicated for women who have urodynamic stress incontinence associated with intrinsic sphincteric deficiency. However, the Food and Drug Administration (FDA) has changed criteria for the use of bulking agents to include patients with Valsalva leak point pressure (VLLP) less than 100 cm H_2O.[14] Additionally, the use of bulking agents is a useful alternative in women with stress incontinence who have multiple medical problems and are poor surgical candidates. Bulking agents can be injected periurethrally or transurethrally and the location of placement can vary. However, the basic concept is to facilitate urethral coaptation by "bulking up" areas of the urethra that appear deficient or patulous. In choosing injectable bulking agents, clinicians look for agents that are easy to use, easy to place, effective (with reproducible results), durable, safe, nonimmunogenic, and nonallergenic. Because few agents satisfy all of these characteristics, newer agents are constantly being developed. A number of bulking agents are currently available on the market.

Collagen Originally receiving premarket approval by the FDA in 1993 for intrinsic sphincteric deficiency, glutaraldehyde cross-linked bovine collagen is probably the most studied periurethral bulking agent. Because allergic reactions, both immediate and delayed hypersensitivity, can occur in about 2% to 5% of patients, candidates for this treatment should be skin-tested 30 days before the actual therapeutic implant is placed. Multiple sites of injection may be required to achieve optimal urethral coaptation and, if symptoms recur, repeat injections may be indicated.

Carbon beads Carbon-coated zirconium oxide beads suspended in a gel matrix received FDA approval in 1999. Because of its larger particle size of 200 to 550 μm, the original product was difficult to inject secondary to needle obstruction. This led to the development of a newer product with a smaller particle size of 95 to 200 μm. One of the advantages of this agent is its resistance to migration due to its particle size. Additionally, because no hypersensitivity reactions occur with this material, skin testing is not required before use.

Ethylene vinyl alcohol copolymers In 2004, the FDA granted premarket approval for use of ethylene vinyl alcohol copolymers as bulking agents. The original product consists of ethylene vinyl alcohol copolymers carried in dimethyl sulfoxide (DMSO).

The advantage of this product is the resistance of ethylene vinyl alcohol to enzymatic degradation and to migration. However, one associated complication was erosion into the urethra, making "fragile urethral mucosal lining" one of the contraindications to the use of this product.

Calcium hydroxylapatite Calcium hydroxylapatite was approved for use in women over age 18 with intrinsic sphincteric deficiency in 2005. The approved product contains calcium hydroxylapatite particles ranging in size from 75 to 125 μm and suspended in glycerin and sodium carboxymethylcellulose. Calcium hydroxylapatite is also a component of bone and teeth, making this product radio-opaque and facilitating postoperative radiographic surveillance. This product also does not require skin testing.

Silicon microparticles Another bulking agent is heat-vulcanized polydimethyl-siloxane, a solid silicone elastomer suspended in poly-vinyl-pyrrolidone carrier gel. It was granted premarket approval in 2006 and has been available since spring 2007.

Other agents Other agents used as urethral bulking agents include autologous carti-lage, human tissue collagen matrix, and autologous myoblasts. Generally, these are reserved for patients with limited bladder neck mobility, although some studies have demonstrated some efficacy in women with urethral hypermobility.[15] Regardless of agent or technique, it is important to ensure that the patient is able to void postpro-cedure. If there is urinary retention, transient use of intermittent self-catheterization is recommended.

Retropubic urethropexy

This group of retropubic urethropexy procedures includes the Burch and MMK oper-ations.[16,17] The Burch technique has long been considered the gold standard for surgical treatment of stress urinary incontinence. Many surgeons employ the Tanagho modification[18] of the Burch procedure, in which sutures are placed in the paravaginal tissue at the bladder neck and proximal urethra, anchored to the iliopectineal ligament (Cooper ligament), and tied down with a suture bridge so as not to compress or over-elevate the urethra. During MMK surgery, but not during the Burch procedure, sutures are used to suspend these tissues from the periosteum of the pubic bone.

With a first-year overall continence rate of 85% to 90% and with a 5-year continence rate of about 70%, the retropubic urethropexy is an effective operation for the surgical treatment of stress urinary incontinence.[19] Complications associated with these procedures include de novo detrusor overactivity, urinary retention, and, in the case of the MMK, osteitis pubis.

The laparoscopic version of the Burch colposuspension has been shown to have objective and subjective cure rates that are lower in the short term (18 month or less) for women with urodynamic stress incontinence when compared with the tension-free vaginal tape (TVT) midurethral sling.[20,21] In contrast, a study with a 4- to 8-year follow-up of patients randomized to laparoscopic Burch colposuspension versus TVT suggests similar long-term efficacy between the two procedures.[22] However, the inves-tigators involved in this study acknowledge that it may have been underpowered. Thus, more studies with adequate sample size comparing these two procedures are needed to be able to make long-term conclusions regarding efficacy.

In women undergoing abdominal sacrocolpopexy for anterior vaginal wall and apical prolapse who do not have stress incontinence symptoms, a recent study has suggested that performing a Burch retropubic urethropexy may significantly reduce the development of symptomatic postoperative stress urinary incontinence.[23,24] In this study, women undergoing abdominal sacrocolpopexy were randomly assigned to receive Burch retropubic urethropexy or not. Three months after surgery, fewer women in the Burch group met one or more of the criteria for stress incontinence (presence of symptoms or positive cough stress test or interval treatment for stress incontinence, Burch 23.8% versus control 44.1%, $P<.001$, n = 322).[23] Two years after surgery, 32.0% and 45.2% of women in the Burch and control groups, respectively, met the criteria for stress incontinence ($P = .026$).[24]

Thus, when discussing surgical options with a patient who has no stress incontinence symptoms and is considering an abdominal sacrocolpopexy, clinicians should mention the findings from the above studies, as well as the availability of efficacious and durable same-day surgical options. However, these results cannot be extrapolated to vaginal procedures nor to other abdominal procedures designed to correct prolapse. Similarly, findings should not be applied to anti-incontinence procedures other than the Burch.

Sling procedures

Midurethral slings The introduction of minimally invasive slings has revolutionized the way we approach surgery for urinary incontinence and has challenged our view of the Burch colposuspension as the gold standard surgical procedure for stress urinary incontinence. The market saw a surge of new sling procedures in the late 1990s and in the early part of this decade. The therapeutic mechanism was based on the integral theory hypothesized by Petros and Ulmsten.[9] In brief, the theory proposed that the control of urethral closure involves the interplay of three structures: the pubourethral ligaments, the suburethral vaginal hammock, and the pubococcygeus muscle, and that laxity of any or all of these support structures results in pelvic floor dysfunction.

There are many variations of these procedures but all involve the midurethral placement of synthetic mesh (currently polypropylene tape) acting as a dynamic fulcrum at the midurethra. Procedures are classified according to the route of placement and can be subdivided into retropubic or transobturator approaches. More recently, yet another variation in the technique and design of the midurethral sling has been introduced—the minimally invasive sling.

Retropubic approach There are several commercial kits available for this procedure. With one technique, separate trocars are placed through a vaginal suburethral incision lateral to the urethra and brought out suprapubically through two skin incisions in a "bottom-up" fashion. Alternatively, needles may be placed suprapubically at the mons pubis, through the space of Retzius, and into the vagina, in a "top-down" approach.

Of these techniques, one of the more commonly studied is one that uses TVT. This technique was introduced to the United States market in 1996. This procedure has proven to be efficacious and durable, and has an acceptable side effect profile, with some considering it to be the new gold standard for the surgical treatment of stress urinary incontinence.[25]

A prospective, observational study conducted at three centers in Sweden and Finland confirmed the long-term safety and efficacy of the TVT device.[26] In this study, the procedure was performed under local anesthesia in 90 women with stress urinary incontinence (defined as having a history of stress incontinence, positive cough stress test at 200 to 300 mL, and urodynamic stress incontinence). Follow-up at 11.5 years (median 141 months, range 127–160 months) included a cough stress test, 24-hour pad weight test, and condition-specific symptom and quality-of-life questionnaires. Of the women available for evaluation, 55 of 61 (90.2%) had both a negative cough stress and pad test. 53 of 69 (77%) were subjectively cured, 14 of 69 (20%) showed improvement, and 2 of 69 (3%) failed treatment. No patients had mesh erosion.

The TVT compares favorably with the Burch colposuspension. A short-term randomized trial comparing the TVT with the Burch was performed by Ward and

Hilton across 14 centers in the United Kingdom and Ireland.[27] Three hundred forty-four women with urinary stress incontinence were randomized to either TVT or Burch. Symptom and quality-of-life questionnaires as well as 1-hour pad tests were performed 2 years after surgery. When all the available data were considered, the TVT was found to be equally efficacious when compared with the Burch (111 of 137 [81%] versus 86 of 108 [80%], $P = .87$). Secondary to patient drop out, the data were analyzed with all withdrawals considered as failures (TVT, 111 of 175 [63%] versus Burch, 86 of 169 [51%], $P = .02$), then with all withdrawals considered as cured (TVT, 149 of 175 [85%] versus Burch, 147 of 169 [87%], $P = .64$). Taken together, these results suggest that the TVT is at least as efficacious as the Burch.

Complications of the TVT procedure include erosion, retention, de novo urge urinary incontinence, urgency, vascular injury, bowel injury, and lower urinary tract injury. The complication rate is variable with a Finnish study of 1455 patients in 38 hospitals reporting a bladder perforation rate of 3.8%, minor voiding difficulties of 7.6%, urinary retention of 2.3%, retropubic hematoma of 1.9%, major vessel injury of 0.07%, and postoperative laparotomy for complication of 0.3%.[28] Bladder perforation has probably become the one of the most common complications associated with the procedure (3%–9%).[27,29–32]

Transobturator approach The transobturator approach to midurethral sling placement was introduced by DeLorme in 2001.[33] One of the goals behind the development of this technique was to reduce the morbidity associated with retropubic passage of a trocar. According to theory, the potential for bladder, bowel, and vascular injury could be reduced by avoiding the space of Retzius. As with the retropubic approach, variations have been developed. Each represents a variation of the needle-and-mesh design. Essentially, a permanent synthetic mesh (usually polypropylene) is also placed at the midurethra. However, in this approach, the mesh is introduced by passing it through the obturator foramen. The two major types of transobturator techniques are distinguished by whether needle placement begins inside the vagina and is directed outward, in an in-to-out approach, or starts outside and is directed inward, in an out-to-in approach. In the out-to-in technique, the trocar, after it courses around the ischiopubic ramus, penetrates the gracilis, adductor brevis muscle, obturator externus muscle, obturator membrane, obturator internus muscle, and periurethral connective tissue, and then exits through vaginal incision.[34]

Although most of the studies regarding the transobturator technique consist of short-term data, the results have been positive thus far. One of the early reports comparing the transobturator and the TVT reported no difference in cure, improvement, or failure between the two procedures.[35] Although the publication of this study was retracted secondary to issues relating to institutional review board approval, it served as an early attestation to the similar efficacy of the two procedures. In fact, other studies have reaffirmed this finding.[36–38]

Although the transobturator approach provides an effective day-surgery technique with potentially lower rates of bladder injury, some retrospective studies have suggested that it may have limited effectiveness for patients who demonstrate urodynamic parameters consistent with intrinsic sphincteric deficiency. One retrospective case series studied 70 women with stress urinary incontinence treated with an out-to-in transobturator midurethral sling by a single surgeon.[39] At a mean follow-up period of 8.1 months (range 6–12 months) after the procedure, 56 of 70 (80%) were completely continent. The data for patients with persistent incontinence symptoms and those who were asymptomatic were analyzed according to VLPPs and MUCPs. Median

VLPP and MUCP in women who had persistent incontinence were lower than those who were asymptomatic after treatment (VLPP$_{cap}$ 32 cm H_2O versus 71 cm H_2O, $P<.001$; MUCP 20 cm H_2O versus 45 cm H_2O, $P<.001$).

Similarly, other retrospective case series have reported that transobturator procedures have lower cure rates in patients with lower VLPPs (77% cure rate with VLPP > 60 versus 25% cure rate with VLPP < 60),[40] or higher relative risk of failure (relative risk 5.89) in patients with lower MUCPs.[41]

The transobturator procedure was developed first as an out-to-in approach. One of the criticisms with this route of trocar passage was that bladder and urethral injury were still potential complications. As a result, the in-to-out approach was developed[42] and promoted with the hope of decreased lower urinary tract injury rates. With the trocar directed away from the urethra and bladder, there should be less likelihood of injuring the bladder and urethra, with some even suggesting that perioperative cystourethroscopy was unnecessary.[43] However, although there was theoretically less lower urinary tract injury with the trocar directed in a medial to lateral fashion (ie, away from the bladder), the trocar tip in this technique was found to be closer to the obturator neurovascular bundle than with the out-to-in method.[44,45] The mean distances from the obturator canal for the in-to-out were 1.3 ± 0.44 cm compared to 2.3 ± 0.41 cm with the out-to-in technique ($P<.001$). Thus, even though each method has its theoretical advantages, the possibility of injury is not entirely eliminated. Clearly prospective randomized comparative studies are needed to clarify the efficacy of each transobturator midurethral sling and to confirm the relative safety of each technique.

Minimally invasive slings The minimally invasive slings, sometimes called *microslings* or *minislings*, constitute the latest addition to the sling revolution. These newer slings, approved by the FDA's 510(K) process, tout the advantage of being less invasive and producing fewer complications. By avoiding trocar passage through the retropubic space, the potential for vascular and lower urinary tract injury should theoretically be reduced. Currently, published data are available for only one minimally invasive sling. This device consists of an 8 × 1.1-cm prolene tape, coated on both ends with polyglactin 910 and poly-p-dioxanon to facilitate mesh incorporation. This mesh is introduced under the midurethra with a curved stainless steel inserter. The manufacturer advertises two mesh configurations, where the prosthetic implant can be fixed in the "hammock" position into the obturator internus muscle or in the U-shaped position behind the pubic symphysis.

There are limited data on the efficacy and safety of this sling. A prospective case series on 100 consecutive patients separated the cohort into two groups. The first 50 patients, the early group, had an objective failure rate at 1 month of 20% (10 of 50), vaginal erosion rate of 10% (5 of 50), and a subjective cure rate at 12 months of 89% (39 of 44). The second 50 patients had an objective failure rate at 1 month of 8% (4 of 50), and a subjective cure rate at 12 months of 94% (43 of 46). Both groups had no lower urinary tract injury.[46]

A prospective multi-institutional study on 95 consecutive patients with stress incontinence 15 months after insertion of this device found 74 of 91 (81%) with objective cure (defined as a negative cough stress test) and 71 of 91 with subjective cure. However, the study also found 9 of 91 (10%) with recurrent urinary tract infections, 9 of 91 (10%) with de novo urge incontinence, and 7 of 91 (8%) with voiding difficulty.[47] As with most technology, it is recommended that data from well-conducted long-term comparative studies on efficacy and safety be obtained before of any new technique be fully adopted.

URGE URINARY INCONTINENCE
Sacral Neuromodulation

The sacral neuromodulation device for an outpatient surgical implantation contains a pulse generator and electrical leads placed into the sacral foramina to modulate innervation to the bladder and pelvic floor. Sacral neuromodulation is generally reserved for women with refractory urgency, frequency, or urge incontinence. The device may also be considered for those with pelvic pain, interstitial cystitis, and defecatory dysfunction, although the FDA has not approved it for these indications. For the most part, this procedure is not considered primary therapy, and women who receive this device have typically exhausted pharmacologic and conservative options. Implantation is typically conducted in a two-stage process. Initially, leads are placed and attached to an externally worn generator. After placement, frequency and amplitude of electrical impulses can be adjusted and tailored to maximize effectiveness. If a 50% or greater improvement in symptoms is noted as determined by a urinary diary, then implantation of a permanent pulse generator is planned. Studies have found improvement rates ranging from 60% to 75%, and cure rates approximating 45%.[48–50]

This procedure is minimally invasive and is typically completed in a day-surgery setting. Accordingly, recovery is rapid. Surgical complications are rare but may include pain or infection at the generator insertion site.

SUMMARY

There is no single "best" procedure for the surgical treatment of incontinence.

All patients are not the same and therapy should be individualized. It is important to establish that the decision to opt for surgical treatment is a quality-of-life decision and that it is patient driven. Urinary incontinence is a spectrum of disease and the specific type of incontinence should be determined before initiating therapy. As practitioners, it is imperative that we evaluate the published literature before widespread adoption of a surgical procedure. Preoperative patient counseling should include a discussion of risks, benefits, patient expectations, and outcomes using the available data.

REFERENCES

1. Abrams P, Cardozo L, Fall M, et al. The standardization of terminology of lower urinary tract function: report from the standardization sub-committee of the International Continence Society. Neurourol Urodyn 2002;21:167–78.
2. Dooley Y, Kenton K, Cao G, et al. Urinary incontinence prevalence: results from the National Health and Nutrition Examination Survey. J Urol 2008;179:656–61.
3. Wilson L, Brown JS, Shin GP, et al. Annual direct cost of urinary incontinence. Obstet Gynecol 2001;98:398–406.
4. Nygaard IE, Lemke JH. Urinary incontinence in rural older women: prevalence, incidence and remission. J Am Geriatr Soc 1996;44:1049–54.
5. Hampel C, Wienhold D, Benken N, et al. Definition of overactive bladder and epidemiology of urinary incontinence. Urology 1997;50(6A Suppl):4–14.
6. Shah AD, Kohli N, Rajan SS, et al. The age distribution, rates, and types of surgery for stress urinary incontinence in the USA. Int Urogynecol J Pelvic Floor Dysfunct 2008;19:89–96.
7. Kinchen KS, Long S, Orsini L, et al. Healthcare utilization among women who undergo surgery for stress urinary incontinence. Int Urogynecol J Pelvic Floor Dysfunct 2004;15:154–9.

8. Wall LL. Urinary stress incontinence. In: Rock JA, Thompson JD, editors. Te-Linde's operative gynecology. 8th edition. Philadelphia: Lippincott-Raven; 1997. p. 1087–134.

9. Petros PE, Ulmsten UI. An integral theory of female urinary incontinence. Experimental and clinical considerations. Scand J Urol Nephrol 1993; 153(Suppl):1–93.

10. Delancey JO. Structural support of the urethra as it relates to stress urinary incontinence: the hammock hypothesis. Am J Obstet Gynecol 1994;170:1713–20.

11. McGuire EJ. Urodynamic findings in patients after failure of stress incontinence operations. Prog Clin Biol Res 1981;78:351–60.

12. Weber AM. Leak point pressure measurement and stress urinary incontinence. Curr Womens Health Rep 2001;1:45–52.

13. Monga AK, Stanton SL. Urodynamics: prediction, outcome and analysis of mechanism for cure of stress incontinence by periurethral collagen. Br J Obstet Gynaecol 1997;104:158–62.

14. McGuire EJ. Urethral bulking agents. Nat Clin Pract Urol 2006;3:234–5.

15. Bent AE, Foote J, Siegel S, et al. Collagen implant for treating stress urinary incontinence in women with urethral hypermobility. J Urol 2001;166:1354–7.

16. Burch JC. Urethrovaginal fixation to Cooper's ligament for correction of stress incontinence, cystocele, and prolapse. Am J Obstet Gynecol 1961; 81:281–90.

17. Marshall VF, Marchetti AA, Krantz KE. The correction of stress incontinence by simple vesicourethral suspension. Surg Gynecol Obstet 1949;88:509–18.

18. Tanagho EA. Colpocystourethropexy: the way we do it. J Urol 1976;116:751–3.

19. Lapitan MC, Cody DJ, Grant AM. Open retropubic colposuspension for urinary incontinence in women. Cochrane Database Syst Rev. 2003;(1):CD002912. Review. Update in: Cochrane Database Syst Rev. 2005;(3):CD002912.

20. Paraiso MF, Walters MD, Karram MM, et al. Laparoscopic Burch colposuspension versus tension-free vaginal tape: a randomized trial. Obstet Gynecol 2004;104: 1249–58.

21. Dean N, Herbison P, Ellis G, et al. Laparoscopic colposuspension and tension-free vaginal tape: a systematic review. BJOG 2006;113:1345–53.

22. Jelovsek JE, Barber MD, Karram MM, et al. Randomised trial of laparoscopic Burch colposuspension versus Tension-free vaginal tape: long-term follow up. BJOG 2008;115:219–25.

23. Brubaker L, Cundiff GW, Fine P, et al. Pelvic floor disorders network. Abdominal sacrocolpopexy with Burch colposuspension to reduce urinary stress incontinence. N Engl J Med 2006;354:1557–66.

24. Brubaker L, Nygaard I, Richter HE, et al. Two-year outcomes after sacrocolpopexy with and without Burch to prevent stress urinary incontinence. Obstet Gynecol 2008;112:49–55.

25. Debodinance P, Delporte P, Engrand JB, et al. Tension-free vaginal tape (TVT) in the treatment of urinary stress incontinence: 3 years experience involving 256 operations. Eur J Obstet Gynecol Reprod Biol 2002;105:49–58.

26. Nilsson CG, Palva K, Rezapour M, et al. Eleven years prospective follow-up of the tension-free vaginal tape procedure for treatment of stress urinary incontinence. Int Urogynecol J Pelvic Floor Dysfunct 2008;19:1043–7.

27. Ward KL, Hilton P, UK and Ireland TVT Trial Group. A prospective multicenter randomized trial of tension-free vaginal tape and colposuspension for primary urodynamic stress incontinence: two-year follow-up. Am J Obstet Gynecol 2004;190:324–31.

28. Kuuva N, Nilsson CG. A nationwide analysis of complications associated with the tension-free vaginal tape (TVT) procedure. Acta Obstet Gynecol Scand 2002;81: 72–7.

29. Meschia M, Pifarotti P, Bernasconi F, et al. Tension-free vaginal tape: analysis of out-comes and complications in 404 stress incontinent women. Int Urogynecol J Pelvic Floor Dysfunct 2001;12(Suppl):S24–7.

30. Agostini A, Bretelle F, Franchi F, et al. Immediate complications of tension-free vaginal tape (TVT): results of a French survey. Eur J Obstet Gynecol Reprod Biol 2006;124:237–9.

31. Karram MM, Segal JL, Vassallo BJ, et al. Complications and untoward effects of the tension-free vaginal tape procedure. Obstet Gynecol 2003;101:929–32.

32. Tamussino KF, Hanzal E, Kolle D, et al. Tension-free vaginal tape operation: results. Obstet Gynecol 2001;98:732–6.

33. Delorme E. Transobturator urethral suspension: mini-invasive procedure in the treatment of stress urinary incontinence in women. Prog Urol 2001;11:1306–13.

34. Whiteside JL, Walters MD. Anatomy of the obturator region: relations to a trans-obturator sling. Int Urogynecol J Pelvic Floor Dysfunct 2004;15:223–6.

35. deTayrac R, Deffieux X, Droupy S, et al. A prospective randomized trial comparing tension-free vaginal tape and transobturator suburethral tape for surgical treatment of stress urinary incontinence. Am J Obstet Gynecol 2004; 190:602–8.

36. Laurikainen E, Valpas A, Kivelä A, et al. Retropubic compared with transobturator tape placement in treatment of urinary incontinence: a randomized controlled trial. Obstet Gynecol 2007;109:4–11.

37. Barber MD, Kleeman S, Karram MM, et al. Transobturator tape compared with tension-free vaginal tape for the treatment of stress urinary incontinence: a randomized controlled trial. Obstet Gynecol 2008;111:611–21.

38. Sung VW, Schleinitz MD, Rardin CR, et al. Comparison of retropubic vs transob-turator approach to midurethral slings: a systematic review and meta-analysis. Am J Obstet Gynecol 2007;197:3–11.

39. Guerette NL, Bena JF, Davila GW. Transobturator slings for stress incontinence: using urodynamic parameters to predict outcomes. Int Urogynecol J Pelvic Floor Dysfunct 2008;19:97–102.

40. O'Connor RC, Nanigian DK, Lyon MB, et al. Early outcomes of mid-urethral slings for female stress urinary incontinence stratified by Valsalva leak point pressure. Neurourol Urodyn 2006;25:685–8.

41. Miller JJ, Botros SM, Akl MN, et al. Is transobturator tape as effective as tension-free vaginal tape in patients with borderline maximum urethral closure pressure? Am J Obstet Gynecol 2006;195:1799–804.

42. de Leval J. Novel surgical technique for the treatment of female stress urinary incontinence: transobturator vaginal tape inside-out. Eur Urol 2003; 44:724–30.

43. Bonnet P, Waltregny D, Reul O, et al. Transobturator vaginal tape inside out for the surgical treatment of female stress urinary incontinence: anatomical consider-ations. J Urol 2005;173:1223–8.

44. Zahn CM, Siddique S, Hernandez S, et al. Anatomic comparison of two transob-turator tape procedures. Obstet Gynecol 2007;109:701–6.

45. Achtari C, McKenzie BJ, Hiscock R, et al. Anatomical study of the obturator foramen and dorsal nerve of the clitoris and their relationship to minimally invasive slings. Int Urogynecol J Pelvic Floor Dysfunct 2006;17:330–4.

46. Neuman M. Perioperative complications and early follow-up with 100 TVT-SECUR procedures. J Minim Invasive Gynecol 2008;15:480–4.

47. Meschia M, Barbacini P, Ambrogi V, et al. TVT-secur: a minimally invasive procedure for the treatment of primary stress urinary incontinence. One year data from a multi-centre prospective trial. Int Urogynecol J Pelvic Floor Dysfunct 2009;20: 313–7.

48. Janknegt RA, Hassouna MM, Siegel SW, et al. Long-term effectiveness of sacral nerve stimulation for refractory urge incontinence. Eur Urol 2001;39:101–6.

49. Schmidt RA, Jonas U, Oleson KA, et al. Sacral nerve stimulation for treatment of refractory urinary urge incontinence. Sacral Nerve Stimulation Study Group. J Urol 1999;162:352–7.

50. Siegel SW, Catanzaro F, Dijkema HE, et al. Long-term results of a multicenter study on sacral nerve stimulation for treatment of urinary urge incontinence, urgency-frequency, and retention. Urology 2000;56:87–91.

Pathophysiology of Pelvic Organ Prolapse

R. Ann Word, MD*, Sujatha Pathi, MD, Joseph I. Schaffer, MD

KEYWORDS

- Prolapse • Protease • Matrix metalloprotease • Collagen
- Elastic fibers • Vagina

Pelvic organ prolapse is a prevalent and disabling condition with suboptimal treatment. Multiple mechanisms have been hypothesized as contributors to the development of prolapse, but none fully explain the origin and natural history of this process. Epidemiologic studies indicate that vaginal birth and aging are two major risk factors for the development of pelvic organ prolapse.[1] Other factors include increased abdominal pressure, increased body mass index, and connective tissue disorders. Hence, there is little doubt that pelvic organ prolapse is multifactorial in etiology and may involve more than one pathology to exhibit full anatomic loss of support. Furthermore, loss of support that evolves decades after vaginal delivery may involve an initial insult compounded by loss of support associated with aging. Currently, it is believed that a complex of pathologies are involved in failure of pelvic organ support. These pathologies include those related to genetics, loss of pelvic floor striated muscle support, and loss of connective attachments of the vaginal wall to striated muscles and structures of the pelvis. In this article, we review the potential mechanisms for loss of pelvic organ support in women and new insights into the role of elastic fibers in the pathophysiology of pelvic organ prolapse.

FAILURE OF PELVIC ORGAN SUPPORT: POTENTIAL MECHANISMS

The pelvic floor comprises several different tissue types that act in concert to provide support and maintain normal physiologic function of the rectum, vagina, urethra, and bladder. All tissue types of the pelvic floor are important for normal support of the

---

Grant support: National Institutes of Health AG 028048.

Division of Female Pelvic Medicine and Reconstructive Surgery, Department of Obstetrics and Gynecology, University of Texas Southwestern Medical Center, 5323 Harry Hines Boulevard, Dallas, TX 75390-9032, USA

* Corresponding author.

E-mail address: ruth.word@utsouthwestern.edu (R.A. Word).

pelvic organs, and failure of one or more of the tissue support systems may be involved in the pathophysiology of pelvic organ prolapse.

Levator Ani

The levator ani is a set of striated muscles comprising three regions. The iliococcygeal portion forms a flat horizontal shelf spanning from one pelvic sidewall to the other. The pubococcygeus muscle arises from the pubic bone on either side, is attached to the walls of the perforating pelvic organs and perineal body, and inserts on the coccyx. The pubococcygeus thereby is important in suspending the vaginal wall to the pelvis. The third portion of the levator ani, the puborectalis, forms a sling around and behind the rectum and extends to the external anal sphincter. Connective tissue covers superior and inferior fascia of the levator muscles. In the healthy state, baseline resting contractile activity of the levator ani muscles elevates the pelvic floor, and compresses the vagina, urethra, and rectum toward the pubic bone, narrowing the genital hiatus and preventing prolapse of the pelvic organs.

It is widely believed that the levator ani muscles sustain either direct or denervation injury during childbirth and that these injuries are involved in the pathogenesis of pelvic organ prolapse. It is hypothesized that nerve injury (due to stretch or compression or both) during the second stage of labor results in partial denervation of the levator ani and, as the denervated muscle loses tone, the genital hiatus opens, thereby leading to prolapse of the pelvic viscera.[2–5]

Experimental evidence for the relationship between denervation-induced injury of the levator ani and pelvic organ prolapse has been difficult to obtain. For example, although pudendal nerve neuropathy has been associated with pelvic organ prolapse,[6] the levator ani muscles are not innervated by the pudendal nerve, but rather by neurons originating from sacral nerve roots S3-S5, which traverse the superior surface of the pelvic floor.[7–10] Thus, pudendal nerve injury may not be related to denervation of levator ani muscles. Investigators who have directly assessed levator ani muscles disagree regarding neuromuscular damage in women with pelvic organ prolapse. Some studies demonstrate histomorphologic abnormalities in the levator ani from women with prolapse and stress incontinence.[8,11] Other studies fail to find histologic evidence of levator ani denervation.[12,13] In addition, full-thickness biopsies obtained from three locations of the levator ani failed to find evidence of atrophy, small-angulated fibers, or type grouping in specimens from parous versus nulliparous cadavers,[14] suggesting that pregnancy and parturition have little or no effect on histomorphology of levator ani muscles. The lack of histologic features of denervation in levator ani muscles from women with prolapse agrees with our own findings using microarray analysis and histomorphology of pubococcygeus muscles from premenopausal women with pelvic organ prolapse compared with age-matched controls.[15] Furthermore, gross disruption of levator ani muscles and its innervation was not observed in squirrel monkeys with or without defects in pelvic organ support.[16] Myogenic changes occurred more frequently in the pubocaudalis compared with the iliocaudalis muscles of this animal model, and a significant association of myogenic alterations in the pubocaudalis was found with aging, but not with pelvic organ prolapse or parity. However, parity was associated with increased apoptosis of fibroblasts in paravaginal attachments.[16]

To determine whether experimental denervation of the levator ani contributes to development of pelvic organ prolapse in squirrel monkeys, Pierce and colleagues[17] compared nulliparous squirrel monkeys without prolapse to those with bilateral levator neurectomy, to parous monkeys without prolapse, and to parous monkeys with prolapse. As expected, significant atrophy of levator ani occurred in denervated animals. However, pelvic organ support was not affected by bilateral denervation of the levator ani. Taken together, experimental evidence does not support a role for denervation-induced injury in the pathophysiology of pelvic organ prolapse. However, loss of skeletal muscle volume and function occurs in virtually all striated muscles during aging. Results obtained from young and old women with pelvic organ prolapse[15] and young and old baboons without prolapse (Marinis and Word, unpublished data, 2003.) indicate that the levator ani undergoes substantial morphologic and biochemical changes during aging, suggesting that loss of levator tone with age may contribute to failure of pelvic organ support in older women, possibly with preexisting defects in connective tissue support. As the striated muscles lose tone, ligamentous and connective tissue support of the pelvic organs must sustain more forces conferred by abdominal pressure. As the connective tissues bear these loads for long periods of time, they stretch and may eventually fail, resulting in clinically recognized prolapse.

INTERACTIONS BETWEEN LEVATOR ANI AND CONNECTIVE TISSUES OF THE PELVIC FLOOR

Ligaments and connective tissues surrounding the pelvic organs support and stabilize the organs in their position above the levator ani. Several connective tissue types are involved in this support system as discussed below.

Bony Pelvis

It has been suggested that women with prolapse have a wider pelvic diameter than women without prolapse[18,19] and, in one study, pelvic organ prolapse was associated with a shorter obstetric conjugate.[18] These findings may represent different types of bony pelvises in women of different racial background. Black women are more likely to have an anthropoid pelvis with a narrow transverse inlet and wide obstetric conjugate.[20] Also, in some,[21] but not all,[22] studies, black women have been characterized as having decreased risk of pelvic organ prolapse. It is possible that certain pelvic shapes may render the connective tissue support system of the pelvic organs more susceptible to stretch injury or trauma. Recently, however, using MRI, postpartum bony and soft tissue pelvic dimensions were measured in 246 postpartum primiparous women with or without pelvic organ prolapse.[23] Although a deeper sacral hollow was significantly associated with fecal incontinence and a wider intertuberous diameter, and pelvic arch was associated with urinary incontinence, there were no significant differences in pelvimetry measurements between women with and without prolapse.[23] The long-term impact of pelvic dimensions on the development of pelvic organ prolapse in parous women is not known.

Arcus Tendineous Fascia Pelvis and Arcus Tendineus Levator Ani

Two prominent lateral connective tissue structures play an important role in muscular and connective tissue support of the pelvic organs. Arising as condensations of the parietal fascia of the obturator internus and levator ani muscle, these aggregations of connective tissue comprise dense regular connective tissue, similar to that of tendons, with fibrous collagen more organized than the visceral connective tissue surrounding the pelvic organs (**Fig. 1**). The arcus tendoneus levator ani provides anchorage for the origin of the iliococcygeus and pubococcyeus muscle inserting at the pubic rami and then crossing over the obturator internus to insert posteriorly at the ischial spine. In contrast, the arcus tendineous fascia pelvis is a condensation of the parietal fascia of the visceral connective tissue that envelops the anterior and

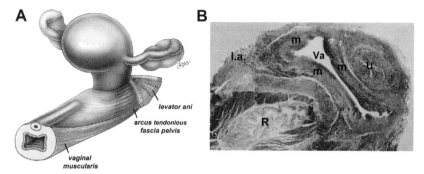

Fig. 1. Connective tissue support of the female reproductive tract (2× magnification). (*A*) The vaginal wall is enveloped in a fibromuscular layer of connective tissue (previously referred to as "endopelvic fascia"). The muscularis of the vaginal wall extends laterally and anteriorly to coalesce with dense connective tissue of the arcus tendineous fascia pelvis. It also interdigitates with fibers of the levator ani laterally. (*B*) Masson's trichrome staining of a section through the mid-vagina. Collagen (blue) and smooth muscle bundles (red) of the vaginal muscularis (m) are immediately adjacent with the pubococcygeus of the levator ani (l.a.). Vaginal muscularis provides connective tissue support for the urethra (U), rectum (R) and vaginal wall.

posterior vaginal wall (see **Fig. 1**). It provides the lateral anchor sites for the anterior and posterior vagina. For many years, it was believed that tendon and the fascia of its corresponding muscle were all one continuous structure. Electron microscopy studies, however, demonstrate that muscle endomysium (fascia) is a separate entity, with its own connective tissues, and is not identical to tendon tissue radiating from the muscle. The arcus tendineous fascia pelvis is, therefore, separate from the fascia of the levator ani and is well developed anteriorly, presenting as a white line emanating from fasciae covering the pubococcygeus and iliococcygeus muscles.

The arcus tendineous fascia pelvis is therefore poised to withstand descent of the anterior vaginal wall and proximal urethra. The ability to prevent descent of the proximal urethra during periods of increased abdominal pressure is crucial in maintenance of urinary continence. Overstretching or tearing of the arcus tendineous fascia pelvis during vaginal delivery is postulated to contribute to pelvic organ prolapse.

Uterosacral Ligaments

There are two main differences between tendons and ligaments. While ligaments and tendons both have bundles of parallel collagen fibers, the fibers in ligaments are arranged in multidirectional layers, whereas the tendon's fibers remain in strictly parallel strands. Ligaments are composed mainly of bundles of white fibrous tissue closely interlaced with one another. Although ligaments are pliant and flexible to allow freedom of movement, they are nevertheless strong, tough, and not able to extend. Elastin between each layer of the ligament allows some movement between collagen and smooth muscle layers for flexibility and change of motion.

The uterosacral ligaments are believed to contribute to pelvic support by suspending and stabilizing the uterus, cervix, and upper vagina to the dorsal body wall. Connective tissues of uterosacral ligaments in women with and without pelvic organ prolapse have been compared.[24–33] The ligament is comprised of about 20% smooth muscle. Using immunohistochemistry, Gabriel and colleagues[25] found that smooth muscle and collagen type I content was similar in uterosacral ligaments from postmenopausal women with or without pelvic organ prolapse. Collagen III expression, however, was significantly increased in ligaments from women with prolapse. In contrast, using a similar technique, Takacs and colleagues[33] found that the fractional area of smooth muscle was decreased and that apoptotic cells were increased in ligaments from women with prolapse. Reisenauer and colleagues[31] found that the distribution of smooth muscle in the uterosacral ligament was abnormal in women with pelvic organ prolapse compared with age-, parity-, and menopause-matched controls. Consistent with the findings of Takacs and colleagues, smooth muscle cell nuclei were smaller.

Brizzolara and colleagues[24] conducted a comprehensive study designed to study gene expression profiles in ligamentous support tissue. In this study, 34 microarrays interrogating 32,878 genes were conducted from 17 women with or without pelvic organ prolapse. Investigators found 249 differentially expressed genes between the two groups and these genes most commonly belonged to immunity and defense pathways. Interleukin-6, thrombospondin 1 and prostaglandin-endoperoxide synthase 2 (COX-2) were increased significantly in ligaments from women with prolapse.[24] Using light microscopy, investigators found no inflammatory infiltrates in the tissue. These studies suggest that the transcriptional program of cells involved in ligamentous support of the pelvic organs is altered in women with prolapse. These alterations most likely lead to altered matrix production, cell shape, and mechanical properties, and aberrant inflammatory and healing processes. The role of stretch and mechanical strain on the ligaments in producing these changes is not known.

Vaginal Wall

Abnormalities in the vaginal wall or in the attachments of the vaginal wall to the pelvic floor muscles may be involved in the pathogenesis of pelvic organ prolapse. The supportive connective tissue of the pelvic floor is a continuous interdependent sheet that envelops the vagina and suspends it to the levator ani muscles of the pelvic floor via the arcus tendineous fascia pelvis (see **Fig. 1**). The connective tissue of the vaginal wall comprises the lamina propria, the vaginal muscularis, and the vaginal adventitia (see **Fig. 1**). Connective tissue of the vaginal wall (formerly referred to as *endopelvic fascia*) coalesces laterally to the arcus tendineous fascia pelvis and superior fascia of the levator ani. In the lower third of the vagina, the vaginal wall is attached directly to surrounding structures—the perineal membrane, and the perineal body. This suspensory system, together with the uterosacral ligaments, prevents the vagina and uterus from descent when the genital hiatus is open. Loss of connective tissue "resilience" is believed to contribute to pelvic organ prolapse during aging.

EVIDENCE THAT THE VAGINAL WALL IS ABNORMAL IN WOMEN WITH PELVIC ORGAN PROLAPSE
Collagen

It has been suggested that abnormal synthesis or degradation of collagen and elastin fibers of the vaginal wall contributes to the pathophysiology of prolapse. The extracellular matrix of connective tissues comprises predominantly fibrillar collagens and elastic fibers embedded in a nonfibrillar ground substance of proteoglycans, glycosaminoglycans, and hyaluronan. Collagen synthesis in pelvic floor connective tissues in women with pelvic organ prolapse has been reviewed comprehensively.[34] Using hydroxyproline assays (an index of cross-linked collagen) and analyses of collagen alpha chains, Jackson and colleagues[35] found decreases in total collagen content in vaginal epithelium from women with prolapse compared with premenopausal controls. The ratios of collagen I to collagen III were similar between the two groups.

These findings agree with those of Soderberg and colleagues,[36] who, using the same assay, found total collagen content of parauthral ligaments to be decreased in young women with prolapse. Histologic methods, such as immunofluorescent techniques with antibodies to collagen subtypes, are not as quantitative as hydroxyproline assays. These techniques have the advantage, however, of localizing collagen subtypes in the connective tissues and can thereby distinguish between vascular and nonvascular matrix in the epithelium, lamina propria, and muscularis of connective tissues. Using immunohistochemical techniques, Kokcu and colleagues[37] and Moalli and colleagues[38] found increased total collagen in vaginal apical biopsies in premenopausal women with prolapse. The discrepancies in findings regarding collagen content in connective tissues of women with prolapse likely stem from differences in technical assessments of collagen content. Newly formed collagen is more extractable and contains more pentosidine cross-links. It is difficult to differentiate between mature and immature collagen using immunohistology. Thus, increased collagen content by immunofluorescence likely represents both mature and newly formed immature collagen, a finding consistent with that of Jackson and colleagues[35] and Soderberg and colleagues,[36] who showed that formed collagen increases in the vaginal wall during aging. Suzme and colleagues[32] found that hydroxyproline content was decreased in the uterosacral ligament of women with pelvic organ prolapse despite histopathological evidence of increased collagen density. Collagen synthesis is increased in fibroblasts from women with prolapse compared with controls[39] and our studies indicate collagen type I and type III mRNA are increased in vaginal muscularis from women with prolapse compared with age-matched controls (Boreham and Word, data not published). Taken together, the data suggest that collagen synthesis is increased in the vaginal wall of women with prolapse, but that the newly formed immature collagen is more susceptible to endogenous proteases and therefore is unlikely to contribute to mature cross-linked collagen that confers strength and durability to connective tissues.

Histomorphology

The normal vaginal wall comprises mucosa (epithelium and lamina propria), a fibroelastic muscularis layer, and an adventitial layer composed of loose areolar tissue, abundant elastic fibers, and neurovascular bundles. Smooth muscle cells of the anterior vaginal wall obtained from the apex of the vagina were identified by immunohistochemistry with antibodies to smooth muscle α-actin.[40] In normal vaginal wall, smooth muscle of the muscularis is well organized in discrete fascicles constituting 45% of total cross-sectional area (**Fig. 2**A). In women with prolapse, smooth muscle bundles are smaller and disorganized. Smooth muscle content in this location of the vagina is decreased significantly (~22%),[40] compared with the normal well-suspended vagina (**Fig. 2**B). In addition, nerve bundles are large and numerous in the deep muscularis of asymptomatic controls, but are smaller and fewer in number in women with pelvic organ prolapse.[41] Although smooth muscle cell density is decreased in the vaginal apex of women with pelvic organ prolapse, there is no evidence that vaginal wall thickness is altered, suggesting that decreased smooth muscle cell volume may be replaced by other cell types or by the extracellular matrix. Furthermore, there is considerable variability in the amount of smooth muscle in this location of the vagina, even in control subjects. Using full-thickness sagittal sections of vaginal wall from fresh female cadavers, we found substantial variability in vaginal wall thickness and smooth muscle cell density along the length of the vaginal wall. In specimens obtained from women undergoing colpocleisis or vaginectomy, smooth muscle cells may be hypertrophied, particularly in midvagina or at the level of maximal bulge.

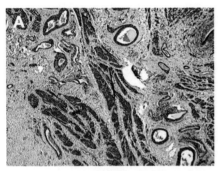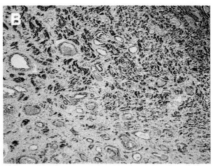

Fig. 2. (*A*) Immunostaining of smooth muscle in vaginal muscularis from control and (*B*) a woman with stage 3 prolapse. Smooth muscle cells and myofibroblasts were identified with an antibody to α-actin. Staining was absent in sections incubated without primary antibody. Magnification 20×. (*Reprinted from* Boreham MK, Wai CY, Miller RT, et al. Morphometric analysis of smooth muscle in the anterior vaginal wall of women with pelvic organ prolapse. Am J Obstet Gynecol 2002;187:56; with permission.)

Contractile Protein Expression

Caldesmon and smooth muscle myosin heavy chain (SM-MHC) are two proteins that serve as molecular markers for smooth muscle cell differentiation. We studied expression, location, and isoform distribution of these proteins in the normal anterior vaginal wall and found caldesmon was predominantly expressed as the high molecular weight isoform (h-caldesmon) and was localized in smooth muscle cells of the vaginal muscularis and vasculature.[42] The predominant isoforms of myosin heavy chain in the normal vagina were SM1 and SM2. Content of caldesmon and SM-MHC were increased in smooth muscle cells of the anterior vaginal wall in women with pelvic organ prolapse. This increase in contractile protein expression was not due to hypertrophy or hyperplasia of smooth muscle cells. Thus, the disproportionate increase in caldesmon expression relative to SM-MHC indicates an abnormal phenotype of smooth muscle cells in the vaginal muscularis of women with pelvic organ prolapse.

Ultrastructural Morphology

Preliminary studies have been conducted to define the ultrastructural morphology of the vaginal muscularis. In agreement with light microscopy studies, smooth muscle cells of asymptomatic controls were organized in fascicles. The cells are closely aligned and contain numerous intermediate junctions indicative of cell-to-cell communication (**Fig. 3**). In contrast, in vaginal muscularis from women with pelvic organ prolapse, smooth muscle cells were dispersed in a sea of collagen surrounding the muscle bundles and interspersed within the bundle, effectively separating the myocytes from direct cell-to-cell communication (see **Fig. 3**). In addition, smooth muscle cells were characterized by (1) a perinuclear halo of dilated, abundant sarcoplasmic reticulum, indicating increased protein synthesis; (2) an indented nucleus; (3) a thick basal lamina; and (4) irregularities of the sarcolemma with numerous caveolae (**Fig. 4**). The cells exhibit classic morphologic features of myofibroblasts, cells characteristically involved in numerous pathologic processes associated with wound healing and inflammation. Intracellular amorphous inclusions were observed specifically in smooth muscle cells in women with prolapse, suggesting a unique type of degeneration in these cells. The inclusions were remarkably common in seven of eight women with prolapse, but absent or rare in normal controls (six of six). Specifically, smooth muscle cells (not fibroblasts or any other cell type) contained large cytoplasmic

Control   ## Stage 3 Prolapse

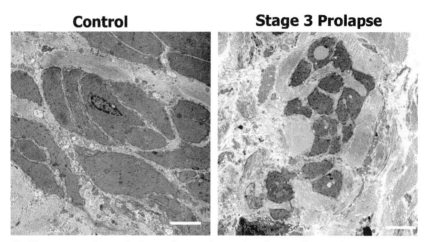

Fig. 3. Ultrastructural morphology of smooth muscle of vaginal muscularis obtained from controls (*left*) or women with pelvic organ prolapse (*right*). Scale bar, 2 μm.

vacuoles filled with proteinaceous material (see **Fig. 4**). It has been proposed that the vacuoles may be filled with either tropoelastin or procollagen (immature collagen or elastin) synthesized and secreted by activated myofibroblasts in response to cellular insult. Macrophages were also observed throughout the deep muscularis in women with pelvic organ prolapse. These cells provide a rich source of metalloproteases and elastases.

Protease Activation in Connective Tissues of the Pelvic Floor

Uninhibited protease activity has been identified as a key underlying cause of matrix degradation during the onset and progression of certain types of degenerative

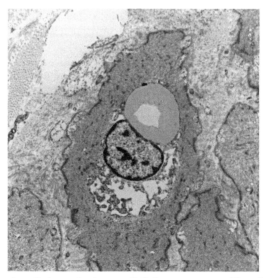

Fig. 4. Smooth muscle cells in vaginal muscularis from women with pelvic organ prolapse. Note perinuclear dilated sarcoplasmic reticulum, irregular sarcolemma, and thickened basement membrane. Large vacuoles are observed either adjacent to the nucleus (shown here) or in the cytoplasm. (Magnification 12,000×.)

diseases. Neutrophil elastase has been shown to disrupt the integrity of the microvascular barrier, and direct infusion of elastase has been shown to contribute to the development of emphysema and aortic aneurysms.[43–47] Up-regulation of matrix metalloproteinase (MMP) 9 (MMP-9)[38] and pro-MMP-2[30] has been reported in the vaginal wall of women with prolapse.

Proteases take part in a multitude of physiologic processes and their action varies from the very broad and indiscriminate (eg, proteases in digestion) to the exceptionally specific cleaving single peptide bonds in a single target protein. Proteolytic enzymes are implicated in regulating a wide range of fundamental biologic processes, such as blood coagulation, cell-cycle progression, development, wound healing, and apoptosis. In the human genome, more than 560 genes are annotated as proteases.[48] An analysis of PubMed, however, reveals no experimental data on the gene products from approximately 27% of these protease genes (ie, >150 genes), and a further 28% of human protease genes have undergone only preliminary characterization.[49] Much effort is needed to explore the physiologic role of genes encoding in a protease because the complexity of the tasks involved for different proteases varies widely. Such approaches as proteomics and genomics will enable investigators to identify proteins responsible for changes in the extracellular matrix of pelvic floor connective tissues that confer loss of support of the pelvic organs. Furthermore, identification of these cellular processes will provide novel targets for therapeutic intervention either for the prevention of pelvic organ prolapse in women at risk for this problem, or for adjunctive therapy in reconstructive surgery.

MMPs represent the most thoroughly studied family of proteases. MMPs, mainly MMP-2, MMP-9, and MMP-12, also process elastolytic activity. MMP-2 and MMP-9 were first identified as 72-kD gelatinase (gelatinase-A) and 92-kD gelatinase (gelatinase-B), respectively, because of their ability to cleave gelatin. MMPs are zinc-dependent endopeptidases that degrade pericellular extracellular matrix proteins, such as collagens, gelatins, and elastin. All three enzymes contain an N-terminal propeptide domain, a catalytic domain, and a hemopexinlike C-terminal domain. They are secreted as inactive proforms, called *zymogens*, and undergo proteolytic cleavage or conformational change to become active enzymes. Activation of pro-MMP-2 occurs at the cell surface through formation of trimolecular complexes with membrane-type 1–MMP and tissue inhibitors of MMP-2. Activation of MMP-9 requires other proteinases, such as MMP-2, MMP-3, MMP-13, or serine proteinases, such as trypsin and plasmin. Serine and cysteine proteases have also been identified as major elastolytic proteases.[50–53] Among cysteine proteases, cathepsins S and K have been considered the most potent elastolytic activities with cathepsin K exhibiting a slightly higher activity than cathepsin S.[54]

MMP-9, a particularly important member of the MMP family, has been associated with degradation of the extracellular matrix (both collagen and elastin) in normal and pathologic conditions. After it is released from the cell, MMP-9 can be found in the extracellular space, but it is also associated with the cell surface through complexes with CD44[55,56] or with a chain of type IV collagen.[57] Furthermore, internalization and catabolism of MMP-9 may result from its interaction with the low-density lipoprotein receptor–related protein.[58] Most studies have focused on transcriptional regulation of MMP-9, but posttranscriptional mechanisms have also been described, including regulation of translational efficiency.[59]

The complexity of MMP activation is compounded by the presence of MMP endogenous tissue inhibitors and, more recently, it has been shown that in vitro active MMPs may be spontaneously inactivated by degradation into smaller fragments by autocatalysis.[60,61] For example, estrogen and progesterone have been shown to increase proteolysis of MMP-13 and thereby inhibit MMP-13 activity in fibroblasts of the arcus tendineous fascia pelvis.[62]

In summary, these results provide compelling evidence that the vaginal muscularis is abnormal in women with prolapse compared with age- and parity-matched controls. Fibromuscular tissue from the prolapsed vagina is characterized by loss of smooth muscle at the vaginal apex, myofibroblast activation, abnormal smooth muscle phenotype, and increased protease activity. It is not known whether these changes are a result of the mechanical forces imposed on the prolapsed tissues, or if these changes in the fibromuscular wall of the vagina play a role in the pathogenesis of prolapse. While epidemiologic studies indicate that vaginal birth and aging are two major risk factors for developing pelvic organ prolapse, the specific effects of pregnancy, parturition, and aging on pelvic floor support mechanisms have not been identified. Studies conducted with vaginal tissues from women with or without pelvic organ prolapse cannot provide information regarding a primary role of these changes in the pathogenesis of the disorder. Factors due to prolonged stretching, mechanical stress, and hypoxia within the vaginal wall may produce secondary effects.

LESSONS LEARNED FROM MOUSE MODELS OF PELVIC ORGAN PROLAPSE

As discussed in the introduction to this article, epidemiologic studies indicate that vaginal birth and aging are two major risk factors for developing pelvic organ prolapse. Nevertheless, the specific effects of pregnancy, parturition, and aging on pelvic floor support mechanisms have not been identified. Progress in this area has been hampered by the lack of readily available animal models to study the disease. Recent findings in mice with null mutations in genes that encode proteins involved in elastic fiber assembly and synthesis suggest that elastic fiber homeostatic networks are important in the pathogenesis of pelvic organ prolapse. In this section, we will briefly review the mouse models and relevant information in women.

LOXL1 Knockout Mice

Recent findings in mice with null mutations in the gene encoding lysyl oxidase–like 1 (*LOXL1*) suggest that lysyl oxidase–like 1 (LOXL1) is crucial for pelvic organ support.[63] *LOXL1* knockout mice are viable and appear grossly normal except for elastic fiber defects in the skin, lung, and postpartum uterus. Interestingly, mice lacking LOXL develop pelvic organ prolapse 1 to 2 days after giving birth. The elastin cross-link was markedly decreased in the postpartum uterus but not in the virgin uterus in *LOXL1* mice.[64] This finding suggested that the failure of the postpartum uterine wall to form fibers might be the reason for pelvic organ prolapse in *LOXL*-null mice.

However, a precise mechanism of elastic fiber remodeling and homeostasis in the pelvic organ associated with pregnancy and parturition is not known. Liu and colleagues[65] published an extension of studies reported previously in *LOXL1*-null mice. They included detailed descriptions of genitourinary pathology and abnormal elastic fibers in the urethra, abnormal bladder function, LOXL1 gene expression in the cervix, and LOXL1 protein in the uterus of young and old mice. By 25 weeks of age, 50% of parous *LOXL1*-deficient mice developed genitourinary prolapse.[66] It should be emphasized that prolapse also occurs in virginal animals as a function of age.

Fibulin-5 Knockout Mice

Fibulin-5 (*Fbln5*) knockout mice exhibit disrupted elastic fiber networks in organs rich in elastin.[67,68] These mice survive into adulthood but develop severe "elastinopathies," including loose skin, vascular abnormalities, and emphysema.[29,30,55] *Fbln5*-null mice also develop pelvic organ prolapse and were reported to be among the first animal models with this condition.[69] Fibulin-5 was first proposed to link elastic fibers to cell surface integrin via its arginyl-glycyl-aspartic acid (RGD) motif, thus providing a bridge between elastic fibers and surrounding cells. MMP-9 is up-regulated in the vaginal wall before the onset of prolapse.[70] Although similarities exist in LOXL1[−/−] and *Fbln5*[−/−] mice, the postpartum bulge in *LOXL1* knockout mice contains a huge, distended bladder. In *Fbln5*[−/−] mice, the bladder appears normal. Furthermore, 91% of *Fbln5*-null female mice develop pelvic organ prolapse by 6 months of age, whereas only 50% of virginal *LOXL1*[−/−] mice develop prolapse by 7 months. Other lysyl oxidases in the vaginal wall supportive tissues may ameliorate the development of prolapse in the absence of parturition-induced degradation of existing elastic fibers. Fibulin-5, on the other hand, may be specific for elastic fiber assembly; or it may have effects on proteins that affect other biologic processes in addition to elastic fiber assembly.

Fibulin-3 Knockout Mice

Efemp1 encodes fibulin-3, an extracellular matrix protein important in the maintenance of abdominal fascia.[71] Recently, we sought to evaluate the role of fibulin-3 in pelvic organ support.[72] Pelvic organ support was impaired significantly in female *Efemp1* knockout mice (*Fbln3*[−/−]), and overt vaginal, perineal, and rectal prolapse occurred in 26.9%. Severity of prolapse increased with age but not parity. Interestingly, fibulin-f was up-regulated in vaginal tissues from *Fbln3*[−/−] mice with and without prolapse. Despite increased expression of fibulin-5 in the vaginal wall, failure of pelvic organ support occurred in *Fbln3*[−/−] animals, suggesting that factors related to aging led to prolapse. Elastic fiber abnormalities in vaginal tissues from young *Fbln3*[−/−] mice progressed to relatively more severe disruption of elastic fibers with age, and vaginal MMP-9 activity was increased significantly in *Fbln3*[−/−] animals with prolapse.

ELASTIC FIBER: LINKING CELLS WITH THEIR MATRIX

Cells within tissues specifically contact other cells. They also contact a complex network of secreted proteins and carbohydrates, the extracellular matrix. Animals contain many different types of extracellular matrices, each specialized for a different function. For example, tendons exhibit great strength, the extracellular matrix in the kidney is designed for filtration, and the uterus expands dramatically during pregnancy. Many tissues, including the uterus, cervix, and vagina, need to be both strong and extensible to function. This is accomplished by a network of elastic fibers in the extracellular matrix, which allows the tissue to stretch and recoil without damage. Elastic fibers are five times more extensible than a rubber band of the same cross-sectional area.[73]

Two distinct entities comprise mature elastic fibers: (1) an abundant amorphous component made up of the protein elastin and (2) microfibrils, proteins that surround elastin (**Fig. 5**). Precursor elastin is secreted from the cell as a soluble monomer called *tropoelastin*. In the extracellular space, lysine residues within tropoelastin are specifically modified to form covalent cross-links between tropoelastin chains. This cross-linked polymer has a high degree of reversible distensibility, including the ability to deform to large extensions with small forces. Cross-linking is initiated by copper-requiring extracellular enzymes, the lysyl oxidases. Microfibrils consist of several proteins, including fibrillin and microfibril-associated glycoprotein. These proteins

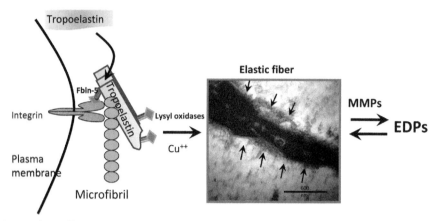

Fig. 5. Elastic fiber assembly and the role of fibulin-5. Tropoelastin is secreted from fibroblasts and smooth muscle cells as a monomer. Fibulin-5 may tether elastin to the cell by interacting with integrins (*orange*) on the cell surface. Cell surface localization would target elastin to the microfibril scaffold (*green*) possibly by interacting with fibulin-2 located in the microfibril. In this way, fibulin-5 may regulate elastic fiber assembly by the microfibril machinery. Thereafter, assembled and coacervated tropoelastin is cross-linked by copper-dependent lysyl oxidases in the extracellular matrix to form mature elastic fibers surrounded by microfibrils (*arrows*). Elastic fibers are extraordinarily stable but may be broken down by activated MMPs or other proteases to form elastin degradative products (EDPs). EDPs are matrikines that amplify proteases to further degrade elastic fibers, tropoelastin, and collagen. Cu^{++}, copper ions; Fbln-5, fibulin-5.

appear before tropoelastin secretion and form a scaffold upon which elastin is deposited before it is displaced to the periphery of the growing fiber (see **Fig. 5**).[74]

Defects in elastic fiber structure result in a myriad of pathologic conditions. Pelvic organ prolapse is just one. Cutis laxa, for example, is a connective tissue disorder resulting from markedly reduced dermal elastin content. With this disorder, skin becomes inelastic and hangs loosely in folds.[75] Pelvic organ prolapse is common in women with cutis laxa. Damage or degradation of elastic fibers leads to emphysema, a degenerative disease of the lungs in which the air sacs lose their elasticity. Mutations in the fibrillin gene have been shown to cause Marfan syndrome, a common genetic disorder with clinical manifestations, including pelvic organ prolapse[76] and aortic dilatation and dissection.[75]

ELASTIC FIBERS AND AGING

Elastin is produced early in life. Production of elastin reaches peak levels in the third trimester of fetal life and steadily decreases during early postnatal development. In undisturbed tissues, elastic fibers may last over the entire human lifespan. In a transgenic mouse line bearing a reporter linked to the elastin promoter, activity of the elastin promoter increases during postnatal development, reaching a peak at 3 months of age in skin, then decreases.[77] In many respects, age-related modifications in elastic fibers (extensively described in all organs and tissues) may be largely interpreted as progressive degradation of a protein polymer produced early in life. In humans, the elastic meshwork grows largely undistorted during postnatal growth, in which fibers seem to enlarge proportionate with tissue growth. Later, in adults and in elderly subjects, elastic fibers gradually become tortuous, frayed, and porous.[78] However, experiments suggest that elastic fiber turnover in the female reproductive tract, unlike elastic fiber turnover in other adult organs, is continuous and accelerates after childbirth.[79,80] This unique adaptation to synthesize and assemble new elastic fibers allows the vagina to expand during pregnancy and recover from childbirth.

FIBULIN-5 AND ELASTOGENESIS

Other proteins, including the emerging family of fibulin proteins, contact elastic fibers in vivo and are thought to promote the formation and stabilization of the fiber.[67,68] The term *fibulin* is derived from the Latin word for *clasp* or *buckle*. Fibulins comprise five family members, each with overlapping, but distinct, patterns of expression. They are particularly prominent in tissues rich in elastic fibers, such as lung, blood vessels, bladder neck, and uterus. Recent studies[67,68] identified fibulin-5 (also known as DANCE [developing arteries and neural crest epidermal growth factor–like protein] or EVEC [embryonic vascular epidermal growth factor–like repeat–containing protein]) as a protein that links elastic fibers to cells and regulates fiber assembly and organization. Fibulin-5 co-localizes with and binds to elastin on the surface of elastic fibers and to cells. Fbln5 binds to cells through interactions with integrin cell surface receptors. Fibulin-5 is essential for formation of new elastic fibers, but apparently not for the maintenance of already existing fibrils.[68] The elastin fiber renewal process that occurs in the female reproductive tract after parturition is unique among adult tissues.[80] The idea that fibulin-5 acts as a bridge between elastin and the cell surface adds an extra level of complexity to the existing model of elastic fiber assembly. Close collaboration between cells and elastin is needed for fiber formation to occur, and molecules that facilitate this have been identified. For example, elastin receptors have been shown to associate with tropoelastin and serve as chaperones to aid in its intracellular transport and extracellular assembly.[74] Fibulin-5 also binds to LOXL1[63] and may coordinate the actions of these molecules by directing elastic fiber assembly at the cell surface.

ELASTIC FIBERS IN THE VAGINAL WALL OF WOMEN WITH PELVIC ORGAN PROLAPSE

In 1975, el-Kholi and Mina,[81] using Verhoeffe's Van Geison stain, studied elastic fibers from the vaginas of 48 women of different age groups with and without vaginal prolapse. Elastic fibers were minimal and showed marked fragmentation in women with pelvic organ prolapse compared with those in age- and parity-matched controls. A more recent investigation failed to find significant abnormalities in vaginal wall elastic fiber staining. According to investigators, the photomicrographs in this report do not support that conclusion. Nevertheless, it is not known whether the reported changes in elastic fibers are a result of the mechanical forces imposed on the prolapsed tissues, or if these changes in the fibromuscular wall of the vagina play a role in the pathogenesis of prolapse. Yamamoto and colleagues[82] compared elastin mRNA expression and elastin synthesis in cultured fibroblasts derived from cardinal ligaments of elderly patients with pelvic organ prolapse with those derived from age-matched control patients. Marked decreases in elastin gene transcripts and elastin synthesis were found in quiescent fibroblasts cultured from women with pelvic organ prolapse. Klutke and colleagues[83] found that desmosine content (an index of cross-linked elastin fibers) was similar in uterosacral ligaments from women with or without prolapse. Desmosine content, however, was significantly decreased in women with complete procidentia. Interestingly, although expression of LOX and LOXL1 mRNA was decreased, fibulin-5 mRNA was increased in uterosacral ligaments from women with prolapse compared with controls.[83] These results differed from those of Jung and colleagues[28] in which fibulin-5 mRNA levels were decreased and

LOXL1 mRNA levels increased in uterosacral ligaments from women with prolapse. Discrepancies in these two studies may stem from differences in the study populations since Jung's investigation was limited to postmenopausal women. Both studies, however, indicate that expression of genes involved in elastic fiber assembly is altered in pelvic floor connective tissues from women with pelvic organ prolapse.

These findings together with the known association between inherited elastinopathies and pelvic organ prolapse suggests that defective elastic fiber assembly is a primary event in the pathophysiology of pelvic organ prolapse. Pelvic organ prolapse is common in women with inherited defects in elastic fiber synthesis or assembly.[76,84] In addition to primary elastinopathies that have been directly linked to alterations in the elastin gene, a number of secondary elastinopathies have been described, caused by functional imbalance of other structural and auxiliary factors regulating elastic fiber deposition (Marfan disease, GM-1-gangliosidosis, Morquio B, Hurler disease, Costello syndrome, Ehlers Danlos syndrome, pseudoxanthoma elasticum). Several investigators have suggested that alterations in collagen synthesis and collagen types are causally related to connective tissue disorders, such as inguinal hernia, pelvic organ prolapse,[85,86] stress urinary incontinence,[87] and benign joint hypermobility syndrome.[86] In this respect, several aspects of collagen and elastic fiber homeostatic pathways are interrelated. Cellular pathways of elastic fiber and collagen synthesis and degradation converge in some areas. For example, the copper-dependent enzyme lysyl oxidase is crucial for cross-linking of elastin and collagen. Several MMPs (ie, MMP-12 and MMP-9) degrade both elastin and collagen. The relative importance of each pathway in the pathophysiology of pelvic organ prolapse is unknown.

SUMMARY

The pelvic floor is a complex dynamic system that supports the vagina and pelvic viscera. In women, failure of pelvic organ support is common. A wealth of literature has established that vaginal parity and aging are important risk factors for pelvic organ prolapse in women. The specific mechanisms by which vaginal delivery and aging lead to failure of pelvic organ support are unknown. For decades, pelvic surgeons have recognized that women with prolapse often exhibit abnormal connective tissues in the pelvic floor. In recent years, new information is accumulating to define the cellular and molecular mechanisms that confer abnormal structural and functional support to the pelvic organs.

By definition, remodeling of connective tissue involves both synthesis and degradation of the extracellular matrix. Remodeling of connective tissue of the pelvic floor in pelvic organ prolapse likely represents aberrations in both synthesis and degradation of matrix components. Early studies by Woessner and Brewer[88] indicate that matrix synthesis and degradation of both collagen and elastin are regulated dramatically in the uterus during pregnancy and postpartum involution. Connective tissues of the pelvic floor also undergo matrix remodeling during pregnancy, parturition, and the puerperium. Recent investigations, together with the phenotype of LOXL1, Fbln-3, and Fbln-5 knockout mice, have led to the idea that pelvic organ prolapse, at least in some women, may represent an elastinopathy brought about by different conditions, including aging and incomplete remodeling of the vaginal wall after parturition. Disturbances in the balance between synthesis/assembly and degradation of matrix components of connective tissues of the pelvic floor may result in slow, but progressive, loss of pelvic organ support. Understanding the basic mechanisms of pelvic organ support will lead to the development of therapeutic strategies to prevent or abrogate pelvic organ prolapse and its associated morbidities, such as urinary and fecal incontinence.

REFERENCES

1. Mant J, Painter R, Vessey M. Epidemiology of genital prolapse: observations from the Oxford Family Planning Association study. Br J Obstet Gynaecol 1997;104: 579.
2. DeLancey JO. Anatomy and biomechanics of genital prolapse. Clin Obstet Gynecol 1993;36:897.
3. Harris T, Bent A. Genital prolapse with and without urinary incontinence. J Reprod Med 1990;35:792.
4. Peschers U, Schaer G, DeLancey J, et al. Levator ani function before and after childbirth. Br J Obstet Gynaecol 1997;104:1004.
5. Shafik A, El-Sibai O. Levator ani muscle activity in pregnancy and the postpartum period: a myoelectric study. Clin Exp Obstet Gynecol 2000;27:129.
6. Snooks SJ, Swash M, Mathers SE, et al. Effect of vaginal delivery on the pelvic floor: a 5-year follow-up. Br J Surg 1990;77:1358.
7. Barber MD, Bremer RE, Thor KB, et al. Innervation of the female levator ani muscles. Am J Obstet Gynecol 2002;187:64.
8. Gilpin SA, Gosling JA, Smith AR, et al. The pathogenesis of genitourinary prolapse and stress incontinence of urine. A histological and histochemical study. Br J Obstet Gynaecol 1989;96:15.
9. Juenemann KP, Lue TF, Schmidt RA, et al. Clinical significance of sacral and pudendal nerve anatomy. J Urol 1988;139:74.
10. Percy JP, Parks AG. The nerve supply of the pelvic floor. Schweiz Rundsch Med Prax 1981;70:640.
11. Hanzal E, Berger E, Koelbl H. Levator ani muscle morphology and recurrent genuine stress incontinence. Obstet Gynecol 1993;81:426.
12. Heit M, Benson JT, Russell B, et al. Levator ani muscle in women with genitourinary prolapse: indirect assessment by muscle histopathology. Neurourol Urodyn 1996;15:17.
13. Koelbl H, Strassegger H, Riss PA, et al. Morphologic and functional aspects of pelvic floor muscles in patients with pelvic relaxation and genuine stress incontinence. Obstet Gynecol 1989;74:789.
14. Dimpfl T, Jaeger C, Mueller-Felber W, et al. Myogenic changes of the levator ani muscle in premenopausal women: the impact of vaginal delivery and age. Neurourol Urodyn 1998;17:197.
15. Boreham M, Marinis S, Keller P, et al. Gene expression profiling of the pubococcygeus in premenopausal women with pelvic organ prolapse. J Pelv Med Surg 2009;4:253.
16. Pierce LM, Baumann S, Rankin MR, et al. Levator ani muscle and connective tissue changes associated with pelvic organ prolapse, parity, and aging in the squirrel monkey: a histologic study. Am J Obstet Gynecol 2007;197:60 e1.
17. Pierce LM, Coates KW, Kramer LA, et al. Effects of bilateral levator ani nerve injury on pelvic support in the female squirrel monkey. Am J Obstet Gynecol 2008;198:585 e1.
18. Handa VL, Pannu HK, Siddique S, et al. Architectural differences in the bony pelvis of women with and without pelvic floor disorders. Obstet Gynecol 2003; 102:1283.

19. Sze EH, Kohli N, Miklos JR, et al. Computed tomography comparison of bony pelvis dimensions between women with and without genital prolapse. Obstet Gynecol 1999;93:229.

20. Longo LD. Classic pages in obstetrics and gynecology. Anatomical variations in the female pelvis and their effect in labor with a suggested classification. William Edgar Caldwell and Howard Carmen Moloy. Am J Obstet Gynecol 1933;26: 479–505. Am J Obstet Gynecol 1977;127:798.

21. Hendrix S, Clark A, Nygaard I, et al. Pelvic organ prolapse in the women's health initiative: gravity and gravidity. Am J Obstet Gynecol 2002;186:1160.

22. Swift S, Woodman P, O'Boyle A, et al. Pelvic organ support study (POSST): the distribution, clinical definition, and epidemiologic condition of pelvic organ support defects. Am J Obstet Gynecol 2005;192:795.

23. Handa VL, Lockhart ME, Kenton KS, et al. Magnetic resonance assessment of pelvic anatomy and pelvic floor disorders after childbirth. Int Urogynecol J Pelvic Floor Dysfunct 2009;20:133.

24. Brizzolara SS, Killeen J, Urschitz J. Gene expression profile in pelvic organ prolapse. Mol Hum Reprod 2009;15:59.

25. Gabriel B, Denschlag D, Gobel H, et al. Uterosacral ligament in postmenopausal women with or without pelvic organ prolapse. Int Urogynecol J Pelvic Floor Dysfunct 2005;16:475.

26. Gabriel B, Watermann D, Hancke K, et al. Increased expression of matrix metalloproteinase 2 in uterosacral ligaments is associated with pelvic organ prolapse. Int Urogynecol J Pelvic Floor Dysfunct 2006;17:478.

27. Goepel C. Differential elastin and tenascin immunolabeling in the uterosacral ligaments in postmenopausal women with and without pelvic organ prolapse. Acta Histochem 2008;110:204.

28. Jung HJ, Jeon MJ, Yim GW, et al. Changes in expression of fibulin-5 and lysyl oxidase-like 1 associated with pelvic organ prolapse. Eur J Obstet Gynecol Reprod Biol 2009;145:117.

29. Kobak W, Lu J, Hardart A, et al. Expression of lysyl oxidase and transforming growth factor beta2 in women with severe pelvic organ prolapse. J Reprod Med 2005;50:827.

30. Phillips CH, Anthony F, Benyon C, et al. Collagen metabolism in the uterosacral ligaments and vaginal skin of women with uterine prolapse. BJOG 2006;113:39.

31. Reisenauer C, Shiozawa T, Oppitz M, et al. The role of smooth muscle in the pathogenesis of pelvic organ prolapse—an immunohistochemical and morphometric analysis of the cervical third of the uterosacral ligament. Int Urogynecol J Pelvic Floor Dysfunct 2008;19:383.

32. Suzme R, Yalcin O, Gurdol F, et al. Connective tissue alterations in women with pelvic organ prolapse and urinary incontinence. Acta Obstet Gynecol Scand 2007;86:882.

33. Takacs P, Nassiri M, Gualtieri M, et al. Uterosacral ligament smooth muscle cell apoptosis is increased in women with uterine prolapse. Reprod Sci 2009;16: 447.

34. Kerkhof MH, Hendriks L, Brolmann HA. Changes in connective tissue in patients with pelvic organ prolapse—a review of the current literature. Int Urogynecol J Pelvic Floor Dysfunct 2009;20:461.

35. Jackson SR, Avery NC, Tarlton JF, et al. Changes in metabolism of collagen in genitourinary prolapse. Lancet 1996;347:1658.

36. Soderberg MW, Falconer C, Bystrom B, et al. Young women with genital prolapse have a low collagen concentration. Acta Obstet Gynecol Scand 2004;83:1193.

37. Kokcu A, Yanik F, Cetinkaya M, et al. Histopathological evaluation of the connective tissue of the vaginal fascia and the uterine ligaments in women with and without pelvic relaxation. Arch Gynecol Obstet 2002;266:75.
38. Moalli PA, Shand SH, Zyczynski HM, et al. Remodeling of vaginal connective tissue in patients with prolapse. Obstet Gynecol 2005;106:953.
39. Makinen J, Kahari VM, Soderstrom KO, et al. Collagen synthesis in the vaginal connective tissue of patients with and without uterine prolapse. Eur J Obstet Gynecol Reprod Biol 1987;24:319.
40. Boreham MK, Wai CY, Miller RT, et al. Morphometric analysis of smooth muscle in the anterior vaginal wall of women with pelvic organ prolapse. Am J Obstet Gynecol 2002;187:56.
41. Boreham MK, Wai CY, Miller RT, et al. Morphometric properties of the posterior vaginal wall in women with pelvic organ prolapse. Am J Obstet Gynecol 2002; 187:1501.
42. Boreham MK, Miller RT, Schaffer JI, et al. Smooth muscle myosin heavy chain and caldesmon expression in the anterior vaginal wall of women with and without pelvic organ prolapse. Am J Obstet Gynecol 2001;185:944.
43. Allaire E, Forough R, Clowes M, et al. Local overexpression of TIMP-1 prevents aortic aneurysm degeneration and rupture in a rat model. J Clin Invest 1998; 102:1413.
44. Curci JA, Liao S, Huffman MD, et al. Expression and localization of macrophage elastase (matrix metalloproteinase-12) in abdominal aortic aneurysms. J Clin Invest 1900;102:2000.
45. Moore G, Liao S, Curci JA, et al. Suppression of experimental abdominal aortic aneurysms by systemic treatment with a hydroxamate-based matrix metalloproteinase inhibitor (RS 132908). J Vasc Surg 1999;29:522.
46. Morris DG, Huang X, Kaminski N, et al. Loss of integrin alpha(v)beta6-mediated TGF-beta activation causes Mmp12-dependent emphysema. Nature 2003;422: 169 [see comment].
47. Senior RM, Tegner H, Kuhn C, et al. The induction of pulmonary emphysema with human leukocyte elastase. Am Rev Respir Dis 1977;116:469.
48. Lopez-Otin C, Matrisian LM. Emerging roles of proteases in tumour suppression. Nat Rev Cancer 2007;7:800.
49. Schluter H, Rykl J, Thiemann J, et al. Mass spectrometry-assisted protease substrate screening. Anal Chem 2007;79:1251.
50. Bank U, Ansorge S. More than destructive: neutrophil-derived serine proteases in cytokine bioactivity control. J Leukoc Biol 2001;69:197.
51. Groutas WC. Inhibitors of leukocyte elastase and leukocyte cathepsin G. Agents for the treatment of emphysema and related ailments. Med Res Rev 1987;7:227.
52. Ottlecz A, Walker S, Conrad M, et al. Neutral metalloendopeptidase associated with the smooth muscle cells of pregnant rat uterus. J Cell Biochem 1991;45:401.
53. Shapiro SD, Campbell EJ, Senior RM, et al. Proteinases secreted by human mononuclear phagocytes. J Rheumatol Suppl 1991;27:95.
54. Stockley RA. Proteases and antiproteases. Novartis Found Symp 2001;234:189.
55. Yu Q, Stamenkovic I. Cell surface-localized matrix metalloproteinase-9 proteolytically activates TGF-beta and promotes tumor invasion and angiogenesis. Genes Dev 2000;14:163.
56. Yu Q, Stamenkovic I. Localization of matrix metalloproteinase 9 to the cell surface provides a mechanism for CD44-mediated tumor invasion. Genes Dev 1999;13:35.
57. Olson MW, Toth M, Gervasi DC, et al. High affinity binding of latent matrix metalloproteinase-9 to the alpha2(IV) chain of collagen IV. J Biol Chem 1998;273:10672.

58. Hahn-Dantona E, Ruiz JF, Bornstein P, et al. The low density lipoprotein receptor-related protein modulates levels of matrix metalloproteinase 9 (MMP-9) by mediating its cellular catabolism. J Biol Chem 2001;276:15498.

59. Jiang Y, Muschel RJ. Regulation of matrix metalloproteinase-9 (MMP-9) by translational efficiency in murine prostate carcinoma cells. Cancer Res 1910;62:2002.

60. Geurts N, Martens E, Van Aelst I, et al. Beta-hematin interaction with the hemopexin domain of gelatinase B/MMP-9 provokes autocatalytic processing of the propeptide, thereby priming activation by MMP-3. Biochemistry 2008;47:2689.

61. Rozanov DV, Strongin AY. Membrane type-1 matrix metalloproteinase functions as a proprotein self-convertase. Expression of the latent zymogen in Pichia pastoris, autolytic activation, and the peptide sequence of the cleavage forms. J Biol Chem 2003;278:8257.

62. Zong W, Meyn LA, Moalli PA. The amount and activity of active matrix metalloproteinase 13 is suppressed by estradiol and progesterone in human pelvic floor fibroblasts. Biol Reprod 2009;80:367.

63. Liu X, Zhao Y, Gao J, et al. Elastic fiber homeostasis requires lysyl oxidase-like 1 protein. Nat Genet 2004;36:178.

64. Molnar J, Fong KSK, He QP, et al. Structural and functional diversity of lysyl oxidase and the LOX-like proteins. Biochim Biophys Acta 2003;1647:220.

65. Liu X, Zhao Y, Pawlyk B, et al. Failure of elastic fiber homeostasis leads to pelvic floor disorders. Am J Pathol 2006;168:519.

66. Lee UJ, Gustilo-Ashby AM, Daneshgari F, et al. Lower urogenital tract anatomical and functional phenotype in lysyl oxidase like-1 knockout mice resembles female pelvic floor dysfunction in humans. Am J Physiol Renal Physiol 2008;295:F545.

67. Nakamura T, Lozano PR, Ikeda Y, et al. Fibulin-5/DANCE is essential for elastogenesis in vivo. Nature 2002;415:171.

68. Yanagisawa H, Davis EC, Starcher BC, et al. Fibulin-5 is an elastin-binding protein essential for elastic fibre development in vivo. Nature 2002;415:168.

69. Drewes PG, Yanagisawa H, Starcher B, et al. Pelvic organ prolapse in fibulin-5 knockout mice: pregnancy changes in elastic fiber homeostasis in mouse vagina. Am J Pathol 2007;170:578.

70. Wieslander CK, Rahn DD, McIntire DD, et al. Quantification of pelvic organ prolapse in mice: vaginal protease activity precedes increased MOPQ scores in fibulin-5 knockout mice. Biol Reprod 2009;80:407–14.

71. McLaughlin PJ, Bakall B, Choi J, et al. Lack of fibulin-3 causes early aging and herniation, but not macular degeneration in mice. Hum Mol Genet 2007;16:3059.

72. Rahn DD, Acevedo JF, Roshanravan S, et al. Failure of pelvic organ support in mice deficient in fibulin-3. Am J Pathol 2009;174:206.

73. Rosenbloom J, Abrams WR, Mecham R. Extracellular matrix 4: the elastic fiber. FASEB J 1993;7:1208.

74. Mecham R, Davis E. Elastic fiber structure and assembly. New York: Academic Press; 1994.

75. Milewicz DM, Urban Z, Boyd C. Genetic disorders of the elastic fiber system. Matrix Biol 2000;19:471.

76. Carley ME, Schaffer J. Urinary incontinence and pelvic organ prolapse in women with Marfan or Ehlers Danlos syndrome. Am J Obstet Gynecol 2000;182:1021.

77. Hsu-Wong S, Katchman SD, Ledo I, et al. Tissue-specific and developmentally regulated expression of human elastin promoter activity in transgenic mice. J Biol Chem 1994;269:18072.

78. Imokawa G, Takema Y, Yorimoto Y, et al. Degree of ultraviolet-induced tortuosity of elastic fibers in rat skin is age dependent. J Invest Dermatol 1995;105:254.

79. Sharrow L, Tinker D, Davidson JM, et al. Accumulation and regulation of elastin in the rat uterus. Proc Soc Exp Biol Med 1989;192:121.
80. Starcher B, Percival S. Elastin turnover in the rat uterus. Connect Tissue Res 1985;13:207.
81. el-Kholi G, Mina S. Elastic tissue of the vagina in genital prolapse. A morphological study. J Egypt Med Assoc 1975;58:196–204.
82. Yamamoto K, Yamamoto M, Akazawa K, et al. Decrease in elastin gene expression and protein synthesis in fibroblasts derived from cardinal ligaments of patients with prolapsus uteri. Cell Biol Int 1997;21:605.
83. Klutke J, Ji Q, Campeau J, et al. Decreased endopelvic fascia elastin content in uterine prolapse. Acta Obstet Gynecol Scand 2008;87:111.
84. Klipple GL, Riordan KK. Rare inflammatory and hereditary connective tissue diseases. Rheum Dis Clin North Am 1989;15:383.
85. Nikolova G, Lee H, Berkovitz S, et al. Sequence variant in the laminin gamma1 (LAMC1) gene associated with familial pelvic organ prolapse. Hum Genet 2007;120:847.
86. Norton PA, Baker JE, Sharp HC, et al. Genitourinary prolapse and joint hypermobility in women. Obstet Gynecol 1995;85:225.
87. Ulmsten U, Ekman G, Giertz G, et al. Different biochemical composition of connective tissue in continent and stress incontinent women. Acta Obstet Gynecol Scand 1987;66:455.
88. Woessner JF, Brewer TH. Formation and breakdown of collagen and elastin in the human uterus during pregnancy and post-partum involution. Biochem J 1963;89:75.

Pessary Use and Management for Pelvic Organ Prolapse

Shanna D. Atnip, MSN, WHNP-BC[a,b,*]

KEYWORDS

- Pessary • Pelvic organ prolapse
- Conservative management • Fitting • Pessary selection

Before the nineteenth century and the advent of surgical treatment for pelvic organ prolapse, vaginal pessaries were the mainstay of therapy for women with symptomatic pelvic organ prolapse. Hippocrates in 400 BC mentioned the use of a half pomegranate in the vagina to reduce prolapse, Soranus used other fruits, and Diocles used pomegranates soaked in vinegar.[1] Later in the fourth century, pledgets of drug-saturated cotton, linen, wool, or sponge were tied to a string and placed tightly against the cervix to hold vaginal tissues in place.[2] In the sixteenth century hammered brass, wax-covered cork or sponge, and a pear- or ring-shaped apparatus made of gold, silver, or brass were sometimes attached to a perineal strap with a belt worn around the waist to support the vaginal tissues.[1,2] After rubber was introduced in the nineteenth century a cup-shaped design with a gold tip in the center permitted cervical secretions to drain. Hodge designed his lever pessary in the late nineteenth century, after which many others designed pessaries to suit their own needs.[1,2]

The advent of asepsis and anesthesia in the late nineteenth century caused a decline in the use of pessary because surgical repair of pelvic organ prolapse became a more viable treatment option.[1] After 1950, silicone and plastic replaced rubber and metal pessaries. Over the course of the twentieth century, women became more educated and determined to have a voice in the choices made concerning their health care. Nonsurgical options for prolapse treatment were sought after by women who did not desire hysterectomy, and a resurgence of the use of pessary for the treatment of pelvic organ prolapse began in the late twentieth and early twenty-first centuries. Pott-Grinstein and Newcomer[3] surveyed 2000 gynecologists in the United States in 2001 and found 86% percent of the 947 gynecologists who returned questionnaires reported prescribing pessaries.

[a] Division of Female Pelvic Medicine and Reconstructive Pelvic Surgery, University of Texas Southwestern Medical Center, 5323 Harry Hines Boulevard, Dallas, TX 75390–9032, USA
[b] Urogynecology Clinic, Parkland Health & Hospital System/WISH, 5201 Harry Hines Blvd., Dallas, Texas 75235, USA
* Division of Female Pelvic Medicine and Reconstructive Surgery, University of Texas Southwestern Medical Center, 5323 Harry Hines Boulevard, Dallas.
E-mail address: satnip@parknet.pmh.org

Obstet Gynecol Clin N Am 36 (2009) 541–563
doi:10.1016/j.ogc.2009.08.010
0889-8545/09/$ – see front matter © 2009 Elsevier Inc. All rights reserved.

Pessaries are an inexpensive, simple, low-risk, and effective conservative treatment for pelvic organ prolapse. Several study authors have concluded that pessaries should be offered as a first-line of therapy for the management of symptoms of pelvic organ prolapse regardless of a patient's age or prolapse severity.[4,5] Unfortunately, the most current Cochrane review in 2004[6] concluded: "... there is no evidence from randomized controlled trials upon which to base treatment of women with pelvic organ prolapse through the use of mechanical devices/pessaries. There is no consensus on the use of different types of device, the indications, nor the pattern of replacement and follow-up care." Although high-quality scientific evidence regarding the use and management of pessary for conservative treatment of pelvic organ prolapse is only beginning to emerge, thousands of years of experience may be used to support and guide decisions about pessary use.

PESSARY INDICATIONS AND PATIENT SELECTION

There are few contraindications to pessary use. The main contraindication is noncompliance with follow-up, which precludes identification of complications. Any condition that could cause neglect of a pessary, such as dementia, should be considered before pessary placement.[7] Active vaginal infection, persistent vaginal erosion or ulceration, or severe vaginal atrophy may be relative contraindications until the conditions improve. Otherwise, the indications for pessary use are outlined in **Box 1**.

Symptomatic Pelvic Organ Prolapse

The most common indication for pessary use is for the relief of pelvic organ prolapse symptoms. Researchers agree that pessary use significantly improves both prolapse and bladder symptoms.[8-12] Fernando and colleagues[12] enrolled 203 women with symptomatic pelvic organ prolapse and prospectively evaluated the symptoms of 97 women after successful pessary fitting who completed baseline and 4-month questionnaires. They found a significant difference in voiding in 39 subjects (40%, $P = .001$); in urinary urgency by 37 (38%, $P = .001$); in urge urinary incontinence by 28 (29%, $P = .015$); in bowel evacuation by 27 (28%, $P = .045$); in fecal urgency by 22 (23%, $P = .018$); and in urge fecal incontinence by 19 (20%, $P = .027$). Clemons and colleagues[9] prospectively found that 73 of 100 women who were successfully fit with pessary had resolved prolapse symptoms from baseline to 2 months, respectively: bulge (90%–3%; $P = .001$); pressure (49%–3%; $P = .001$); discharge (12%–0%; $P = .003$); and splinting (14%–0%; $P = .001$). Unlike Fernando and colleagues[12] and Clemons and colleagues,[9] Komesu and coworkers[11] found in 2007 that although other prolapse symptoms were improved or resolved with pessary use, there was little effect of pessary on bowel-related symptoms.

Box 1
Pessary indications

1. Symptomatic pelvic organ prolapse
2. Surgery not desired or recommended
3. Diagnostic tool, prediction of surgical outcome
4. Correcting stress urinary incontinence
5. Pregnancy complications

Surgery Not Desired or Not Recommended

Women expect to be given options for the treatment of their pelvic organ prolapse. For a variety of reasons, a woman may believe conservative management is her best option. Some fear surgery or lack confidence in surgical results, others find time away from career or family make surgery inconvenient, and still others need to get past a particular event before surgery is practical for them. Many surgeons do not recommend childbearing after reconstructive surgery, and often a hysterectomy is part of the reconstructive procedure. Despite having prolapse, which can be significant even in young women, many women choose to delay surgery until childbearing is complete. Pessary can be a very good temporary treatment to improve quality of life.

Surgery may not be recommended for women with medical conditions that increase the risk of operative and postoperative complications. These women are often very happy to have pessary as a treatment option. Clemons and colleagues[13] showed that age greater than 65 and severe comorbidity were significant predictors of continued pessary use after 1 year in women with pelvic organ prolapse. Cundiff and colleagues[14] surveyed members of the American Urogynecologic Society (AUGS) and found that 77% of respondents use pessary as a first-line therapy, but 12% reserved them only for patients who declined or were not candidates for surgery.

In patients whose prolapse has become edematous and ulcerated because of rubbing on clothing, a pessary may be beneficial to allow the ulcer to heal and edema to recede so the patient can undergo surgical correction. Another indication for temporary use of pessary is urinary retention secondary to anterior vaginal wall prolapse and urethral obstruction.[15] A pessary "unkinks" the urethra, which can lead to improved voiding.

Diagnostic Tool and Prediction of Surgical Outcome

There are times that a woman complains of symptoms that she believes are linked to prolapse but are not typical prolapse symptoms. Often physical findings do not match the patient's symptoms, such as the patient with stage 1 or mild stage 2 prolapse who complains of severe bulge symptoms. In these cases, before surgery is offered, a pessary can be used as a diagnostic tool to simulate surgical results. Many patients with prolapse complain of pelvic and low back pain. These symptoms can have numerous etiologies. In 2002, Heit and colleagues[16] studied 152 women with pelvic organ prolapse and did not find an association between pelvic organ prolapse and pelvic or low back pain. They concluded that pelvic organ prolapse was not a cause of pelvic or low back pain. In patients with symptoms that cannot be directly associated with prolapse, a trial of pessary for a few weeks or a month can help to predict the symptom relief a patient may or may not expect with surgery and aids in the preoperative counseling of the patient.

Women planning reconstructive surgery may present with an elevated postvoid residual (PVR). It is useful to have a preoperative screening tool with the potential for predicting postoperative voiding function. Lazarou and colleagues[17] retrospectively reviewed the records of 24 women who planned reconstructive surgery, had a PVR greater than 100, and were fit with a pessary before surgery. They found that 75% (19) of women with a PVR greater than 100 had normal PVRs after pessary placement. Only 1 of the 19 had a PVR greater than 100 at 3 months post reconstructive surgery. The study concluded pessary reduction of PVR preoperatively for patients with urinary retention had good sensitivity, specificity, and positive predictive value for postoperative cure of urinary retention.

In 1985, Bhatia and Bergman[18] were able to predict retropubic urethropexy would cure stress urinary incontinence in women who became continent during urodynamic evaluation with a well-fit Smith or Hodge vaginal pessary preoperatively. They concluded the pessary simulated the anticipated results of the anti-incontinence surgery by correcting the anatomic defect without occluding the urethra or urethrovesical junction. Many providers use pessary or other devices to reduce pelvic organ prolapse during urodynamics to simulate a surgical repair. Mattox and Bhatia[19] wanted to ascertain if these devices could create variance in the urodynamic data. They used a ring pessary, Smith or Hodge with and without a knob, and the lower half of a medium Graves speculum taped in place or a hand-held speculum. The variance in the functional urethral length or the maximum closure pressure was not significantly different despite the device used for reduction of prolapse.

Prediction of postoperative incontinence in women who are continent preoperatively is also a useful screening tool. Clemons and colleagues[9] found 21% of the women who were successfully fitted with either ring or gellhorn pessary developed de novo stress urinary incontinence. Prolapse can kink the urethra and create a bladder neck obstruction.[20] Pessary supports the prolapsed vagina and may potentially expose this occult stress urinary incontinence. Pessary placement may be useful in predicting which of these continent patients require concurrent anti-incontinence surgery at the time of reconstructive surgery to prevent postoperative stress urinary incontinence.

Correcting Stress Urinary Incontinence

Many women with pelvic organ prolapse also have stress or mixed urinary incontinence. Donnelly and colleagues[10] showed that 50% of women treated with incontinence pessaries were satisfied with their results and continued pessary use. Komesu and colleagues[11] fit women with stress or mixed incontinence with a ring with a knob or a dish with a knob pessary. The women who continued the pessary for 6 to 12 months had significantly less urine leakage related to coughing, sneezing, or laughing ($P = .01$) and had smaller amounts of leakage ($P = .01$) than women who discontinued the pessary as measured by their answers on the Pelvic Floor Distress Impact Questionnaire. In Clemons and coworkers'[9] prospective study, women who had urinary symptoms at baseline in addition to prolapse had 45% improvement in stress incontinence, urge incontinence improved in 46%, and voiding difficulty improved in 53% after 2 months.

In 2004, Donnelly and colleagues[10] retrospectively evaluated women who were offered incontinence pessaries to manage their incontinence. Of the 106 women who were fit and took the pessary home to try, 55 used the pessary for at least 6 months. Nygaard[21] studied 18 women with exercise incontinence in 1995 in a prospective, randomized trial using a Hodge pessary with support, versus a super tampon, versus nothing. She found that 58% of participants achieved continence, and the tampon achieved continence more frequently than pessary (8 of 14 compared with 5 of 14).

Bhatia and colleagues[22] used urodynamic studies to show that Smith and Hodge pessaries increased urethral functional length and maximal urethral closure pressure. They found these pessaries stabilize the urethrovesical junction without causing obstruction. To date there have been no studies to determine the mechanism of action of pessaries with a knob attached designed to apply pressure beneath the urethra for support.

In 2006, a Cochrane review of mechanical devices for urinary incontinence concluded there is little evidence from controlled trials to judge if pessary use is better than no treatment. There was also insufficient evidence favoring one device over another and no evidence to compare mechanical devices with other forms of treatment.[23] The recently concluded ATLAS trial, a National Institutes of Health funded randomized trial of pessary versus behavioral therapy versus combined therapy for treatment of stress urinary incontinence is expected to provide high-quality evidence regarding the role of pessary in the management of stress urinary incontinence.[24]

Pregnancy Complications

Miller[1] describes the use of pessary to treat uterine retrodisplacement that may occur in 15% of pregnancies and that can lead to uterine incarceration in the hollow of the sacrum after 12 weeks gestation. A lever-type pessary (like the Smith or Hodge) may help to displace the cervix posteriorly resulting in anteverting the uterus allowing it to rise out of the pelvis.

Pregnancy complicated by preterm cervical dilation (incompetent cervix) is usually treated with a surgical cervical cerclage in the United States to prolong pregnancy. Miller[1] references multiple studies from the 1970s and 1980s done in Europe that show pessary may be a nonsurgical alternative to surgical cerclage. Although no randomized prospective placebo-controlled trials exist, in 2006 a Norwegian prospective cohort study of a cerclage pessary as a nonsurgical alternative found of 32 women with sonographically detected cervical shortening before 30 weeks, the mean gestational age at delivery was 34 weeks with birth weights of average 2255 g. They conclude the cerclage pessary may be useful in the management of cervical incompetence.[25]

The prevalence of prolapse during pregnancy is unknown. It is supposed that pregnant women with pre-existing prolapse have a decrease in the prolapse as the uterus grows and moves out of the pelvis, and pessary use until then may be needed. In rare cases, the prolapse does not recede and the weight of the uterus causes further descent of the cervix outside the vaginal opening where ulceration, infection, and urinary retention can develop.[26–28] Some case reports recommend treatment with bed rest and Trendelenburg positioning,[27] and others have tried pessary use with mixed results. Piver and Spezia[29] saw excellent maternal and fetal outcomes, whereas Brown's[26] three case reports all ended in preterm birth.

Other uses for pessaries continue to be suggested. Women periodically complain of "vaginal wind" that can occur with a gaping vagina and weak pelvic floor musculature. There is one report of using a cube pessary to treat this complaint successfully.[30] Many would like to promote the use of pessary as preventive of worsening prolapse, or to use pessary post reconstructive surgery to prevent recurrence, but there is no evidence for this. Jones and colleagues[31] postulated that continued use of pessary may result in some degree of recovery of the levator ani muscles, which are weakened in women with prolapse. They measured genital hiatus before and 3 months after pessary use and found a reduction in the genital hiatus. Whether this muscle recovery is long term and could prevent progression of prolapse, or is simply a physiologic response to the reduced tension stressor on the muscle, still needs to be established.

PESSARY SELECTION

In the past, multiple materials including fruit, metal, porcelain, rubber, and acrylic have been used to manufacture pessaries. Fortunately, today almost all pessaries are made of medical-grade silicone, which provides many advantages. Silicone pessaries are pliable and have a long shelf life, lack odor and secretion absorption, are biologically inert and nonallergenic and noncarcinogenic, and they can be boiled or autoclaved for sterilization. Because most pessaries are made of silicone, pessary style and size are the main considerations when selecting a pessary.

A wide range of pessary styles and sizes are available and new styles continue to be designed (**Fig. 1**). There is limited evidence for the use of any particular style of pessary for a specific patient characteristic, compartment of prolapse, or presence of incontinence. Clinicians continue to rely on guidelines of the pessary manufacturers, expert opinion, personal experience, and provider or patient preferences for one style or another.

Generally, pessaries have been classified as either a support pessary, a space-filling pessary, or an incontinence pessary. Support or lever pessaries, such as the ring or

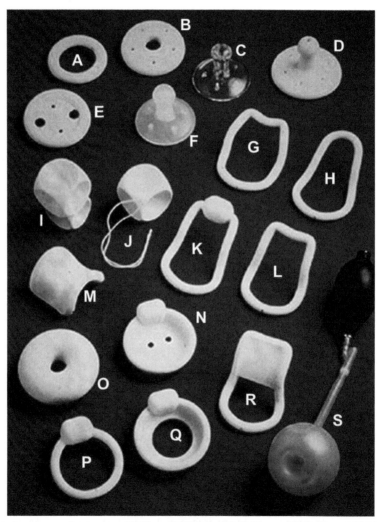

Fig.1. Various types of pessaries. (*A*) Ring. (*B*) Shaatz. (*C*) Gellhorn. (*D*) Gellhorn. (*E*) Ring with support. (*F*) Gellhorn. (*G*) Risser. (*H*) Smith. (*I*) Tandem cube. (*J*) Cube. (*K*) Hodge with knob. (*L*) Hodge. (*M*) Gehrung. (*N*) Incontinence dish with support. (*O*) Donut. (*P*) Incontinence ring. (*Q*) Incontinence dish. (*R*) Hodge with support. (*S*) Inflatoball (latex). (*Courtesy of* Milex Products, a division of Cooper Surgical, Trumbull, Connecticut.)

Hodge use a spring mechanism and are thought to rest in the posterior fornix and behind the symphysis pubis, which provides support of the prolapsing structures. These pessaries have traditionally been thought to be best for less severe prolapse not extending past the hymenal ring. Space-filling devices, such as the gellhorn and cube, use suction between the device and the vaginal walls or, in the case of the donut, merely occupy the vaginal space as long as the pessary diameter is larger than the genital hiatus. Space fillers have traditionally been thought useful for larger prolapse beyond the hymen.[1,7,32–36]

In the AUGS survey in 2000, 78% of 348 respondents said they tailor the pessary style to the support defect. Support pessaries were more commonly used for anterior and apical defects (ring), whereas space-filling pessaries were more common for posterior defects (donut) and procidentia (gellhorn). Twenty-two percent used the same pessary, usually a ring, for all support defects.[14] Nine hundred forty-seven gynecologist's surveyed in 2001[3] thought the gellhorn, donut, cube, and ring to be the most effective pessaries for uterine prolapse; the cube, gellhorn, donut, and inflatoball best for vault prolapse; gehrung, ring, donut, and cube best for cystocele; cube, inflatoball, donut, and gellhorn best for rectocele; and the incontinence ring or dish, ring, Smith, gehrung, and Hodge best for incontinence. Overall, pessaries were thought to be the least effective for rectocele and enterocele and rarely effective for urge incontinence. Among the gynecologists, the ring was most commonly used and believed to be the easiest to wear and remove, the gellhorn was thought to be the most effective for prolapse, the donut the most difficult to wear, and the gellhorn the most difficult to remove.[3] In a randomized crossover trial comparing ring with support with gellhorn pessary, both were found to be equivalent in relieving symptoms of protrusion and voiding dysfunction.[37] Most current studies used the ring (with or without support) or gellhorn as their first-line pessaries for pelvic organ prolapse.[4,5,12,36,38–43] The cube or donut pessaries were used by a few as an alternative when other pessaries were unsuccessful.[12,33,36,40,41,43] The most common pessaries used for pelvic organ prolapse with incontinence or incontinence alone were the ring (or ring with support); the incontinence ring (with or without support); the incontinence dish (with or without support); and the Hodge with support.[10,24,44–46]

Choosing a pessary size is also subjective. Nager and colleagues[47] looked at using pelvic organ prolapse quantification examination parameters to determine the size of incontinence ring or dish pessary for urinary incontinence. Women with a shorter vaginal length were less likely to be successfully fitted, but specific pelvic organ prolapse quantification examination measures were not helpful in determining incontinence pessary size. They concluded that the trial and error method of incontinence pessary fitting cannot be made more scientific with specific vaginal measures. A ring pessary sizer was devised with the hope of making the choice of pessary size more objective for the clinician and less inconvenient for the patient.[48] The sizer was able to correctly estimate within one size of the ring in 84% (31) of cases. In current studies, the average number of pessaries tried was about two to three over one to three fitting sessions with most requiring only one session.[11,31,41,42,49] Those unable to retain a pessary after the first fitting were more likely to be unsuccessful with subsequent fittings,[42] but persistence may pay off. Clemons and coworkers[38] found 22 of 49 women who were unsuccessful at the first visit became successful on the second visit, and the gellhorn is more likely to require refitting than the ring. The most common sizes of the ring (incontinence and with or without support) used are the numbers 2, 3, 4, and 5.[41,49] According to one manufacturer the most commonly used gellhorn sizes are 2.25, 2.50, 2.75, and 3 inches. In general, younger women require larger pessaries, whereas older women use smaller ones.

Identification of the best candidates for pessary success would help to better determine who to offer pessary to and eliminate the influence of biases on who will or will not be successful. It could save both provider and patient time and save the patient from the potential discomfort of pessary refitting. It would also be a useful tool in counseling patients in their treatment options.

Predictors of pessary fitting success depend a lot on the definition of success. Researchers define success differently. Some claim success if after a visit the pessary is retained and comfortable. Most researchers define successful pessary fit as a comfortable pessary that is retained and the patient continues to use on at least one follow-up visit.[9,41,42] Several studies agree that 63% to 86% of women with pelvic organ prolapse[4,9,39–42] and 89% to 93% with urinary incontinence can be successfully fit with pessary.[10,47]

Unfortunately, there is less agreement in the recent studies about the characteristics of women that predict success. In a prospective observational study of 100 women in 2004, Clemons and colleagues[38] found a short vaginal length (≤ 6 cm) and a wide vaginal introitus (measured by at least four fingerbreadths accommodated) were associated with unsuccessful pessary fitting. Wu and colleagues[41] found in a prospective trial that women who were younger, had a greater stage of prolapse, had prior pelvic surgery, had less parity, and had urinary incontinence had less successful pessary fittings. In several retrospective studies, researchers found predictors of unsuccessful fitting to be prior reconstructive pelvic surgery,[4,40,42] stress urinary incontinence,[40,41] and cystocele or rectocele.[40] Hanson and colleagues[39] found local and systemic hormone replacement predicted successful fitting, whereas Maito and colleagues[42] found mild posterior prolapse (<+1) was a single predictor of success. Other researchers found no difference in fitting success based on age, obesity, vaginal length, genital hiatus, compartment of prolapse, stage of prolapse, or hormone use.[4,40–42] Agreement on common characteristics that can be used to identify the best candidates for pessary have yet to be determined.

Culligan's[50] opinion is that "the vast majority of patients can be treated with one of only two basic types—the ring and the gellhorn. In most cases, if a gellhorn pessary does not work, the likelihood of finding a successful pessary device drops precipitously." Weber and Richter[7] offer the ring first (ring when cervix present, ring with support when cervix absent), and the gellhorn if there is more advanced prolapse and less perineal support. Currently, selection of pessary depends most on the provider's ability to insert or fit a particular style of pessary and the patient's satisfaction. Becoming adept at several styles of pessary seems to work well.[51]

PESSARY FITTING

Pessary fit not only depends on appropriate pessary selection and patient characteristics, but is also dependent on provider training and experience. Despite pessary being considered a first-line therapy for pelvic organ prolapse,[4,5] there is often little time spent in residency training programs teaching providers the use and management of pessary.[3] Fortunately, it is not difficult to learn and the skill improves rapidly with experience. Success or failure of pessary as a treatment option depends a great deal on an adequate fit and the patient's satisfaction with her pessary.

After the initial evaluation of the patient and the decision to fit a pessary, the initial pessary style and size is selected using a combination of the vaginal width and length. The size is selected by performing a pelvic examination and determining the vaginal width at the posterior vaginal vault by spreading the index and middle fingers horizontally as if checking for cervical dilatation in a laboring woman. Then, determine the length of the vagina by rotating the fingers vertically and measure from the posterior fornix to the symphysis pubis. If a selection of sizes is available, one can visually compare the pessaries with a mental image of the vaginal vault size and shape, and then try the pessary that most closely fits the visual image. Pessaries tried but not sent home with the patient can be autoclaved and reused. For those with less ability to visualize, there are fitting kits available with most sizes of the ring and gellhorn pessaries. Some practices prescribe the pessary for purchase at medical supply stores. This method is likely not to succeed because the correct size is not often the first one tried.

It is important to show the patient what the pessary looks like before insertion and describe how it is positioned in her body using pelvic models, pictures, or one's hand as a model. Let her hold it to see how it feels, folds, or bends. Wash the pessary with soap and water to remove the cornstarch used in packaging. Apply water-based lubricating gel at the vaginal introitus or on the leading edge of the pessary to ease insertion. Avoid getting lubricants on the gloved hand holding the pessary. This makes it very difficult to control the pessary and could make insertion difficult. Use gentle pressure downward on the posterior vaginal wall or the oblique angle where the opening is the largest to avoid pressure against the urethra and to ease the pessary behind the symphysis into the vaginal apex beneath the cervix (if present).

After insertion, ask the patient to valsalva or cough. It is common for a well-fit pessary to descend to near the introitus, but it recedes with relaxation. If it is nearly or completely expelled, a larger size or different style should be tried. If the pessary is uncomfortable or the patient feels lower abdominal discomfort, the pessary is likely too large and a smaller size or different style should be tried. If properly sized, the patient is not able to feel the pessary. In general, most pessaries should not fit tightly against the vaginal wall, but should be able to be gently rocked back and forth or a fingertip fit between the pessary and vaginal wall. The patient should be able to walk around comfortably, squat, and sit without feeling any discomfort. If a patient describes a vague sensation of irritation or is not sure it is uncomfortable, it is possible she is experiencing irritation from manipulation during the session. Clinical judgment should be used to determine if removal or refit is necessary. It is helpful to have the patient sit on the toilet and valsalva gently or void (with a measuring "hat" on the toilet to avoid having the pessary fall into the toilet) to be sure the pessary remains in place after leaving the office. If using an incontinence pessary it helps to try to recreate the patient's normal pattern of activity like running in place, bending, jumping jacks, or straining. Also check to see the patient can void and if necessary check a PVR to make sure there is no obstruction.[39]

If it is necessary to try several pessaries, one may wish to use lidocaine gel around the introitus, especially if it is very atrophic, sclerosed, and tears easily. It may also be helpful to have the patient empty the bladder or bowels if one is having difficulty. With very atrophic or scarred vaginal tissue, it may be necessary to estrogenize the tissue and then try fitting at another time. It is also helpful during a fitting session to record the pessary styles and sizes tried. This helps to avoid unnecessary future attempts with failed pessaries. If one pessary does not hold a very large bulge, consider placing two pessaries (donut and gellhorn or two rings), which has been described as successful in hard to fit patients.[52,53]

SPECIFIC PESSARY FEATURES, FITTING, AND REMOVAL
Ring

The ring pessary comes with and without a support diaphragm in the center and with or without a knob for incontinence. It has two semicircular plastic inserts imbedded in the silicone, which make it rigid yet allows it to fold into a half-circle shape making it smaller for introduction into the introitus. It is the easiest pessary for the provider and the patient to insert and remove, unless a patient has very weak hands from arthritis or neuromuscular disease and cannot fold the device. It can be used for any type of prolapse or incontinence. In some patients, intercourse may be possible with the ring and the ring with support. Sizes range from 0 to 13 (**Fig. 2**).

To insert, the "bend" in the pessary is located and the pessary folded. (Two indentations on the ring indicate the fold line, and the two large holes in the ring with support indicate the axis for folding.) It is directed with the arc pointing downward using gentle pressure on the posterior vaginal wall and gradually advanced into the canal when it is released (approximately two thirds into the vagina) and advanced past the cervix into the posterior fornix with the index finger. It may help to elevate the outer edge of the pessary behind the symphysis so the pessary sits parallel to the vaginal axis. The incontinence ring pessary is fit in the same way, but the knob adds an additional centimeter to the size of the pessary. The knob should be situated so it is suburethral behind the symphysis, ideally at the level of the urethrovesical junction (**Fig. 3**).

Removal is accomplished with the index finger inserted and the leading edge of the rim hooked. The patient should valsalva gently while the provider applies traction bringing the pessary to the introitus. The pessary is then rotated to an oblique angle and gently pulled through the introitus. If the genital hiatus is too small to easily allow the pessary out this way, use the thumb and forefinger of the opposite hand in an upside down V-shape above the introitus to put pressure on the pessary sides to fold it as it is pulled out. **Fig. 4** shows ring with support pessary in situ.

Gellhorn

The gellhorn has a wide, convex, perforated base with either a long or short stem and a knob. The convex surface of the base develops suction between the pessary and the vaginal wall, which makes it stay in place without using the symphysis to keep it in place. The base sits almost perpendicular (or obliquely) to the vaginal axis with the cervix (or apex) resting in the convexity while the stem lays almost parallel (or obliquely) to the axis with the knob end of the stem resting on the posterior wall and perineal body. The gellhorn is often cited as being difficult for the patient and the provider to insert and remove, but experienced providers and patients rarely find this is a big problem. It is useful for all types of prolapse and despite its unusual appearance is preferred equally by women compared with the ring pessary.[37] It is not possible to have intercourse with the pessary in place, but many women remove it to engage in sexual activity. Sizes range from 1.50 to 3.75 inches (**Fig. 5**).

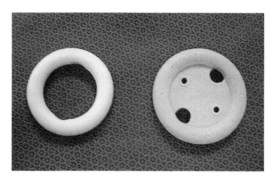

Fig. 2. Support pessary: ring and ring with support.

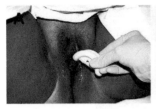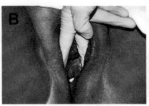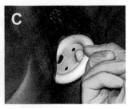

Fig. 3. (*A*) Insertion of ring with support pessary. (*B*) Valsalva shows small amount of pessary. (*C*) Removal of ring with support.

The gellhorn does not fold like the ring. For insertion, the stem is used to hold the gellhorn with the convex base perpendicular to the introitus. The base as the leading edge is then inserted at an oblique angle avoiding the urethra. Gentle downward pressure on the posterior vaginal wall is used to ease the pessary beneath the posterior pubic rami. Using a corkscrew motion the pessary is pushed upward into the vagina with the base perpendicular to the cervix (or apex) and the stem parallel to the vaginal axis. Then the index finger is used to push the knob up along the vaginal axis to finally place the base against the apex or cervix. The knob may be slightly visible with valsalva or with the labia separated. If it extends too far out of the introitus, a short-stem gellhorn can be used (**Fig. 6**).

To remove the gellhorn, the patient performs valsalva while the provider's thumb and index finger are used to grasp the knob firmly. With gentle downward and lateral traction, the suction can be released and the pessary removed at an oblique angle. Alternatively, while the knob is grasped with one hand, the index finger of the other hand sweeps behind the base to release the suction and the pessary is removed at an oblique angle. Attempting to pull the gellhorn straight down and out is usually impossible; the suction must be broken before it comes out. If the pessary is too high to reach even during valsalva, a ring forceps can be used to grasp the pessary and pull it down so the knob can be grasped. **Fig. 7** shows gellhorn in situ.

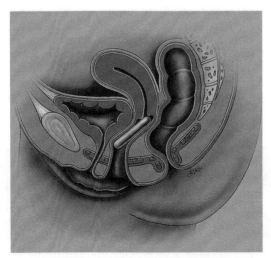

Fig. 4. Ring with support pessary in situ. (*Courtesy of* Lindsay Oksenburg, Dallas, TX.)

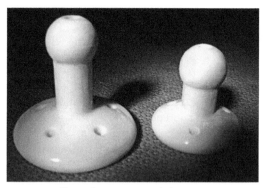

Fig. 5. Space-filling pessary: gellhorn long stem and short stem.

Donut

The donut pessary was a favorite in the nineteenth century after rubber was invented and the "red rubber donut" was produced. Women were still using these pessaries late in the twentieth century, but they have been replaced by the silicone pessary version. The use of donut pessaries has fallen into a last resort category in many practices. In several of the studies cited previously, a donut was used in the rare occasion when the ring or gellhorn was unsuccessful. To retain it, the genital hiatus must be of sufficient size to admit it yet smaller than the pessary itself. The inflatoball pessary is a donut but made of latex rubber that can be inflated once inside the vagina. It is useful for women with big prolapse but a relatively small hiatus. It cannot be used in women with latex allergies and it absorbs odor so must be cleaned every 1 to 3 days. The donut can be difficult for providers to insert and remove and rare women remove the pessary themselves unless an inflatoball is used. Intercourse is not possible with it because it is a "space filling" pessary. Sizes range from 2 to 3.75 inches (**Fig. 8**).

Insertion requires a large amount of lubrication of the introitus. The pessary is held vertically at an oblique angle to the introitus. Gentle downward pressure on the posterior wall to avoid the urethra and to get beneath the inferior pubic rami is used until the pessary can be rotated upward along the vaginal axis into place at the apex. **Fig. 9** shows donut pessary in situ.

Removal is difficult because the rounded edges make it hard to grasp. If the index finger can be inserted into the center hole, apply downward traction with pressure on the posterior vaginal wall. Be sure to have the introitus well lubricated with a water-based lubricant. Some use a tenaculum to assist in removal or deflation of the donut with a large-bore needle and syringe before removal. Both methods reduce the life of the pessary.

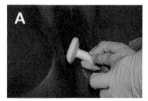
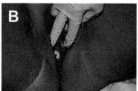
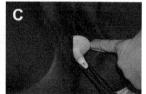

Fig. 6. (*A*) Insertion of gellhorn pessary. (*B*) Gellhorn with valsalva. (*C*) Use of ring forceps for difficult gellhorn removal.

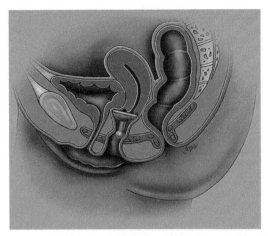

Fig. 7. Gellhorn pessary in situ. (*Courtesy of* Lindsey Oksenberg, Dallas, TX.)

Cube

The cube is similar to the donut in that it is a space-filling pessary and is used as a last resort pessary by most. It has six convex sides that create suction along the vaginal walls to hold it in place. It is relatively difficult to insert and remove for both patient and provider, and intercourse is not possible with it in place. Sizes range from 0 to 7 (**Fig. 10**).

The introitus needs to be well lubricated to insert the cube. The pessary is compressed as much as possible and inserted with downward pressure on the posterior wall while gently guiding the pessary to the apex. There is often a silicone string attached to help locate the pessary for removal. It must be situated like a tampon string so it is accessible later. It can be tucked between the labia for comfort. **Fig. 11** shows cube pessary in situ.

To remove, the string is used to locate the edge of the pessary. The string cannot be solely used to pull the cube out; it will break before the suction releases. An attempt to

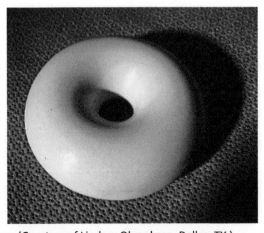

Fig. 8. Donut pessary. (*Courtesy of* Lindsey Oksenberg, Dallas, TX.)

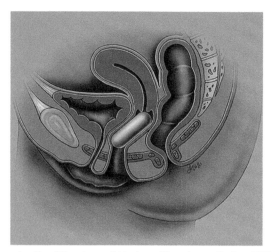

Fig. 9. Donut pessary in situ. (*Courtesy of* Lindsey Oksenberg, Dallas, TX.)

sweep the vaginal wall with the index finger between it and the pessary is made to break the suction, and then the edge of the cube is grasped and pulled out. Ring forceps are often needed to grasp the pessary to provide the traction needed for removal.

There are numerous other pessaries that are used all over the world other than those described. Practitioners find that when they become experienced using any particular pessary, they are able to fit that pessary in most cases. Pessary fitting is successful if the patient's symptoms are relieved, she is comfortable, and both the patient and provider are satisfied with the ease of use.

PESSARY WEAR AND CARE

Whether a patient continues to wear a pessary after the initial fitting period is influenced by how satisfied she is with this treatment. The education she receives in caring for the pessary and convenience of use are very important, and convenience of

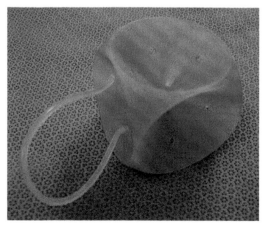

Fig. 10. Cube pessary.

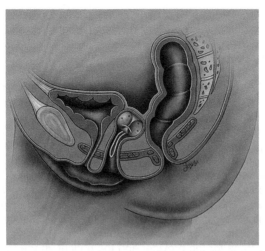

Fig. 11. Cube pessary in situ in woman with no uterus. (*Courtesy of* Lindsey Oksenberg, Dallas TX.)

follow-up care, sexual activity, and complications or side effects of use. Using life table analysis, Wu and coworkers[41] found that 66% of women who continued pessary use after 1 month were still users after 12 months and 53% were still users after 36 months. This is similar to Clemons and coworkers,[13] who found 73% continued use at 1 year and 64% at 2 years using life table analysis.

Common reasons for discontinuation include (1) inadequate symptom relief, (2) inconvenience or the inability or dislike of caring for pessary, (3) persistent incontinence, (4) expulsion, and (5) discharge or erosion.[5,12,31,43,54,55] The characteristics of women satisfied with pessary use include greater than or equal to age 65, and those who are poor surgical risks.[13] Characteristics of women more likely to be dissatisfied include the presence of de novo stress urinary incontinence (occult incontinence),[9] desire for surgery before pessary trial, and stage 3 or 4 prolapse.[13] Clemons and coworkers[13] found that one third of patients who wanted surgery initially but agreed to a pessary trial changed their mind about surgery, so a pessary trial may be warranted even in women who desire surgery.[13]

Attaining a good fit is the first step to successful pessary use. The second step is educating the patient in how to wear and care for the device. Most women are willing and able to remove and clean their pessary. Sometimes they are afraid or embarrassed to try and think it will be too hard for them. Some older women or women of certain cultural backgrounds have never explored their genital area and have not used tampons so are less comfortable inserting an object into the vagina. Women are often surprised at their ability to perform this task and are comfortable performing pessary care. With a little encouragement from an empathetic health care provider, the patient can be empowered to be an active partner in the health care relationship.

Self-care consists of removal of the pessary for cleaning periodically and replacing it. There is no research on how often the pessary should be removed for cleaning. It should be individualized and tailored to the woman's lifestyle. Some women prefer to remove the pessary daily for hygienic purposes; others find that burdensome and prefer a once weekly schedule. If there are no complications at the follow-up visit, the schedule can be flexible. When the pessary is removed, it is considered good practice to leave it out overnight and replace it the next morning. The pessary may also be removed for intercourse if desired or left in place, unless the woman wears a space-filling pessary. Studies have shown that frequency and satisfaction with sexual function improve with pessary use[12] and sexually active women were more likely to continue pessary use.[55]

Most researchers teach pessary users self-care when possible.[9,39,41,43] Unfortunately, in the AUGS member survey, only 53% of respondents teach all patients self-care, and 45% only teach those using a support pessary. In Sulak and coworkers'[43] retrospective review, 96 of the 107 pessary users were fit with a gellhorn and all were taught self-care. There seems to be a bias that women are unable to remove space-filling pessaries; however, in practice this is not true. The dexterity in a woman's hands or other physical limitations might not be overcome, but fear and lack of knowledge can.

Patients may be influenced to perform self-care once they realize frequent office visits are necessary if no self-care is performed. Manufacturer recommendations and expert opinions are typically used in developing follow-up schedules for pessary users. There is no consensus on the best regimen.[9,14,31,32,36,41,50,56] Often the return schedule is burdensome for the provider and the patient. In the survey of gynecologists, the most common follow-up regimen was 1 week after fitting, then 1 month, and then every 3 months for long-term follow-up.[3] There is only one prospective observational study where a more relaxed follow-up schedule was used.[41] In this study patient's were asked to return 2 weeks after fitting unless there was a problem, then return every 3 months for a year, then every 6 months in subsequent years. All the patients in this study were offered self-care but most declined. There were no serious complications from this more relaxed schedule leading researchers to the conclusion that recommendations for frequent pelvic examinations with pessary use can be safely relaxed. A reasonable schedule for follow-up should be individualized and based on the patient's willingness to perform self-care. **Table 1** is a sample follow-up schedule.

At the follow-up visit it is important to ask about symptoms of vaginal bleeding, discharge, or odor that might indicate infection or erosion. Any change in bowel or bladder symptoms or abdominal discomfort might be an indication that a different size is required. The patient is asked about any difficulty removing or replacing. The pessary is checked for position and fit, then removed and washed with soap and water. A careful inspection of the vaginal vault is performed looking for erythema or erosion. Finding an impression on the vaginal wall or cervix of the drain holes in the pessary is not uncommon. A "lesion" may appear perfectly round and match the size of the holes in the pessary. The gellhorn can produce a raised 2-mm "lesion" that is the size of the center hole in the pessary base. Neither "lesion" is cause for alarm. When the pessary is replaced, the "lesion" resolves and another might appear in another area by the next visit. After the vault inspection, the patient is encouraged to learn self-care if not already done.

Table 1		
Pessary follow-up schedule after pessary fitting		
Visit	**Self Care**	**Provider Care**
Visit 1	2–4 wk	1–2 wk
Visit 2	3 mo	1–2 mo
Visit 3	6 mo	3 mo
Visit 4	Yearly	Every 3 mo

Some practices teach pessary care on the initial fitting visit, whereas others wait until the second visit. Much depends on the patients' willingness to learn, the time available, and the purpose for using pessary. One may want the pessary to remain in place for a few weeks initially if using the pessary for diagnostic purposes so the patient can evaluate her symptom relief. It is helpful when teaching pessary use to have pictures depicting the pessary within the vaginal vault. Often women are afraid the pessary will get lost and are surprised at how the pessary actually sits in the vagina. Sometimes a woman complains that the pessary has rotated or that she put it in wrong. Providing reassurance is helpful. There is no wrong way of putting the pessary in, as long as it is comfortable and relieving symptoms. Describing the vagina as a pouch, and telling the patient "the pessary cannot go anywhere," may be helpful and pictures alleviate her fears.

The teaching can be done in the examination room after fitting. First have her wash her hands. Dry fingers make holding and inserting the pessary much easier. Lubricate the leading edge of the pessary or the vaginal introitus if necessary. Have the patient handle the pessary and become comfortable with it. Next, she needs to find a comfortable position: standing with knees bent in a semi-squatting position; standing with one foot on a stool, bench, or chair; or lying with the head and shoulders elevated on pillows. If standing, a wall can be used to lean against to stabilize the patient. Encourage the patient to try different positions; there is no wrong way. Using a pessary of the same style to demonstrate how to hold the pessary while she is practicing helps her to visualize what she is being asked to do.

To teach insertion of a ring pessary, ask the patient to fold the pessary like a taco and insert it upward into the vagina with the arch pointing downward. Ask her to hold the fold of the pessary until most of the pessary is inside, and then release it. Next, she should use her index finger to gently push the pessary into place. It is very helpful to give positive reinforcement at this point. While sitting on a stool, have the patient separate her legs to allow a check for pessary position. Occasionally it may need to be pushed up a little further.

To teach removal, the patient should get into a comfortable position as described previously, place the index finger deeply into the vagina, hook her finger under the rim, and then pull downward and out. Again, demonstrating with a like pessary helps.

To teach insertion of a gellhorn, ask the patient to grasp the knob of the stem, and then place the base edgewise, almost parallel to the introitus. Avoid the urethra by pushing firmly against the posterior wall while using a corkscrew motion to move the pessary under the symphysis and up into the vault. Once the flat disk is in the vagina, she can push the pessary upward as far as it goes. Again, check for proper placement and provide positive feedback.

To teach gellhorn removal, have the patient valsalva to bring to stem closer to the introitus and within reach. She can then grasp the knob and use gentle traction downward and laterally toward the thigh until the suction releases and the pessary comes out parallel to the introitus. Practice improves her ability quickly.

Most other pessaries can be taught in a similar fashion. The pessary manufacturer also provides information in each package describing how to insert and remove that particular pessary.

Often, the patient cannot comfortably reach her pessary for removal. A short piece of dental tape can be tied to most pessaries like a tampon string to facilitate removal. The dental tape does not absorb odors and is strong enough to pull the pessary out without tearing it. Dental tape threaded through the knob of the gellhorn and tied can provide a lever effect to break the suction when removing the pessary.

Occasionally, a pessary falls out during a bowel movement. If this is the only time it falls out, the pessary may still be considered a good fit. Initially, the patient should retrieve the pessary and wash it with soap and water and then replace it. In the future she can place her hand wrapped in tissue against the vagina and perineum to provide support during valsalva to prevent expulsion.

If the patient experiences discomfort, she should first check that the pessary is in the proper position. If the discomfort continues, the pessary should be removed and brought to the next clinic visit. If she cannot remove the pessary, she needs to be seen as soon as possible. It is not uncommon for patients who have lost or gained weight or regained tissue compliance with local estrogen therapy to find the pessary is uncomfortable or falls out. Refitting with a larger or smaller pessary usually resolves the problem.

Caring for the vaginal tissues is important during pessary use to prevent irritation or erosion from the pessary. In postmenopausal women, even with oral hormone replacement, the vagina is often found to have thin, atrophic vaginal epithelium. Those with a thin vaginal epithelium have a higher rate of vaginal abrasions, which may lead to pessary discontinuance.[41] Hanson and coworkers[39] found the highest pessary success rate was in menopausal women using local estrogen with or without systemic hormone-replacement therapy. The estrogen cream tends to get better overall vaginal coverage compared with the estrogen tablet, which needs vaginal moisture to dissolve so may not be the best choice for women with significant atrophy. The finger application method for use of vaginal estrogen cream is preferred by many women to the use of an applicator because of the mess made by the leakage of the excess cream when warmed by the body. A silicone ring with slow-release estradiol is a good option for a woman who has difficulty using the creams or has a contraindication to estrogen that is absorbed systemically. The ring can be placed on top of the pessary and left in place for 3 months. It can be replaced when the patient returns for routine provider care. The North American Menopause Society published a position statement in 2007 stating the progestogen is generally not indicated when low-dose vaginal estrogen is administered locally for vaginal atrophy.[57] This allayed some concerns regarding the need for annual endometrial surveillance or progesterone withdrawal routinely when using local estrogen. Another option for tissue care may be a gel designed to provide pH balance to the vagina, which may help control discharge and odor.

Some discoloration of the pessary during use is common but does not affect the performance of the pessary. The pessary should be replaced if it becomes worn or torn. Silicone pessaries can last many years without needing to be replaced. Menstruating women find the pessary is discolored more easily, so daily cleaning is helpful. Some women choose not to wear the pessary while menstruating, but others use tampons with the pessary in place, especially if it is a ring.

It is time consuming to teach the patient self-care, but the time spent is well worth it in the long run. Nurses in the clinic can be very good at teaching patients insertion, removal, and pessary maintenance. An educated patient is much more satisfied with pessary treatment and better able to inform her provider of problems that arise.

COMPLICATIONS AND CONSIDERATIONS

There are some complications that may affect the patients' satisfaction if not addressed. Most of these issues are not dangerous and not difficult to deal with. Increased vaginal discharge is relatively common for pessary users who do not perform self-care. Most often it is not problematic but some patients develop a very heavy discharge with odor. The pessary can trap secretions caused by desquamation, which break down and cause increased creamy, sometimes green-colored discharge and odor. In a historical cohort study, 32% of pessary users versus 10% of controls were Gram stain positive for bacterial vaginosis with a relative risk of 3.3 (odds ratio 4.37; 95% confidence interval, 2.15–9.32; $P = .0002$).[58] More research needs to be done, but acidification of the vaginal pH can help to restore the pH balance of the vagina. A monthly douche with water and a small amount of vinegar or irrigation of the vagina with a vinegar-water solution during pessary follow-up visits may be helpful for women with significant discharge and odor. Observation of pregnant pessary users for bacterial vaginosis is important in preventing adverse pregnancy outcomes. Alnaif and Drutz[58] advise pessary removal 10 days before vaginal surgery to allow normalization of the vaginal flora, and treatment of bacterial vaginosis before surgery to prevent cuff cellulitis and pelvic inflammatory disease.

The most common true complication of the pessary is vaginal erosion or ulceration. Signs of erosion are a heavier and more odiferous vaginal discharge. The patient cannot feel an ulcer so inspection of the vault at each visit is essential. Ulceration rates vary between 2% and 24%.[9,39–41] The ring pessaries in these studies were less likely than the gellhorn or cube to cause erosion and erosion was less likely to occur in women performing self-care. In Wu and coworkers' study,[41] five of six cube users developed erosion of the vaginal wall. The numbers of pessary erosion in this study was directly related to the vaginal epithelial thickness at the time of pessary fitting. Erosion or ulceration is often treated by removing the pessary for 2 to 3 weeks and using estrogen vaginal cream nightly.[35,50] After healing, the provider should determine if the pessary is the correct size and style to avoid future problems. Some patients refuse to have the pessary out for any amount of time because of discomfort with the bulge out, or because ulcerations occur when the bulge rubs the clothing. In this case a different style or size pessary could be placed and estrogen cream used nightly. If the ulceration persists, biopsy of the site may be required. There is one case report of sucralfate (aluminum salt of sucrose oscasulfate that binds preferentially to the ulcerated area and promotes healing, usually used in peptic ulcer) being used for a pessary ulcer.[59]

Pessary use rarely results in severe complications. In a review of the literature from 1950 to 2007, 39 major complications requiring surgical intervention were identified.[60] These included 8 vesicovaginal fistulas, 5 urologic complications, 4 rectovaginal fistulas, 3 bowel complications, and 19 impacted pessaries. This emphasizes the importance of regular follow-up, but 2 of the 39 cases occurred in elderly women who were receiving appropriate follow-up. All cases were related to gellhorn or gellhorn-like pessaries. Keeping a list of pessary users with their follow-up schedules in the office may be useful so if a patient is hospitalized, has a stroke, or has a change in mental status, the hospital or caregiver may be informed of the patient's pessary use.[51]

Other considerations include the potential effect of pessary use on pap smears. A report in 1997 described 23 postmenopausal women who wore vaginal pessaries and showed cytologic atypia in the form of severe inflammatory changes in squamous cells, and atypical metaplasia and reparative changes with a background pattern of acute inflammation and prominent superficial maturation of the squamous cells. These changes were not found in users of oral estrogen, and were found to completely reverse with removal of the pessary and use of estrogen cream. Actinomyces was also found in half of the 23 patients.[61] In 1992, a case series report of 96 pessary users over 20 years in two institutions revealed 68 cases of cervical cancer and 28 cases of vaginal cancer that were linked to pessary use. The pessaries used during the study period were made of two types of rubber but the researchers could not link the cancers to chemical carcinogenesis. They concluded the cancers were likely associated with chronic inflammation injuries related to the foreign body.[62] Atypical cells in the pap smear of a postmenopausal woman who wears pessary should not be dismissed. Removal of the pessary and use of estrogen cream a week before a pap smear may be helpful in clarification of cytology results. Otherwise, normal smears may be read as atypical.

Occult incontinence unmasked with pessary use is an issue that affects patient satisfaction significantly. The use of periurethral bulking agents, or in some cases outpatient mid-urethral sling surgery, may be a good solution if the patient is distressed by the leakage but wants to continue pessary use.[63]

SUMMARY

Pessary use is the only nonsurgical option available for pelvic organ prolapse. Indications for pessary use include symptomatic pelvic organ prolapse, the patient either does not desire or is not a candidate for surgery, use as a diagnostic tool to predict surgical outcome, correcting stress urinary incontinence, and in pregnancy for incarcerated uterus and preterm cervical dilation. Despite the lack of randomized controlled trials comparing surgery with pessary, a long history of clinical use suggests pessaries are a satisfactory treatment option for many women.

There are no patient characteristics identified by researchers that consistently help in selection of appropriate pessary size or style for a particular woman. Subjective methods for selection include trial and error, expert opinion, and the provider's past experience. Providers continue to use these methods to produce continuation rates that demonstrate patient satisfaction.

After fitting, the second most important part of pessary use in any practice is patient education for self-care. Women who care for the pessary themselves experience fewer complications. Complications from pessary use are usually mild, such as vaginal discharge or erosion of the vaginal mucosa. Treatment is usually simple and effective. Severe complications requiring surgical intervention and cancer related to pessary use are rare.

Offering a nonsurgical option for treatment of pelvic organ prolapse is important because of the morbidity, mortality, and potential failure of reconstructive surgery. It is a low-risk option that is not difficult to learn and can greatly enhance the patient's quality of life. Adding pessary to the treatment armamentarium includes purchasing two to three styles of pessaries in the most common sizes and identifying candidates who desire a nonsurgical treatment option. Experience comes with trial and error, persistence, and practice.

ACKNOWLEDGMENTS

I would to thank Pam Martinez and Carla Richardson for their assistance with this chapter.

REFERENCES

1. Miller DS. Contemporary use of the pessary. Gynecol Obstet 1991;39:1–12.
2. Shah SM, Sultan AH, Thakar R. The history and evolution of pessaries for pelvic organ prolapse. Int Urogynecol J 2006;17:170–5.
3. Pott-Grinstein E, Newcomer JR. Gynecologists' patterns of prescribing pessaries. J Reprod Med 2001;46(3):205–8.

4. Mutone MF, Terry C, Hale DS, et al. Factors which influence the short-term success of pessary management of pelvic organ prolapse. Am J Obstet Gynecol 2005;193:89–94.
5. Powers K, Lazarou G, Wang A, et al. Pessary use in advanced pelvic organ prolapse. Int Urogynecol J 2006;17:160–4.
6. Adams E, Thomson A, Maher C, et al. Mechanical devices for pelvic organ prolapse in women. Cochrane Database Syst Rev 2004;(2):CD004010. CD004010.pub2. DOI:10.1002/14651858. Last assessed as up-to-date: October 26, 2005.
7. Weber AM, Richter HE. Pelvic organ prolapse. Obstet Gynecol 2005;106: 615–34.
8. Barber MD, Walters MD, Cundiff GW. Responsiveness of the Pelvic Floor Distress Inventory (PFDI) and Pelvic Floor Impact Questionnaire (PFIQ) in women under-going vaginal surgery and pessary treatment for pelvic organ prolapse. Am J Obstet Gynecol 2006;194(5):1492–8.
9. Clemons JL, Aguilar VC, Tillinghast TA, et al. Patient satisfaction and changes in prolapse and urinary symptoms in women who were successfully fitted with a pessary for pelvic organ prolapse. Am J Obstet Gynecol 2004; 190:1025–9.
10. Donnelly MJ, Powell-Morgan S, Olsen AL, et al. Vaginal pessaries for the management of stress and mixed urinary incontinence. Int Urogynecol J 2004; 15:302–7.
11. Komesu YM, Rogers RG, Rode MA, et al. Pelvic floor symptom changes in pessary users. Am J Obstet Gynecol 2007;197:620.e1–6.
12. Fernando RJ, Thakar R, Sultan AH, et al. Effect of vaginal pessaries on symptoms associated with pelvic organ prolapse. Obstet Gynecol 2006;108:93–9.
13. Clemons JL, Aguilar VC, Sokol ER, et al. Patient characteristics that are associ-ated with continued pessary use versus surgery after 1 year. Am J Obstet Gyne-col 2004;91:159–64.
14. Cundiff GW, Weidner AC, Visco AG, et al. A survey of pessary use by members of the American Urogynecologic Society. Obstet Gynecol 2000;95(6):931–5.
15. Micha JP, Rettenmaier MA, Clark M, et al. Successful management of acute renal failure with a vaginal pessary: a case report. Gynecol Surg 2008;5: 49–51.
16. Heit M, Culligan P, Rosenquist C, et al. Is pelvic organ prolapse a cause of pelvic or low back pain? Obstet Gynecol 2002;99(1):23–8.
17. Lazarou G, Scotti RJ, Mikhail MS, et al. Pessary reduction and postoperative cure of retention in women with anterior vaginal wall prolapse. Int Urogynecol J 2004; 15:175–8.
18. Bhatia NN, Bergman A. Pessary test in women with urinary incontinence. Obstet Gynecol 1985;65:220–6.
19. Mattox TF, Bhatia NN. Urodynamic effects of reducing devices in women with genital prolapse. Int Urogynecol J 1994;5:283–6.
20. Bump RC, Fantl JA, Hurt WG. The mechanism of urinary continence in women with severe uterovaginal prolapse: results of barrier studies. Obstet Gynecol 1988;72:291–5.
21. Nygaard I. Prevention of exercise incontinence with mechanical devices. J Reprod Med 1995;40:89–94.
22. Bhatia NN, Bergman A, Gunning JE. Urodynamic effects of a vaginal pessary in women with stress urinary incontinence. Am J Obstet Gynecol 1983;147:876.
23. Shaikh S, Ong EK, Glavind K, et al. Mechanical devices for urinary incontinence in women. Cochrane Database of Syst Rev 2006;2:CD001756.

24. Richter HE, Burgio KL, Goode PS, et al. Non-surgical management of stress urinary incontinence: ambulatory treatments for leakage associated with stress (ATLAS) trial. Clinical Trials 2007;4:92–101.

25. Acharya G, Eschler B, Gronberg M, et al. Noninvasive cerclage for the management of cervical incompetence: a prospective study. Arch Gynecol Obstet 2006; 273:283–7.

26. Brown HL. Cervical prolapse complicating pregnancy. J Natl Med Assoc 1997; 89(5):346–8.

27. Daskalakis G, Lymberopoulos E, Anastasakis E, et al. Uterine prolapse complicating pregnancy. Arch Gynecol Obstet 2007;276:391–2.

28. Ziv E, Levavi H, Ovadia J. Severe edema of the uterine cervix-an unusual cause of acute urinary retention in pregnancy. Int Urogynecol J 1995;6:180–3.

29. Piver MS, Spezia J. Uterine prolapse during pregnancy. Obstet Gynecol 1968;32: 765.

30. Jeffery S, Franco A, Fynes M. Vaginal wind: the cube pessary as a solution. Int Urogynecol J 2008;19:1457.

31. Jones K, Yang L, Lowder JL, et al. Effect of pessary use on genital hiatus measurements in women with pelvic organ prolapse. Obstet Gynecol 2008; 112(3):630–6.

32. Bash KL. Review of vaginal pessaries. Obstet Gynecol Surv 2000;55(7): 455–60.

33. Zeitlin MP, Lebherz TB. Pessaries in the geriatric patient. JAGS 1992;40(6): 635–41.

34. Roehl B, Buchanan EM. Urinary incontinence evaluation and the utility of pessaries in older women. Care Manag J 2006;7(4):213–7.

35. Trowbridge ER, Fenner DE. Practicalities and pitfalls of pessaries in older women. Clin Obstet Gynecol 2007;50(3):709–19.

36. Handa VL, Jones M. Do pessaries prevent the progression of pelvic organ prolapse? Int Urogynecol J 2002;13:349–52.

37. Cundiff GW, Amundsen CL, Bent AE, et al. The PESSRI study: symptom relief outcomes of a randomized crossover trial of the ring and Gellhorn pessaries. Am J Obstet Gynecol 2007;196:405.e1–8.

38. Clemons JL, Aguilar VC, Tillinghast TA, et al. Risk factors associated with an unsuccessful pessary fitting trial in women with pelvic organ prolapse. Am J Obstet Gynecol 2004;190:345–50.

39. Hanson LM, Schulz JA, Flood CG, et al. Vaginal pessaries in managing women with pelvic organ prolapse and urinary incontinence: patient characteristics and factors contributing to success. Int Urogynecol J 2006;17:155–9.

40. Nyguyen JN, Jones CR. Pessary treatment of pelvic relaxation: factors affecting successful fitting and continued use. JWOCN 2005;32(4):255–61.

41. Wu V, Farrell SA, Baskett TF, et al. A simplified protocol for pessary management. Obstet Gynecol 1997;906:990–4.

42. Maito JM, Quam ZA, Craig E, et al. Predictors of successful pessary fitting and continued use in a nurse-midwifery pessary clinic. J Midwifery Womens Health 2006;51(2):78–84.

43. Sulak PJ, Kuehl TJ, Shull BL. Vaginal pessaries and their use in pelvic relaxation. J Reprod Med 1993;38(12):919–23.

44. Realini JP, Walters MD. Vaginal diaphragm rings in the treatment of stress urinary incontinence. J Am Board Fam Pract 1990;3:99–103.

45. Noblett KL, McKinney A, Lane FL. Effects of the incontinence dish pessary on urethral support and urodynamic parameters. Am J Obstet Gynecol 2008;198:592.e1–5.

46. Nygaard I, Zinsmeister AR. Treatment of exercise incontinence with a vaginal pessary: a preliminary study. Int Urogynecol J 1993;4:133–7.
47. Nager CW, Richter HE, Nygaard I, et al. POP-Q measures do not predict incontinence pessary size. Int Urogynecol J 2009;20:1023–8.
48. Qureshi NS, Appleton F, Jones AB. Ring pessary sizer: a pilot study to objectively measure size of a ring pessary required by a patient. Gynecol Surg 2008;5: 247–9.
49. Mainprize TC, Robert M. Long-term assessment of the incontinence ring pessary for the treatment of stress incontinence. Int Urogynecol J 2002;13:326–9.
50. Culligan PJ. Pessary devices: a stepwise approach to fitting, teaching, and managing. In: Culligan PJ, Goldberg RP, editors. Urogynecology in primary care. London: Springer; 2007. p. 89–93.
51. Carcio H. The vaginal pessary: an effective yet underused tool for incontinence and prolapse. Adv Nurse Pract 2004;12:47–54.
52. Myers DL, LaSala CA, Murphy JA. Double pessary use in grade 4 uterine and vaginal prolapse. Obstet Gynecol 1998;91(6):1019–20.
53. Singh K, Reid WMN. Non-surgical treatment of uterovaginal prolapse using double vaginal rings. BJOG 2002;108(1):112–3.
54. Bai SW, Yoon BS, Kwon YJ, et al. Survey of the characteristics and satisfaction degree of the patients using a pessary. Int Urogynecol J 2005;16:182–6.
55. Brincat C, Kenton K, Fitzgerald MP, et al. Sexual activity predicts continued pessary use. Am J Obstet Gynecol 2004;191:198–200.
56. Poma PA. Nonsurgical management of genital prolapse: a review and recommendations for clinical practice. J Reprod Med 2000;45(10):789–97.
57. The North American Menopause Society. The role of local vaginal estrogen for treatment of vaginal atrophy in postmenopausal women: 2007 position statement of the North American Menopause Society. Menopause 2007;14(3):355–6.
58. Alnaif B, Drutz HP. Bacterial vaginosis increases in pessary users. Int Urogynecol J 2000;11:219–23.
59. Lentz SS, Barrett RJ, Homsley HD. Topical sucralfate in the treatment of vaginal ulceration. Obstet Gynecol 1993;81:869–71.
60. Arias BE, Ridgeway B, Barber MD. Complications of neglected vaginal pessaries: case presentation and literature review. Int Urogynecol J Pelvic Floor Dysfunct 2008;19(8):1173–8.
61. Christ ML, Haja J. Cytologic changes associated with vaginal pessary use with special reference to the presence of actinomyces. Acta Cytol 1978;22(3): 146–9.
62. Schraub S, Sun XS, Maingon PH, et al. Cervical and vaginal cancer associated with pessary use. Cancer 1992;69:2505–9.
63. Walters MD, Jannetta LT. Combination of pessary and periurethral collagen injections for nonsurgical treatment of uterovaginal prolapse and genuine stress urinary incontinence. Obstet Gynecol 1997;90(4):691–2.

Vaginal Surgery for Pelvic Organ Prolapse

Stephen B. Young, MD

KEYWORDS

- Pelvic organ prolapse • Reconstructive surgical procedures
- Hysterectomy • Vaginal • Cystocele • Rectocele

The art and science of vaginal reconstructive surgery has evolved during the past 2 centuries. The first vaginal hysterectomy was performed for malignancy by Langenbeck in 1813,[1] although there is much controversy surrounding this. The surgical treatment of prolapse developed through multiple varied operations in the second quarter of the nineteenth century. Early procedures were somewhat or fully obliterative. The more prominent were largely occlusive and included élytrorhaphie—removing long vertical vaginal strips and placing several supportive sutures, cauterization of the vagina, episiorrhaphy—where dependent parts of the labia majora were removed and the raw surfaces united resulting in almost complete vulvar occlusion, perineorrhaphy, and cervical amputation, finally full cervical removal with bladder displacement.[1] In America, the first vaginal hysterectomy for prolapse was performed by Samuel Choppin in New Orleans in 1861.

Before the introduction of general anesthesia and aseptic technique, these early procedures were limited. Operations had to be brief as pain was not fully alleviated. A general imprimatur reigned against entering the peritoneal cavity for fear of peritonitis.

Gradually, over the next 100 years, as the theory of pelvic organ prolapse etiology and pathophysiology developed, and more definitive curative surgical procedures could be performed safely, the operations that became popular in the early part of the twentieth century were established. These include procedures such as the standard anterior colporrhaphy with Kelly plication suture for cystocele and urinary incontinence.

For several decades, vaginal hysterectomy has been generally accepted as the approach of choice for removal of the benign uterus. Ribeiro and colleagues,[2] in an randomized control trial (RCT) published in 2003 concluded, "vaginal hysterectomy presents superior results in terms of operative time and inflammatory response

Division of Urogynecology & Reconstructive Pelvic Surgery, Department of Obstetrics & Gynecology, UMass Memorial Medical Center, University of Massachusetts Medical School, 119 Belmont Street, Worcester, MA 01605, USA
E-mail address: youngs01@ummhc.org

Obstet Gynecol Clin N Am 36 (2009) 565–584
doi:10.1016/j.ogc.2009.08.013
0889-8545/09/$ – see front matter © 2009 Elsevier Inc. All rights reserved.

obgyn.theclinics.com

when compared with total abdominal and laparoscopic hysterectomy and should be the first option for hysterectomy."

This article is meant to be a pragmatic how-to guide in the performance of standard vaginal reconstructive operations. The sequencing mirrors that which occurs in the operating room. It will deal exclusively with techniques for the vaginal approach to pelvic organ prolapse correction. Most of the procedures described are based closely on the teachings of Dr David Nichols.

EXAMINATION UNDER ANESTHESIA

With the patient in lithotomy position but not yet Trendelenburg, separation of the lateral vaginal walls with two medium Breisky-Navratil retractors will afford a quality view of the anterior compartment. One may note the presence of any anterior prolapse and determine if it is caused by a midline, transverse (superior), and/or lateral (paravaginal) defect. Cervico-uterine prolapse can be seen and uterine mobility noted by tenaculum traction. Bimanual exam is used to determine uterine size, shape, and mobility; presence, location, and size of myomata; and pelvic capacity. Of particular importance is the adequacy of the subpubic arch. A narrow subpubic arch will compromise the operator's ability to perform meaningful vaginal surgery. Adnexal masses can be palpated. Next, with a Deaver retractor elevating the anterior compartment, the posterior wall can be assessed. Any possible weakness can be further defined with a digital rectal exam. Importantly, the presence and extent of defects in the vaginal outlet and perineum should be judged. Vaginal outlet relaxation, perineal deficiency, and possible introital scars can be corrected at the end of the procedure with a careful perineorrhaphy.

There is a significant difference in the prolapse findings on examination under anesthesia (EUA) and those in an ambulatory setting. Although one can be more thorough in both observation and palpation, still, the absence of the Valsalva effort removes the active component that manifests and maximizes the clinical prolapse. Significant differences have been reported in the findings of EUA versus those of ambulatory pelvic exam.[3,4]

The completion of the EUA is the appropriate moment to strategically plan the order of procedures and surgical tailoring to achieve vulvovaginal dimensions that will afford optimal coital function.

VAGINAL HYSTERECTOMY
Simple

A Lone Star Self-retaining Retractor (Lone Star Medical Products, Stafford, TX) with yellow and blue stays is extremely useful for exposure. Over a weighted speculum, the cervix can be grasped with two Jacobs tenaculae and infiltrated at the vaginal/ epithelial junction with local anesthetic such as 0.5% bupivacaine with 1:200,000 epinephrine solution. With the goal of leaving the vagina as long as possible, a full-thickness circular incision is made around the cervix using either a curved Mayo scissor or scalpel. With scissors slightly open, achieving a full-thickness incision is confirmed by the ability to easily push the vaginal skin cephalad. Hemostasis is obtained and the posterior peritoneum is grasped with a Debakey forceps between the uterosacral ligaments and incised, thus entering the posterior cul-de-sac. Digital exam of the posterior peritoneal surfaces reveals the characteristics of the uterosacral ligaments, the size and freedom of the posterior uterine surface, and the presence of any cul-de-sac or uterine adhesions or masses. One is now ready to begin securing the uterine pedicles (**Fig. 1**).

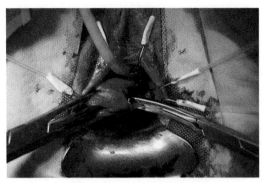

Fig. 1. The left uterosacral ligament is grasped with a Zeppelin clamp.

Using a Zeppelin, Masterson, or Heaney clamp, the uterosacral and cardinal ligament pedicles, as they insert onto the cervix, are separately grasped, cut, suture-ligated with 0-Vicryl, and held. This is usually an optimal time to enter the anterior cul-de-sac. The curved Mayo scissor held perpendicular to the cervix is used to incise its anterior covering connective tissue (supra-cervical septum) from 11 to 1 o'clock. It is usually necessary to sever the more vascular connections immediately lateral (bladder pillars). This can be done with cautery. At 12 o'clock, the Mayo scissor, now held closed parallel and immediately anterior to the cervix, will slide cephalad, posterior to the bladder and just anterior to the peritoneum of the anterior cul-de-sac. An index finger will confirm location and a Deaver will maintain exposure. Often the anterior peritoneum is not yet easily accessible. Although the anterior cul-de-sac itself may not be opened, the bladder and ureters are now elevated out of harm's way. The ureters can be palpated most easily after the anterior peritoneum is opened (see the section "Ureteral palpation").

Attention is returned to the uterine pedicles where the uterine vessels can now be secured. The same Zeppelin and 0-Vicryl suture ligature technique is used, but the pedicles are not held. After another pedicle or two on each side, the adnexae come into view with a normal-size uterus. Their pedicles are secured and the uterus handed off. A free tie of 0-Vicryl, 1 cm proximal to the instrument will, with instrument "flashing," compress the pedicle before the suture ligature. The needle is placed centrally, behind the instrument, and both treads passed around the instrument's tip and tied behind its heel. If further adnexal traction is required, an additional distal 2-0 Vicryl suture can be placed and held.

Ancillary Techniques for the Large Uterus

Uterine myomata very often complicate vaginal hysterectomy. Simply by the nature of their size, making the uterus larger than the pelvic canal or by their awkward location in relationship to the placement of hysterectomy pedicles, fibroids can be singular or multiple, small or very large; submucosal, intramural, subserosal or pedunculated; located at almost any position on the uterus or cervix; and may appear in a host of different degenerative conditions. The presence of uterine myomata alone does not form a contraindication to vaginal hysterectomy. However, when fibroids make a uterus larger than 12 to 14 weeks gestational size, a careful plan of action is indicated in accomplishing the vaginal approach to hysterectomy. It is difficult to state an absolute size above which one ought not consider vaginal hysterectomy. One always has to consider the size of the passageway (the pelvis) in relationship to the passenger (fibroid uterus), as well as the location and size of the individual myomata. Is it one large fibroid or are there multiple small myomata? With experience in the ancillary maneuvers of intramyometrial coring (Lash procedure), cervical amputation, bivalving, wedging, and myomectomy, a considerably enlarged uterus can be reduced in size such that it is easily and safely deliverable vaginally. Before any of these maneuvers are performed, securing of the uterosacral, cardinal, and uterine vascular pedicles are essential prerequisites. Once the uterine vessels are secured and, hopefully, the anterior and posterior cul-de-sacs have been entered, large myomas of the corpus and fundus may soon limit the securing of more apical pedicles. At this point a Lash procedure with or without cervical amputation will convert a very large, globular fibroid uterus into a more manageable ovoid-shaped structure. Using a Beaver blade, a continuing circular incision is carried up from the lower uterine segment, at least 1 cm in from the serosa and parallel to it, toward the fundus. Gentle traction is applied on the inner uterine specimen with triple-tooth Lahey-type tenaculae. This should be done slowly as danger lies just outside the serosa. Deviating somewhat too medial and entering the endometrial cavity, however, is not a problem. A cautery on cutting function may be intermittently substituted for the Beaver knife. But here, even greater care must be used. As one progresses, the fundus in the midline will become palpable. At this point, the uterine specimen is usually deliverable and the ovarian suspensory ligaments and fallopian tubes can be clamped.

In a very large uterus with multiple myomata, the Lash with or without cervical amputation may not be adequate to reduce the uterus to a deliverable size. Individual myomas encountered along the way can easily be shelled-out via their pseudocapsule and handed off. If the posterior or anterior uterine aspect is particularly dominant, a large wedge may be excised. If all these maneuvers still leave an undeliverable specimen, the remaining uterus can be cut in half vertically or bivalved. This affords two more manageable pieces.

VAGINAL ADNEXECTOMY

After removal of the uterus and cervix, and the intestinal contents packed with the patient in Trendelenburg position, Breisky retractors will normally demonstrate the adnexa at 3 and 9 o'clock. Maintaining minimal traction on an additional distal suture on the adnexal pedicle eases its removal. After gently grasping the ovary with a Babcock, a free adnexa can be safely removed with a LigaSure (ValleyLab, Boulder, CO) type of device, an endoloop and transfixation suture, or a clamp/cut/suture process using an instrument such as the infundibulopelvic (IP) Zeppelin clamp. Filmy adhesions may be sharply lysed. It is often less of a technical challenge to remove the ovary separate from its Fallopian tube.

URETERAL PALPATION

One must become beware of the path of the ureter. Upon entering into the anterior cul-de-sac, this is an ideal point to palpate the ureter through part of its pelvic course. One ought to locate it again before placing the first anterior colporrhaphy suture and at any point during the entire surgery where one may be within close proximity to it (2 cm). **Fig. 2** depicts a ureteral palpation technique. Gynecologists are concerned about avoiding the ureter near the uterine vessels during vaginal hysterectomy. A site where it is even in closer proximity to operative maneuvers is at the initial suturing of an anterior colporrhaphy where it may be within 0.9 cm.[5]

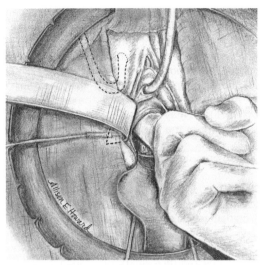

Fig. 2. Ureteral palpation technique during vaginal surgery. One method is to begin identi-fication from within or just outside of the anterior cul-de-sac. The dominant index finger tip begins just lateral to the tractioned Foley balloon (urethrovesical junction). It moves 3 to 4 cm cephalad and lateral, at a 30° angle toward the same shoulder, to the area of the ipsi-lateral uretero-vesical junction. The ureter is felt by gentle index fingertip palpation as its volar aspect slides down in an arc posterior and lateral from 10:30 o'clock on the right side, slowly toward a vaginal Deaver tip at 9:00. One often senses one's fingertip run over the ureter as a nonpulsatile, somewhat mobile, cylindrical tube—quite akin to a cooked spaghetti strand, as it approaches the Deaver. Alternatively, it may snap at the edge of the Deaver tip or just over its anterior surface. It is generally felt 2 to 4 cm away from the vaginal incision. If not palpable this way, it may be felt between two index fingers, one inside and one outside the anterior vaginal wall. They are placed as high as they can get and gently, slowly brought down—frequently encountering the ureter along their way (*From* Young SB, Kambiss SK. Anterior wall support defects. In: Bent AE, Cundiff GW, Swift SE, editors. Os-tergard's Urogynecology and Pelvic Floor Dysfunction. 6th edition. Philadelphia: Lippincott, Williams & Wilkins; 2008; with permission.)

VAGINAL VAULT SUSPENSION

Whichever method one chooses to suspend the vaginal vault following a hysterectomy is, perhaps, less important than actually performing some definitive culdeplasty proce-dure. The vaginal apex, preferably anterior and posterior apices, should be secured with delayed-absorbable or permanent suture to an intact component of the uterosac-ral-cardinal connective tissue complex. As connective tissue breaks may exist in the more distal vaginal ends of the cardinal-uterosacral ligament condensation, as part of prolapse etiology, it seems logical to use more cephalad portions of these structures to suspend the vaginal cuff.

McCall (New Orleans) Culdeplasty

Suspending the vaginal apex to the uterosacral ligaments was first published by Miller[6] in 1927. McCall[7] described his culdeplasty procedure while in New Orleans in 1957. He sutured the vaginal cuff to the uterosacral ligament remnants after vaginal hysterec-tomy as a means of maintaining normal support of the vaginal apex. This procedure was modified over the next several decades at the Mayo clinic and elsewhere and now has many different variations. McCall culdeplasty modifications are aimed at physiologically maintaining vaginal length and axis and closing the cul-de-sac.

Delayed-absorbable and/or permanent sutures sew the distal uterosacral ligament (USL) to the posterior vaginal apex and peritoneum. A single suture secures both uterosacral ligaments and posterior vaginal apices and reefs across the posterior peritoneum between the ligaments, obliterating the posterior cul-de-sac in the process. A wedge of mid-posterior vaginal wall apex can be excised if redundant. Two or more McCall sutures may be placed "internally"—intraperitoneally and through the "internal" aspect of the vaginal apices. An additional "external McCall stitch" is placed similarly, but is brought through the full-thickness of the vaginal skin into the apical lumen on both sides.

High Uterosacral Suspension

Although the McCall culdeplasty is effective in maintaining apical length and axis,[8,9] it is not known as a definitive therapeutic reconstructive operation for uterine descent with accompanying vaginal vault prolapse or posthysterectomy vaginal vault prolapse with enterocele. The high uterosacral suspension is such an excellent procedure that we ordinarily use it both therapeutically, for posthysterectomy vaginal vault prolapse-enterocele and prophylactically, to suspend the apex immediately following vaginal hysterectomy.

By placing gentle traction on the held uterosacral ligament pedicle in 180° opposite direction, the intermediary portion of the uterosacral ligament can be palpated, usually running 1.5 cm medial and posterior to the ipsilateral ischial spine. The middle third of the uterosacral ligament is chosen as the fixation point because it has been shown to be both stronger and farther from the ureter than the distal (vaginal) third.[10,11] The separation between this intermediary portion of the uterosacral ligament and both the lateral aspect of the rectum and the ipsilateral ureter can be palpated. A long Allis clamp can be placed on the distal end of the uterosacral ligament for stabilization and assistance in suturing. With the patient in moderate Trendelenburg position and the bladder emptied, the bowel is packed away with 1-inch peritoneal moist pack and excellent exposure obtained using a Light-Mat on a Deaver retractor anteriorly and a Miyazaki lighted retractor posteriorly. The Deaver holds away the packing and bladder while the Miyazaki guards the rectum. A headlamp is an optional feature to give even more illumination to the pelvis.

We use a 0-PDS and a 0-Prolene on a CT-2 needle held in the strong jaws of a 14-inch Nolan needle driver, sewing from anterior to posterior, going through and not around the intermediary portion of the uterosacral ligament, and retrieve the needle with a separate long, straight needle driver. The suture is passed from anterior to posterior on each side. The packing and lighted retractors are removed. Any redundant posterior peritoneum or enterocele sac can be excised. Similarly, if the posterior vaginal cuff is redundant, a wedge can be removed with cautery without compromising significant vaginal length. The eight ends of these four sutures are sewn, one PDS and one Prolene each, to the right and left posterior and anterior cuffs. The PDS is sewn from inside the incision out to the vaginal lumen and back in, going through the full thickness of the vaginal wall. The Prolene sutures are rather sewn in a manner that obtains purchase on the fibromuscular layer of the vagina and spares the lumen, also from inside to inside. The addition of a free #5 Mayo-needle on the suture arm without one makes these maneuvers simpler. These four sutures can then be held, to be tied after completion of an anterior colporrhaphy. The Velcro strips that come in the laparoscopy drapes, which we use in vaginal surgery, will adhere to each side of the Lone Star Retractor. The suspension sutures will remain straight in the Velcro straps, avoiding the otherwise ever-present tangling.

Just before tying the suspension sutures it is useful to have the bladder empty, mild Trendelenburg, and wet gloves. We tie the Prolene suspension sutures first, as the knot moves the most easily and is least apt to catch. Then the PDS sutures are tied. If free mesh has been placed in the anterior compartment, for example in recurrent cystocele repair, the PDS suspension sutures can be brought through the apical aspect of the mesh before tying. The sutures are held and not cut. Cystoscopy with Indigo Carmine (1 amp IV), will demonstrate projective blue flow from both ureteral orifices if patent. If one or both ureters fail to produce dye-stained urine, one should serially remove sutures, including anterior colporrhaphy and vault suspension until the dye appears. Ureteral stenting is sometimes indicated. We then examine the cuff to see if additional cuff closure is necessary between the suspension sutures. If it is, cutting all but the lateral two suspension sutures and tractioning them will make the cuff more accessible for closure.

CYSTOSCOPY WITH DYE

The bladder should be thoroughly viewed during any incontinence or anterior and/or apical vaginal reconstructive operation. A 70° or 30° cystoscope will work well to view the internal anatomy and function of the trigone, ureteral orifices, and the remainder of the bladder mucosa. Intravenous indigo carmine (5 mL) may take from 3 to 15 minutes to appear, in a projectile manner, from the ureters. Ibeanu and colleagues[12] have recently shown that the indigo carmine dye from the ureteral orifices need not be projectile to have confidence that the ureters are functional.

Enterocele Repair

The problem of posthysterectomy vaginal vault prolapse and enterocele can be addressed either abdominally with a sacrocolpopexy or vaginally with an enterocele repair and vault suspension. The vaginal approach will be discussed here. One can approach a posthysterectomy vaginal vault prolapse and enterocele either apically with an elliptical incision around the cuff or via the Nichols' approach—transperineally, using a curved-Mayo scissor dissection of the superficial posterior vaginal skin from the underlying connective tissue and old obstetrical scar, working cephalad to gain entry into the rectovaginal space.

Whichever approach is chosen, dissection in the superior aspect of the rectovaginal space will reveal the possible enterocele sac. A small or even moderately sized enterocele, particularly in a woman with obesity and one or more previous pelvic operations, may be quite difficult to differentiate from the anterior rectal wall or other surrounding tissues. Gentle manipulation of this potential sac with a Russian forceps, while the opposite index finger is flexed in the rectal ampulla, will usually assist in identification. Sharp entry into the sac is confirmed with two small Breisky retractors showing bowel. The neck, or narrowest portion of the peritoneal hernia, is easily noted. Superficial to that, the redundant peritoneum of the enterocele can be dissected and removed. A thorough high uterosacral ligament vaginal vault suspension performed at this point will elevate the vaginal cuff and peritoneal neck and also effectively close it.

Alternatively, one can place a formal peritoneal purse-string suture for closure of the enterocele sac at its neck. Prior to the high uterosacral ligament vaginal vault suspension becoming a dominant vaginal reconstructive operation, enterocele sacs were typically ligated at their neck, after identification, incision, and dissection, with a delayed-absorbable or permanent purse-string suture. Before placing the purse-string suture, one would carefully palpate both ureters. Then, the surgeon could be sure to purposefully avoid them during purse-string placement. In a purse-string suture, 8 to 10 bites through the peritoneum and the subperitoneal retinaculum are taken all at the same level, ending with the last bite very near the first. The ends are held. If a uterosacral suspension has been done, these culdeplasty sutures would be tied before tying the purse-string. At this point, a cystoscopy with dye would demonstrate ureteral patency.

Sacrospinous Fixation

There are advantages to performing vaginal sacrospinous fixation (SSF) for apical prolapse: it restores a functional vagina with a normal, horizontally inclined upper vaginal axis (albeit deviated, particularly if SSF is unilateral) resting on the levator plate.[13] Because it is an extraperitoneal procedure, compared with abdominal sacrocolpopexy and requires less operative time, it has a lower rate of postoperative ileus, intestinal obstruction, incisional pain, and other transabdominal surgical risks. A disadvantage of the SSF is its 23% rate of postoperative anterior compartment prolapse.

When performing SSF, we recommend placing the sutures into the sacrospinous ligament (SSL) under direct visualization rather than by palpation. Following completion of a hysterectomy, if indicated, we make a V-shaped incision in the perineum. The skin and posterior vaginal wall are dissected from the perineal body until the avascular rectovaginal space is entered. After making matching parallel incisions in the cephalad direction on the posterior wall, the redundant segment is excised. At this time, we open, mobilize, and resect, then close any enterocele sac.

This procedure may be performed either unilaterally or bilaterally; a right SSF will be described. The right rectal pillar separates the rectovaginal space from the right pararectal space and has two layers of condensed areolar tissue. The SSL is located deep within the coccygeus muscle, which runs through the pararectal space from the ischial spine to the sacrum. Easy exposure of the coccygeus muscle–SSL complex depends on how thick the rectal pillar is and whether it is fused or exists as two distinct layers.

The right rectal pillar is perforated 1.5 fingerbreadths posteromedial to the ischial spine. If the pillar is weak or thin, it may be easily pierced with one's fingertip; otherwise, we use scissor tips or tonsil forceps. We insert our middle and index fingers through a "window" in the rectal pillar into the right pararectal space. The medial tip of the middle finger should touch the medical surface of the ischial spine. Exposure is achieved with a Breisky or Nichols retractor anteriorly and another medially. Extra viewing and suturing space may be secured with a Vital Vue suction/irrigation light laterally. To pass the suture, one may use either a Capio transvaginal suture-capturing device (Boston Scientific, Natick, MA), Nolan or other heavy needle-driver, Miya hook ligature carrier (Zinnanti Surgical, Woodland Hills, CA), Deschamps ligature carrier, or Shutt suture punch (Conmed Linvatec, Largo, FL). Regardless of which instrument is used, we pass the sutures through—rather than around—the ligament, 2 fingerbreadths medial to the ischial spine, to avoid the posterior gluteal vessels, the lateral sciatic nerve, and the pudendal neurovascular complex. Using the Miya hook, two sutures may be passed simultaneously. One absorbable and one nonabsorbable are recommended. After passing the sutures through the SSL, we catch them with a nerve hook and cut the loop in the center and pair each end with its respective free suture.

One method of bringing the softer, more mobile vagina to the surface of the coccygeus muscle and ligament is the "pulley-stitch." We sew the anterior ends of the sutures to the undersurface of the posterior vaginal apex. The vaginal suture end is tied to itself, making the posterior apex a fixed point. The posterior limb of the sacro-spinous stitch is left free. We then begin the upper portion of the posterior vaginal skin closure, closing the upper 2 inches. Using traction on the posterior limb of the suture, we pull the vaginal apex directly into the coccygeus muscle and sacrospinous ligament and use a square knot to fix it in place. With a simple square knot, the second or "safety" stitch can be readily tied. Posterior colporrhaphy and perineorrhaphy, if indicated, are then completed. The vagina may then be lightly packed with gauze for 24 hours.

ANTERIOR COLPORRHAPHY
Incision

The anterior wall is elevated with Allis clamps in the midline at any point where one can grasp it atraumatically. Intracutaneous infiltration with a 0.5% bupivacaine/1:200,000 epinephrine, using a 30-gauge needle is carried out until the peri-incisional area is fully blanched. The anterior wall is incised from apex to 1 cm short of the urethral meatus and proximally to the apex. If a mid-urethral sling is to be placed, the incision should stop 1 cm proximal to the urethrovesical crease.

If anterior colporrhaphy is performed with vaginal hysterectomy, circumferential cervico-vaginal incision can be followed by midline anterior full-thickness incision between two Allis clamps halfway toward the urethral meatus. Early proximal dissec-tion (either full or split-thickness, **Fig. 3**) at this point demonstrates local anatomy to ease safe anterior cul-de-sac entry. Following hysterectomy and culdeplasty, one returns to the anterior dissection.

Absent hysterectomy, the same full-thickness curved Mayo scissor midline vertical incision directly into the vesicovaginal space is used and extended from apex anteri-orly to 1 cm short of urethral meatus, as the two Allis clamps grasp and advance along the cut-edge. Retracting the skin edges with blue Lone Star stays will improve exposure.

Dissection

Now in the vesicovaginal space (VVS) with excellent exposure and lighting, the next step is dissection. It may be effectively performed via two alternative depths (see **Fig. 3**). The bladder may be dissected from the full-thickness anterior vaginal wall, developing and remaining in the VVS. This is the anterior equivalent of the Goff posterior colporrhaphy dissection.[14] Alternatively, the dissection from the VVS may split the anterior vaginal wall between the epithelium and the muscular-adventitial layer, as it is performed posteriorly in the split-thickness Bullard modification (preferred by this author).[14] This technique leaves a distinct layer of vaginal fibromus-cularis/adventitia between bladder and vaginal epithelium for separate repair. This dissection path, if continued laterally, just under the ischiopubic rami, gains entry into the retropubic, paravesical space for the vaginal paravaginal repair.

Sharp technique throughout is advised whether using full- or split-thickness dissec-tion depth. One or two Allis clamps hold the vaginal skin edge above (distal to) the line of dissection. The operator's nondominant hand holds the clamp(s) with that index finger at the outside location of the vagina where it is being dissected inside. The dominant hand holds a curved Mayo scissors and that index finger stabilizes the fulcrum of the scissors. In a real sense, the outside index finger communicates data to its inside counterpart regarding depth of dissection. There are many technical features that can only be adequately exchanged in the operating room. In general, we find it best to keep the scissors parallel and next to the curve of the inner vaginal

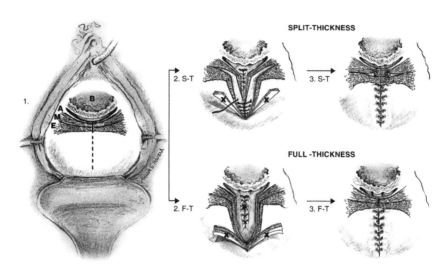

Fig. 3. Two depths of anterior dissection/repair. 1. Layers of the anterior vaginal wall and bladder on schematic cross-section; from vaginal lumen going into bladder lumen (B) in the following manner: E, vaginal epithelium; M, vaginal muscularis; A, vaginal adventitia merging into bladder adventitia, bladder muscularis, bladder mucosa. The solid line represents the full-thickness (F-T) vaginal incision into the VVS, whereas the dotted line shows the incision's continuation towards the apex. 2. S-T. In the split-thickness (S-T) or Bullard anterior dissection, a plane is sharply dissected between the E and the M, whose A/P and lateral limits are individually determined. A large prolapsing bladder may be inverted with a 3-0-polygalactin purse-string and imbricated with one or more running or interrupted suture lines in the bladder serosa. Repair strength comes from 2-0 polydioxanone running suture of M. Medially redundant E (x) is trimmed. 3. S-T. E closure with running 2-0 polygalactin. 2. F-T. Dissection plane in this full-thickness (F-T) Goff dissection is between vaginal A and bladder A (shared by both organs). As in 2.S-T, prolapsing bladder is imbricated. F-T medial vagina is excised (x). 3. F-T. Repair strength comes from F-T 2-0 polydioxanone interrupted sutures. (*From* Young SB, Kambiss SK. Anterior wall support defects. In: Bent AE, Cundiff GW, Swift SE, editors. Ostergard's Urogynecology and Pelvic Floor Dysfunction. 6th edition. Philadelphia: Lippincott, Williams & Wilkins; 2008; with permission.)

wall, as one cuts and pushes with very little use of spreading, using traction and countertraction, looking to find and enlarge (develop) a potential plane. Traction on whatever tissue is being dissected off the vagina (vaginal muscularis or bladder) toward the contralateral side reveals small sites of vaginal attachment to incise. The assistant uses a Russian-type atraumatic forceps to give gentle countertraction, thereby demonstrating the exact connective tissue/skin attachment site to incise. The countertraction on attached connective tissue frequently creates a triangulated appearance, with the narrow end attached to the inside vaginal skin to be cut. Immediately after a definite plane is established (white, hypovascular, shiny), the flexed dominant index fingertip is inserted into that plane, to that point where the plane ends and the fingertip is extended against the vaginal undersurface. This will deepen and enlarge the dissected plane. This act is in complete counterdistinction to wrapping a Ray-tec sponge around one's index finger and with or worse, without an open plane, bluntly pulling the vaginal muscularis or bladder off the epithelium; such a rough, blunt dissection act ought to be avoided.

The dissection may be ended halfway to the level of the ischiopubic rami, or carried laterally part or all the way to the rami. We prefer to carry sharp dissection laterally out to the level of the medial aspect of the ischiopubic rami, apically to the anterior fornix or cuff, and distally to the periurethral connective tissue. The distal dissection limit must often be modified if a concomitant anti-incontinence procedure is to be performed. Similarly, one may not wish to disturb a well-supported anterior vault. There is, at least a theoretical issue over performing a central repair, especially apically, when a paravaginal defect may have been missed. The anterior colporrhaphy may be seen to aggravate an ongoing lateral defect. Could this be one of the many possible factors responsible for the high (29%) rate of recurrent pelvic organ prolapse (POP) surgery?[15] There exists, therefore, an ethical and clinical imperative to get the site or sites of anterior wall defect on clinical exam and EUA "right the first time."

Venous bleeding can be encountered anywhere during anterior compartment dissection, but can be most troublesome lateral to the urethrovesical junction. The minor vessels of the incision or the more apical dissection can be fully controlled with cautery or hemostat/forceps and cautery. However, the larger paraurethral venous sinuses, especially those proximate to the anterior aspect of the inferior pubic ramus, require more attention. Figure-of-eight sutures may effectively surround these low-pressure complexes, and the knots are brought down gently. We use 2-0 polyga-lactin on a UR-6 (5/8 circle urologic) needle passed on a Heaney needle driver in this tight space to surround the bleeding sinus while making the acute curve complete short of the bone. Direct pressure on several ray-tec sponges for 2 to 5 minutes may stop the ooze. If that fails, a very effective technique uses triangular strips of Gel-foam-100 (Pharmacia & Upjohn, Bridgewater, NJ), placed narrow-end first with a dressing forceps into "the bloody angle" between the ramus, pubic bone, and bladder and is almost uniformly successful.

Repair

Regardless of the depth of dissection and repair about to be performed, exposure in the VVS allows optional plication and imbrication of a large prolapsing bladder and its adventitia. This reduces the width of the VVS, but adds little strength to the repair. It may be first plicated with a purse-string or other type running 2-0 polygalactin or polyglycolic acid suture and imbricated with an interrupted or running second and sometimes third layer of the same material. The strength of the repair comes from the next layer. In the Goff full-thickness repair, the weakened distended excess medial vaginal wall is excised. Then, the repair's strength comes from suturing the undersurface of the more lateral full-thickness anterior vaginal wall where the muscular-adventitial tissue has been left connected to the epithelium. Using Bullard's split-thickness technique, the dissected muscular-adventitial vaginal layer over the bladder is carefully examined. Generally, poor tissue and specific tears related to pathophysiology or dissection are noted and strategies for correction developed. Individual, site-specific tears are repaired with interrupted 2-0 polydiaxonone. The entire dissected layer can be brought together and reinforced in the midline using one or two layers of interrupted or running 2-0 polydiaxonone. Skin redundancy can be trimmed and the edges of the vaginal epithelium brought together with running 2-0 polygalactin.

PARAVAGINAL REPAIR

George White published in 1909[16] and Cullen Richardson and colleagues in 1976[17] established that a major aspect of vaginal support consists of lateral connective tissue attachments from the lateral sulci of the anterior vaginal wall to the arcus tendineus fascia pelvis (ATFP). Disruptions of these attachments can be corrected with high success rates using the paravaginal repair be it via vaginal,[18,19] abdominal,[20,21] or laparoscopic approaches.[22,23]

VAGINAL PARAVAGINAL REPAIR

The vaginal paravaginal repair uses permanent sutures around the ATFP, under direct observation within the retropubic/paravesical space by careful dissection from the vesicovaginal space. Maximum exposure and lighting are critical. Use of the Lone Star retractor with yellow and blue hooks, a laparoscopy drape with two Velcro straps on the medial thighs, catheterized bladder, empty rectum, and a weighted speculum are all important. Additional lighting instruments that we use include the Vital Vue Gyn-tip (United States Surgical, a division of Tyco Healthcare, LP) and the Miyazaki lighted retractor (Marina Medical, Hollywood, FL).

The lateral limit of the anterior colporrhaphy dissection, the ischiopubic ramus, is the beginning of the paravaginal dissection. First the ischial spine is palpated laterally under the apical end of the ramus. Naturally, its anterior facet feels different than it usually does from a posterior perspective. Running one's dominant index finger medially, anterior, and cephalad, the operator comes to the inferolateral pubic bone. It is not quite as distinct as the anterior aspect of the spine, and feels like a rough corner. These two points are critical because they mark the boundaries of the linear archus tendineus to which one will reattach the vaginal anterior lateral sulcus.

At 1 to 2 cm anterior to the spine, slight lateral, perpendicular pressure on a closed curved Mayo scissor, just under the ramus and over the volar aspect of the nondominant index fingertip very gently opens a small window into the retropubic space (RPS). This window is enlarged minimally with cautious scissor and finger-tip dissection, before gently placing serially sized Breisky or Deaver retractors anteriorly and a Miyazaki lighted retractor medially—all *very deliberately* just within the window. Proof that the dissection is correctly in the RPS is obtained by demonstrating the pelvic sidewall, retropubic fat, and the fatty cylindrical obturator neurovascular bundle descending at the far limit of the exposure. The ATFP is prepared for suturing by carefully retracting the bladder medially with the Miya lighted retractor and the ureter and anterior abdominal wall anteriorly with a Deaver (preferably wrapped with a Lite-Mat). A posterior Breisky is optional. One tries to obtain optimal exposure before placing arcus sutures. Nevertheless, one must be extremely cautious with forward movement of the retractor tips. If the long retractor tips are adjusted forward, without direct observation by the surgeon, they are at high risk of endangering large veins.

Damaged paravaginal attachments result in an ATFP that is quite variable to palpation and appearance. Palpating between the two landmark limits of the arcus will show whether it is present or has been torn away from the sidewall. In the latter case, we suture in the same manner as if it were present. The line (arcus) that is or was between the two bony prominences, serves as a series of points, 1 cm apart. Each point marks the center of a circle around which a 0-grade permanent suture is sewn, having a diameter of 2 cm, and is passed perpendicular to the ATFP. The CT-1 type needle pass may begin with a 1-cm 90° curve on either the obturator internus or levator ani side, turning widely around the real or surmised arcus and turning back 90° widely to include a 1-cm pass through the other muscle. We begin suturing 1.5 cm anterior to the spine (**Fig. 4**) and move up 1 cm apart toward the pubic bone with each successive vaginal paravaginal repair (VPVR) stitch. Four to six sutures are placed on each side in a complete bilateral paravaginal defect. We use a Nolan needle driver and long straight needle driver for needle retrieval. Alternatively, some prefer the Capio Suture Capturing Device (Boston Scientific, Natick, MA). Gentle traction in the opposite

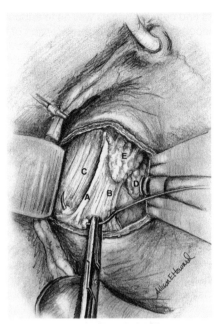

Fig. 4. Vaginal paravaginal repair: First suture. A, Arcus tendineus fasica pelvis (ATFP); B, obturator internus muscle; C, levator ani muscle; D, obturator neurovascular bundle; E, retropubic fat. (*From* Young SB, Kambiss SK. Anterior wall support defects. In: Bent AE, Cundiff GW, Swift SE, editors. Ostergard's Urogynecology and Pelvic Floor Dysfunction. 6th edition. Philadelphia: Lippincott, Williams & Wilkins; 2008; with permission.)

direction on the arcus suture should give the sense of a secure purchase. Any doubt mandates a second slightly deeper throw while placing mild traction on the first throw. The ATFP sutures are kept parallel in Velcro straps. Before sewing the arcus sutures to the vagina and bladder, we perform the anterior muscularis plication and other anterior compartment procedures as indicated.

The ATFP sutures are then sewn to the connective tissue layers of the bladder and the vagina at matching levels. For each of these two points, we locate halfway between the ramus and the midline. Sewing the vagina and bladder to the ATFP at points too lateral results in an inadequate lift. Choosing points too medial yields a very dramatic anterolateral elevation of a vagina that one cannot close. But sewing and tying at the midpoints yields dramatic anterolateral lift and tension-free skin closure. Any remaining slight excess epithelium is trimmed and the vagina closed with running 2-0 polyglycolic acid or polygalactin suture.

TRANSVERSE DEFECT REPAIR

Following vaginal hysterectomy, the anterior vaginal wall is shorter than the posterior wall because of cervical excision. The connective tissue supports of the proximal anterior vagina will also be weakened if there is a transverse defect (TD). This leaves a large anterior apical gap and an even larger area without a muscular-adventitial layer. Repair of the TD (TDR) is performed as part of the culdeplasty. When supporting the apex and orienting the vault more horizontally over the levator plate with the high (or deep) uterosacral ligament vaginal vault suspension (HUS), one must remember the importance of lifting the anterior as well as the posterior vault. It is important to repair a transverse defect and cervical gap as well as to support the proximal anterior wall. Many techniques accomplish this.[24,25] Is the inclusion of the anterior apical skin in the HUS adequate to close the cervical gap and repair the transverse defect? Do we not often leave a significant anterior apical gap in women suffering from transverse defect?

The technique that follows is one possible method to repair a TD, close the cervical gap, and help suspend the anterior apex. One or two 0-polydiaxonone or polypropylene sutures support, close, and elevate the anterior and posterior lateral apices to the mid-cardinal ligament bilaterally, while a midline suture connects both anterior and posterior apices, right and left sides (**Fig. 5**). During a preliminary vaginal hysterectomy, the cardinal ligament pedicle must be taken in a manner similar to preparing the uterosacral ligaments for HUS. Essentially, this means palpation and pedicle preparation such that the cardinal ligament pedicle will be free of vessels, yet its support value maximized. After completion of the anterior repair, a running suture is used to close the anterior wall. It is tied with 2 cm left open at the midline apex. The TDR suture picks up the fibromuscular layer and the undersurface of the right anterior lateral apex. The ureter is repalpated. A Breisky retractor will expose the cardinal ligament pedicle. Then the suture is placed through the cardinal ligament from up to down, 2 cm proximal to the ligature. It is then sewn, similarly to the right posterior lateral apex. After the contralateral TDR stitch has been placed, the midline suture obtains purchase on both

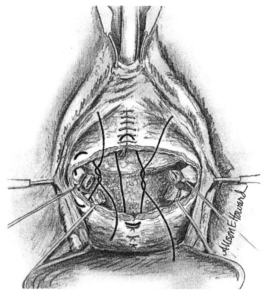

Fig. 5. Transverse defect repair. The first TDR stitch starts anteriorly. It is placed 1 to 2 cm from either lateral apex: 1 cm from the cut-edge, starting inside. Next, a secure bite is taken, at least 2 cm up from the cut-edge of the cardinal ligament pedicle. The anterior lateral apical bite is repeated as a mirror image at the posterior lateral apex, ending inside opposite the suture's anterior entry point. Before anterior and cardinal bites, the ureter can be re-palpated. After placing one suture on each side, a central suture is placed 1 cm off both midline and cut-edge, securing both anterior and posterior apices. Simulation of tying by crossing the three TDR stitches will define the need for a second lateral suture on one or both sides. (*From* Young SB, Kambiss SK. Anterior wall support defects. In: Bent AE, Cundiff GW, Swift SE, editors. Ostergard's Urogynecology and Pelvic Floor Dysfunction. 6th edition. Philadelphia: Lippincott, Williams & Wilkins; 2008; with permission.)

sides of anterior and posterior apices. If a posterior apical wedge has been excised, this must be considered. The HUS, with or without wedge excision, may have already been performed and wedge closure completed. This should not compromise TDR exposure and will facilitate its posterior apical suture site choice. Even in the absence of a transverse defect, these three sutures help support the apex and close the anterior apical gap left from cervical excision.

Once satisfied with all support and anterior work, the sutures are tied and held to facilitate removal should cystoscopy reveal a ureteral problem. Thorough intravesical evaluation for sutures and ureteral patency via IV indigo carmine is important following every major anterior and/or apical operation. Failure to see projectile blue dye from one or both ureteral orifices mandates investigation.

To our knowledge this is a new modification for anterior apical support and transverse defect repair. We have found no studies of any kind either describing this technique or quantifying its results in the literature since 1966.

PUBOURETHRAL LIGAMENT PLICATION

When performing an anterior colporrhaphy, what is the surgeon to do when the patient complains of stress urinary incontinence and demonstrates urethral hypermobility (UHM) but no urodynamic stress incontinence on urodynamic evaluation? One can repeat the cough stress test. If it remains negative, one may feel hard-pressed to perform a definitive anti-incontinence procedure. This is a good opportunity to perform the single-suture pubourethral ligament plication (PULP), which will decrease UHM and may eliminate SUI. Following an anterior vaginal dissection, the plication is performed. Condensations of pelvic connective tissue between proximal urethra and pubic bone are thoroughly secured with serial Allis clamps anterolaterally at 45°. A single far-near, near-far delayed absorbable suture around both Allis clamps will plicate this pubourethral connective tissue creating a proximal suburethral strap. The lateral bites are deep and the medial bites are superficial. A midline, paravaginal, or any other indicated reconstructive procedure may be performed. Then, redundant vaginal skin is excised and the anterior wall closed with a running 2-0 polygalactin or polyglycolic acid suture. We do not consider this an anti-incontinence procedure; rather a urethral stabilizer.

POSTERIOR COLPORRHAPHY

One ought to clearly know preoperatively the extent to which the rectocele referable symptoms cause patient bother, the posterior compartment pelvic organ prolapse quantification (POP-Q) measurements and stage, and, if possible, the patient's desire for future coital function. A careful rectal exam with two Breisky retractors gently separating the lateral vaginal walls, performed after completion of the anterior, apical, and/or incontinence portions of the operation will demonstrate the size, extent, and often the etiology of the rectocele.

The surgical description that follows is modified from the two-incision, transverse dissection, Bullard-type of posterior colporrhaphy.[14] The hymeneal remnants at 4 to 5 and 7 to 8 o'clock are grasped with Glassman or Allis clamps, such that when crossed, the introitus admits three moistened fingers without tightness. The perineal skin incision is marked between the two clamps as a "V" when the perineum is only mildly deficient and the vaginal outlet mildly relaxed. It is marked as a "U"-shaped incision, excising more perineal skin, when there has been more damage to the outlet and perineum. The incision line may be infiltrated with local anesthetic and vasoconstrictor. We use 0.5% bupivacaine in epinephrine 1:200,000 in a control syringe, through a 30-gauge needle, intracutaneously. The incision is usually made with a #10 scalpel blade; the second scalpel pass is angled inward at 45 degrees to begin dissection of the perineal skin flap. For the remainder of the posterior dissection, a curved Mayo scissors—directed transversely between the undersurface of the superficial perineal and posterior vaginal epithelium—is used to sharply take all the old obstetrical scar and fibromuscular layer off the epithelium. The scissor tips are held closed and gently advanced transversely in an attempt to get between these two layers (**Fig. 6**).

At the medial aspects of the two previously placed Allis-type clamps, the perineal incision is carried cephalad, up the posterior vaginal wall, creating matching parallel incisions, no less than 1 cm medial to the posterior lateral sulci to allow adequate vaginal caliber for comfortable coitus. This perineal and distal posterior skin flap is held in Allis, or better still, a Krobach clamp. The surgeon's nondominant hand holds this instrument up vertically, with the middle-finger gently pushing on the luminal side of the posterior skin, at the point of dissection. This facilitates entry of the scissor tip into the split-thickness (Bullard) plane. The scissor tip is removed and only its lower blade reinserted, always remaining transverse (**Fig. 7**). At a point as close as possible to the distal end of the skin flap, the scissor tips are brought together, anatomically freeing all but the superficial epithelium. This dissection continues until an area is fully freed. Then the two matching parallel posterior incisions are carried further up the posterior compartment. As these incisions progress, the Allis clamps are moved up to points just lateral to the furthest extent of the two incisions. As the transverse dissection and two incisions progress cephalad, the connective tissue usually becomes a bit looser and entry into the bluish-tinged rectovaginal space is obtained. The scissors may now be directly cephalad and opened widely revealing the damaged

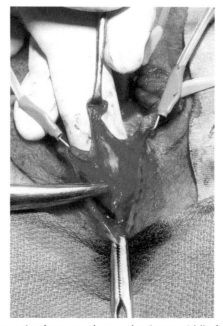

Fig. 6. Bi-digital proprioception between the nondominant middle finger and the dominant index finger at the fulcrum of the dissection scissor appreciates the proper thickness of posterior skin to achieve and thus, the amount of pressure to place on the scissor tips.

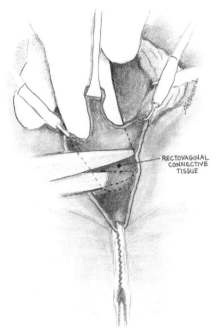

Fig. 7. The lower scissor blade is inside the connective tissue to be cut and the transversely placed scissor is elevated distally as far as possible, leaving maximal connective tissue in situ.

rectovaginal connective tissue (septum), as shown in **Fig. 8**. Placement of a self-retaining Rigby retractor intravaginally, while an intrarectal index finger is partially flexed, will clearly define the details, directions, and limits of the connective tissue defects.

For repair, we usually close all site-specific defects and then run a vertical plication suture, obtaining apical purchase on the uterosacral or other strong apical tissue. As the plication progresses, we pick up the best available connective tissue with each bite and carry it down for anchoring into the perineal body, thus reestablishing posterior continuity between Delancey levels I, II, and III. For connective tissue plication, we use 2-0 polydiaxonone suture on a CT-2 needle.

The redundant posterior vaginal skin is consequently removed in the dissection and the skin is closed, again from apical connective tissue to perineal body, with continuous 2-0 polygalactin suture.

As the posterior colporrhaphy is completed and the perineum sits open, awaiting reconstruction, we consider the history, particularly concerning coital dysfunction symptoms: looseness, lack of coital sensation, inability to hold partner in vagina; or alternatively acoital status secondary to whatever reason and importantly, the desire for coital activity in the future. A posterior colporrhaphy and perineorrhaphy may be performed a bit more aggressively, leaving a slightly narrowed vaginal tube and introitus and a long thick perineum. This would likely result in diminished risk of POP recurrence, while making future coitus difficult or impossible. I believe that a fully competent middle-aged or older woman, who is no longer coitally active, ought to be given the right to make a permanent judgment regarding her coital future—if she desires. This result may be achieved without using obliterative procedures (covered by Wheeler elsewhere in this issue).

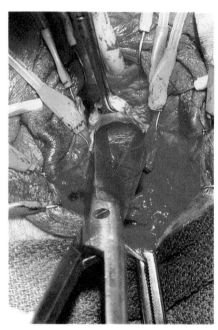

Fig. 8. Rectovaginal space entry is confirmed by directing the scissor tips cephalad and pointing anteriorly. Spreading the tips reveals the bluish-tinged open rectovaginal space with the rectovaginal septal connective tissue posteriorly.

For the standard perineorrhaphy in a coitally active woman (or anyone who wants to maintain that option) we plan the vagina and introitus to comfortably accommodate her partner. We try to leave the vagina from hymeneal remnant to apex of a cylindrical-shape that easily admits three-fingerbreadths.

"Crown-stitches" of 2-0 or 0-polydiaxonone are placed in a mirror image manner, from inside/deep perineal to outside/subcutaneous vulva and back in the opposite way, thus bringing back the retracted ends of the perineal body musculature (bulbocavernosus and transverse perineal muscle) into the new perineal body (**Fig. 9**). The size and number of these crown-stitches and the needle used (CT-1, CT, or CT-X) will determine the extent of perineal enlargement, lengthening the posterior vagina and controlling introital width. We use between two and five of the sutures. They are placed as the hands of a clock, held and tied after all are placed. Crossing the stitches without tying demonstrates their effect and allows one to determine if they should be made using smaller or larger bites and where the next crown-stitches should be placed. They must not be tied tightly.

If there remains a deep perineal gap after the crown stitches are tied, this can be closed with interrupted 2-0 polygalactin. The skin can be approximated with 4-0 monocryl subcuticular interrupted sutures.

The vaginal approach to pelvic organ prolapse repair is a superb and natural approach to the effective performance of reconstructive procedures. Through the works of Dr David Nichols and others beginning 40 years ago, as well as the Vaginal Surgeons Society (established in 1974, for many years now the Society of Gynecologic Surgeons), the discipline of vaginal surgery has become a mainstay of benign gynecologic therapy. Over the years, the vaginal approach has proven to be a safe

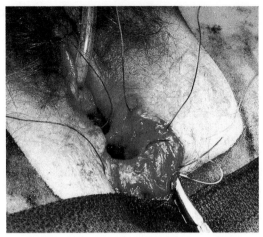

Fig. 9. Wide bites with a large needle better secure and reconstitute the retracted ends of the perineal musculature. In a right-handed surgeon, to maximize the effectiveness of the left side bite, the wrist must be open (fully pronated).

and efficacious method of alleviating the disabling effects of pelvic floor dysfunction. Currently, our gastroenterology and general surgery colleagues are beginning to find the "natural orifice" in achieving their own intra-abdominal therapeutic goals, while affording their patients the benefit of avoiding an "unnatural" incision.

REFERENCES

1. Ricci JV. The development of gynecologic surgery and instruments. San Francisco(CA): Norman Publishing; 1990.
2. Ribeiro SC, Ribeiro RM, Santos NC, et al. A randomized study of total abdominal, vaginal and laparoscopic hysterectomy. Int J Gynaecol Obstet 2003;83:37–43.
3. Barber MD, Cundiff GW, Weidner AC, et al. Accuracy of clinical assessment of paravaginal defects in women with anterior vaginal wall prolapse. Am J Obstet Gynecol 1999;181(1):87–90.
4. Segal JL, Vassallo BJ, Kleeman SD, et al. Paravaginal defects: prevalence and accuracy of preoperative detection. Int Urogynecol J Pelvic Floor Dysfunct 2004;15(6):378–83.
5. Hofmeister FJ. "Cinefluorography" [video]. Marquette University Medical School, Milwaukee Hospital, Milwaukee County Hospital, Minnesota.
6. Miller NF. A new method of correcting complete eversion of the vagina: with or without complete prolapse; report of two cases. Surg Gynecol Obstet 1927;44:550–5.
7. McCall ML. Posterior culdeplasty: surgical correction of enterocele during vaginal hysterectomy; a preliminary report. Obstet Gynecol 1957;10:595–602.
8. Montella JM, Morrill MY. Effectiveness of the McCall culdeplasy in maintaining support after vaginal hysterectomy. Int Urogynecol J 2005;16:226–9.
9. Chene G, Tardieu AS, Savary D, et al. Anatomical and functional results of McCall cludoplasty in the prevention of enteroceles and vaginal vault prolapse after vaginal hysterectomy. Int Urogynecol J 2008;19:1007–11.
10. Elkins TE, Hopper JB, Goodfellow K, et al. Initial report of anatomic and clinical comparison of the sacrospinous ligament fixation to the high McCall culdeplasty

for vaginal cuff fixation at hysterectomy for uterine prolapse. J Pelvic Surg 1995;1: 12–7 [discussion: 383].

11. Buller JL, Thompson JR, Cundiff GW, et al. Uterosacral ligament: description of anatomic relationships to optimize surgical safety. Obstet Gynecol 2001;97: 873–9.

12. Ibeanu OA, Chesson RR, Echols KT, et al. Urinary tract injury during hysterectomy based on universal cystoscopy. Obstet Gynecol 2009;113:6–10.

13. Young SB, Zylstra S. Managing vaginal vault prolapse with Sacrospinous fixation. Contemp Ob Gyn 1995;40(7):64–72.

14. Nichols DH, Randall CL, editors. Vaginal surgery. 3rd edition. Baltimore(MD): Williams & Wilkins; 1996. p. 283–4.

15. Olsen AL, Smith VJ, Bergstrom JO, et al. Epidemiology of surgically managed pelvic organ prolapse and urinary incontinence. Obstet Gynecol 1997;89(4): 501–6.

16. White GR. Cystocele, a radical cure by suturing lateral sulci of vagina to white line of pelvic fascia. JAMA 1909;21:1707–10.

17. Richardson AC, Lyons JB, Williams NL. A new look at pelvic relaxation. Am J Obstet Gynecol 1976;126:568–73.

18. Weber AM, Walter MD. Anterior vaginal prolapse: review of anatomy and techniques of surgical repair. Obstet Gynecol 1997;89:311–8.

19. Young SB, Daman JJ, Bony LG. Vaginal paravaginal repair: one-year outcomes. Am J Obstet Gynecol 2001;185:1360–7.

20. Richardson AC. Paravaginal repair. In: Hurt WG, editor, Urogynecologic surgery, 5-3. Maryland(MD): Ashland Publishers; 1992. p. 73–80.

21. Richardson AC, Edmonds PB, Williams NL. Treatment of stress urinary incontinence due to paravaginal fascial defect. Obstet Gynecol 1981;57:357–62.

22. Weber AM. New approaches to surgery for urinary incontinence and pelvic organ prolapse from the laparoscopic perspective. Clin Obstet Gynecol 2003;46(1): 44–60.

23. Miklos JR, Moore RD, Kohli N. Laparoscopic pelvic floor repair. Obstet Gynecol Clin North Am 2004;31(3):551–65.

24. Cruikshank SH, Kovac SR. Anterior vaginal wall culdeplasty at vaginal hysterectomy to prevent posthysterectomy anterior vaginal wall prolapse. Am J Obstet Gynecol 1996;174(6):1863–9 [discussion: 1869–72].

25. Shull BL, Bachofen C, Coates KW, et al. A transvaginal approach to repair of apical and other associated sites of pelvic organ prolapse with uterosacral ligaments. Am J Obstet Gynecol 2000;183:1365–74.

Abdominal, Laparoscopic, and Robotic Surgery for Pelvic Organ Prolapse

Colleen D. McDermott, MD, FRCSC[a],
Douglass S. Hale, MD, FACOG, FACS[a,b],*

KEYWORDS

- Pelvic organ prolapse • Uterosacral • Sacral colpopexy
- Sacral colpoperineopexy • Paravaginal
- Laparoscopic • Robotic

APICAL SUPPORT
Sacral Colpopexy/Colpoperineopexy

Support of the anterior vaginal wall and, to a lesser extent, the posterior vaginal wall is related to the position of the vaginal apex.[1,2] Correction of apical support is therefore considered to be the foundation of prolapse surgery. The sacral colpopexy is an abdominal procedure that resuspends the vaginal apex to the anterior longitudinal ligament overlying the sacrum using graft material, and has often been cited as the "gold standard" surgery for pelvic organ prolapse.

Reduction of uterovaginal prolapse by anchoring the posterior uterine fundus to the anterior longitudinal ligament was first described by Arthure and Savage in 1957.[3] This technique was an attempt to prevent recurrent enteroceles that were forming after standard vaginal procedures used to correct apical prolapse.[3] The addition of graft material between the vagina and sacral promontory to reduce vaginal tension was subsequently described by Huguier and Scali in 1958 and then by Lane in 1962.[4,5] A decade later, Birnbaum described proximal placement of the graft at the S3 to S4 vertebral level to recreate the natural angulation of the vaginal plane.[6] Unfortunately,

[a] Female Pelvic Medicine and Reconstructive Surgery, Indiana University/Methodist Hospital, Urogynecology Associates, 1633 North Capitol Avenue, Suite 436, Indianapolis, IN, 46202, USA
[b] Department of Obstetrics and Gynecology, Division of Urogynecology, Indiana University, Urogynecology Associates, 1633 North Capitol Avenue, Suite 436, Indianapolis, IN 46202, USA
* Corresponding author. Department of Obstetrics and Gynecology, Division of Urogynecology, Indiana University, Urogynecology Associates, 1633 North Capitol Avenue, Suite 436, Indianapolis, IN 46202.
E-mail address: DHale@Clarian.org (D.S. Hale).

Obstet Gynecol Clin N Am 36 (2009) 585–614
doi:10.1016/j.ogc.2009.09.004
0889-8545/09/$ – see front matter © 2009 Elsevier Inc. All rights reserved.

this approach was complicated by severe hemorrhage in the presacral space. This complication led to the suggestion by Sutton that the proximal end of the graft be attached at the S1 to S2 vertebral level where one could adequately visualize the middle sacral vessels before graft placement[7] without significantly distorting the natural axis of the vagina.[8] Issues with regard to recurrent posterior vaginal wall prolapse following sacral colpopexy led to the evolution of the sacral colpoperineopexy with extension of the posterior graft down to the level of the perineal body.[9]

The colpopexy graft has evolved from a single graft, to a cone, to Y-shaped graft, to a double-strap configuration (**Fig. 1**). Compared with the Y-shape, the double-strap configuration has the advantage of individual wall tensioning without overcorrecting the urethrovesical junction.

Graft material may be either biologic (autologous, allograft, xenograft) or synthetic. Biologic grafts are thought to have the advantage of reduced erosion rates, but the disadvantage of reduced longevity. There is only one case series on sacral colpopexy using autologous fascia lata. This study reported no complications and postoperative pelvic organ prolapse quantification (POP-Q) scores at stage II or higher in all patients.[10] The use of cadaveric fascia lata in sacral colpopexy has been reported in two studies showing contrary results in anatomic cure rates (17% vs 95%,[11,12]). This disparity may represent a difference in graft harvesting and preparation, both of which have been shown to affect graft strength and viability. On the other hand, synthetic graft materials have the advantage of durability but the disadvantage of increased graft erosion rates. Nonabsorbable synthetic mesh has been classified as types I to IV based on pore size and filament type.[13] Despite the risk of mesh erosion, several investigators have reviewed and support the use of type I polypropylene mesh for sacral colpopexy, demonstrating excellent anatomic cure rates with few complications.[14–16] Comparative studies between cadaveric fascia lata and polypropylene mesh used in sacral colpopexy have shown superiority in anatomic cure rates with use of synthetic mesh material.[17,18]

Procedure

Abdominal sacral colpopexy is done in one of three ways: open laparotomy, traditional laparoscopy, or robotic-assisted laparoscopy. Selection of a particular approach is

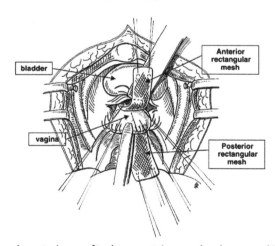

bladder

Anterior rectangular mesh

vagina

Posterior rectangular mesh

Fig. 1. Anterior and posterior graft placement in sacral colpopexy. (*From* Costantini E, Mearini L, Bini V, et al. Uterus preservation in surgical correction of urogenital prolapse. Eur Urol 2005;48(4):642–9; with permission.)

dependent on the surgeon's level of comfort and expertise, the need for concomitant procedures, and various patient factors such as age, body mass index, previous prolapse or incontinence surgery, and comorbidities that may limit the duration of anesthesia.

For all three approaches, the patient is placed in protective stirrups in the dorsal supine lithotomy position, allowing the surgeon to have access to the patient's abdomen and vagina. A laparotomy can be performed through a Pfannenstiel or midline incision. Once the peritoneal cavity has been entered, the small bowel and sigmoid colon are packed away from the surgical field. A hysterectomy may be performed if indicated, and the vaginal cuff is closed. The right ureter, iliac vessels, and aortic bifurcation are identified. A peritoneal incision is made over the sacral promontory and the presacral space is developed with the use of blunt and sharp dissection, identifying the anterior longitudinal ligament and the middle sacral vessels. Other critical anatomic landmarks are the sacral foramina, the sympathetic chain, and superior hypogastric nerve plexus. Some surgeons recommend incising the peritoneum down to the pelvic cul de sac, whereas others open the rectovaginal and vesicovaginal spaces separately from the presacral space. Opening the entire space allows for retroperitoneal placement of the graft, thereby obliterating the cul de sac by wrapping the graft around the rectosigmoid colon. This approach has the combined benefit of eliminating the potential for small bowel herniation below the graft, preventing small bowel adhesion to the exposed graft material, and providing rectal support in cases of rectal prolapse. If the surgeon chooses not to completely retroperitonealize the graft, a concomitant culdoplasty is considered.

The vagina is then elevated in a cephalad position with the use of a vaginal probe (sponge stick, end-to-end anastomosis sizer, or customized vaginal retractor; **Fig. 2**) and the peritoneum overlying the vaginal apex is incised allowing for dissection into the vesicovaginal space, separating the bladder from the anterior vaginal wall. This dissection is carried down to the superior aspect of bladder trigone (4–8 cm). The rectovaginal space is entered, dissecting the rectum away from the posterior vaginal wall until the superior aspect of the rectovaginal septum is identified. The width of both the anterior and posterior vaginal dissections should be a minimum of 4 cm. The posterior graft and then the anterior graft are attached as widely as possible on their respective vaginal walls along the length of the dissected areas. This procedure

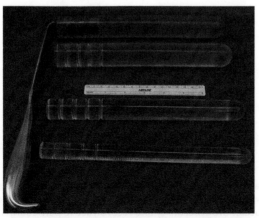

Fig. 2. Customized lucite stents for vaginal or rectal manipulation during graft placement.

is done with 3 to 4 pairs of typically nonabsorbable sutures. Each pair of sutures should be approximately 2 cm apart. Separation of the anterior and posterior grafts laterally should not exceed 2 cm, as wider separation may predispose these areas to future prolapse.

Attention is then turned back to the presacral space that was previously dissected. A total of 2 to 4 nonabsorbable sutures are anchored in the midline of the anterior longitudinal ligament. Although somewhat attenuated, the anterior longitudinal ligament is usually present at the vertebral level of S1 to S2. The anterior and posterior grafts are drawn toward the sacrum, at which point the surgeon should remove the vaginal probe and perform a vaginal examination to ensure adequate vaginal tension and prolapse reduction. The previously placed sacral sutures are passed through both leaves of the graft and tied down. The peritoneum overlying the presacral space is then closed.

A variation of the this procedure, the sacral colpoperineopexy, incorporates extension of the posterior graft down to the level of the perineal body to recreate a full-length rectovaginal septum for correction of posterior wall defects and perineal descent (**Fig. 3**). One of three approaches is used for posterior graft placement. The graft may be attached through an initial vaginal approach whereby the posterior vaginal wall is opened and the dissection extends laterally to the level of the levator ani muscles and superiorly to the level of the peritoneal cavity. The graft is anchored along the pelvic sidewall into the fascia overlying the levator ani muscles. Three sutures typically are placed on each side. The graft is also secured to the perineal body with deep sutures for strong fixation. The peritoneal cavity is entered, and the proximal portion of the graft is placed within the cavity. A perineorrhaphy is completed and followed by the abdominal portion of the procedure, whereby the graft is retrieved and fixed to the posterior vaginal wall. Alternatively the perineal body may be approached abdominally, and the distal portion of the graft can be attached to the vaginally reconstructed perineal body at the completion of the procedure. Both approaches allow for narrowing of the vaginal introitus and reconstruction of the perineal body. Because these fixations involve a combined abdominal-vaginal procedure, copious pelvic irrigation with

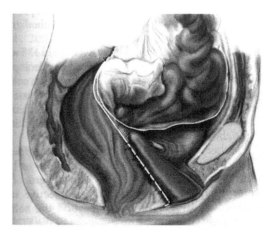

Fig. 3. Posterior graft attachment down to perineal body in sacral colpoperineopexy (no anterior graft shown). (*From* Karram M, Walters MD. Surgical treatment of vaginal vault prolapse and enterocele. Urogynecology and reconstructive pelvic surgery. 3rd edition. Philadelphia: Mosby Elsevier; 2007. p. 262–87; with permission.)

antibiotic solution is recommended following sacral graft attachment to dilute any bacteria that may have been introduced during the vaginal portion of the procedure. Finally, attachment to the perineal body may also be achieved solely through an abdominal approach when a perineorrhaphy is not required; however, strong distal fixation is more difficult to attain.

Traditional and robotic-assisted laparoscopic sacral colpopexy/colpoperineopexy use the same surgical principles as the open laparotomy approach. These 3 approaches primarily differ by the degree of invasiveness and instrumentation used to attach the graft materials. A traditional laparoscopic approach will typically use 4 abdominal incisions including a 12 mm infraumbilical port for placement of the laparoscope, a 12 mm right lower quadrant port used to pass and tie sutures, and 2 left lower quadrant 5 mm ports for instrumentation, although many port variations exist (**Fig. 4**). Incisions for the robotic approach are somewhat different, and include a 12 mm infraumbilical port for the camera, two 8 mm ports located 2 cm below and 8 cm lateral to the umbilicus for the robotic arms, and another 12 mm port placed in either the right upper or lower quadrant for passage of sutures (**Fig. 5**). Some surgeons will also use a fourth robotic arm for retraction purposes; this is also an 8 mm port and is often placed in the left lower quadrant. Once the ports are placed, the robot is positioned and docked.

Both traditional and robotic-assisted laparoscopy require the use of carbon dioxide gas to achieve a pneumoperitoneum and steep Trendelenberg positioning to assist with adequate visualization of the pelvis. To attain suitable lateral retraction of the sigmoid colon, a temporary suture can be passed through the medial cut edge of the peritoneal incision over the sacrum and pulled through the left upper abdominal wall using a suture grasper. This suture is anchored at the abdominal surface throughout the procedure, and provides a hammock that pulls the sigmoid away from the pelvis and presacral space. Alternatively, sigmoid epiploicae can be sutured to the left lateral sidewall and released at the end of the procedure.

Graft attachment to the anterior and posterior vaginal walls is essentially the same for both an open and a minimally invasive approach. Traditional laparoscopy commonly uses extracorporeal knot tying, whereas robotic-assisted laparoscopy uses intracorporeal knot tying for suture placement. Laparoscopic graft fixation to the anterior longitudinal ligament with two to four permanent sutures is highly recommended, although many surgeons will often use spiral staples. There are currently no trials comparing suture fixation to staple fixation; however, one cadaveric study showed that nonabsorbable sutures had a stronger biomechanical resistance than

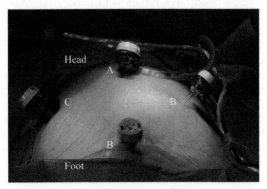

Fig. 4. Typical laparoscopic port placement for pelvic floor reconstructive surgery. A, 12 mm laparoscope port; B, 5 mm instrument port; C, 12 mm suture port.

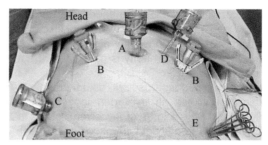

Fig. 5. Robotic-assisted laparoscopic port placement. A, 12 mm camera port; B, 8 mm robotic arm port; C, 12 mm suture port; D, 5 mm additional instrument port; E, hammock suture used to assist with left lateral retraction of sigmoid (passed through medial cut edge of peritoneum overlying the sacrum and pulled through anterior abdominal wall).

staples, and that more than one staple was required to avoid mesh detachment when placed under tension.[19] The advantage of staples over sutures is primarily the speed at which they are placed.

Surgical outcomes

Abdominal sacral colpopexy/colpoperineopexy Nygaard and colleagues[14] have previously summarized postoperative outcomes following abdominal sacral colpopexy in 98 studies between 1966 and 2004. Lack of postoperative apical prolapse was seen in 78% to 100% of patients after this procedure. When the definition was broadened to include no evidence of any postoperative prolapse, 58% to 100% of patients were considered a surgical success. The median rate for prolapse recurrence requiring reoperation was 4.4% (range, 0%–18.2%), with the majority being for anterior or posterior recurrences. The follow-up period generally ranged from 6 months to 3 years for all studies. Beer and colleagues[20] also performed an extensive review of 37 studies related to abdominal sacral colpopexy with mesh. These investigators identified an objective cure rate of 85% to 99% and a subjective cure rate of 32% to 100%. Anatomic outcomes following abdominal sacral colpoperineopexy are less defined. One study followed a small cohort of patients after abdominal sacral colpoperineopexy in which postoperative defecography showed significant correction of posterior vaginal wall defects and improvement in perineal descent with straining.[9] A more recent study demonstrated significant improvement in POP-Q measurements 12 months after abdominal sacral colpoperineopexy in 169 patients.[21]

Patients with prolapse often have issues with urinary retention or incontinence. Reduction of the vaginal apex and anterior wall with sacral colpopexy will cure issues of urinary retention in approximately 90% of patients with this preoperative symptom.[22] Patients with prolapse and symptomatic stress urinary incontinence should be investigated with preoperative urodynamics performed with and without prolapse reduction.[14] Those with proven urodynamic stress incontinence should then be asked to consent a concomitant incontinence procedure at the time of sacral colpopexy. There are no studies comparing various incontinence procedures at the time of sacral colpopexy, such that a pubovaginal autologous fascial sling, Burch urethropexy, or midurethral synthetic sling are each justifiable procedures in the treatment of urodynamic stress incontinence, and may be considered as surgical adjuvants at the time of abdominal sacral colpopexy.[23–29]

Women with prolapse who do not have symptoms of stress incontinence are less straightforward. The surgeon may choose one of three approaches to such a patient: routine use of an incontinence procedure, postoperative assessment with the possibility of a second surgery for incontinence, or preoperative urodynamics with prolapse reduction in an attempt to identify those patients who are at risk of developing postoperative incontinence and who may benefit from an incontinence procedure.[14] The Colpopexy and Urinary Reduction Efforts (CARE) trial randomized women with prolapse but no symptoms of stress incontinence to abdominal sacral colpopexy with or without concomitant Burch urethropexy.[30] Significantly more women in the control group (no Burch) had new symptoms of stress incontinence at 3 months, 1 year, and 2 years after sacral colpopexy. Another study followed a cohort of patients for 15 years after abdominal sacral colpopexy and Burch urethropexy.[31] No patients who were continent before surgery developed de novo stress incontinence. These studies suggest that a concomitant incontinence procedure at the time of abdominal sacral colpopexy in women with no preoperative stress incontinence is beneficial and should be recommended.[30]

When assessing postoperative bladder function, most studies have not distinguished between recurrence and de novo urinary incontinence.[20] Women enrolled in the CARE trial were assessed 1 year after surgery for irritative, obstructive, and stress incontinence symptoms.[32] Both irritative and obstructive symptoms significantly decreased after sacral colpopexy, regardless of whether a Burch urethropexy was performed. In addition, patients who had a concomitant Burch urethropexy had lower rates of postoperative stress incontinence (25% vs 40.1%) and urge incontinence (14.5% vs 26.8%).

Postoperative bowel function is more difficult to ascertain and has been less defined in the literature. Results are further obscured by the fact that many studies follow cohorts of patients who have sacral colpopexy with and without concomitant posterior repair. Sacral colpopexy has the potential to improve defecation by elevating the posterior vaginal wall and improving anal outlet obstruction, or it may worsen defecation by significantly disrupting the rectovaginal septum.[14] Worsening symptoms of bowel evacuation and outlet obstruction,[33,34] as well as de novo constipation and defecatory dysfunction rates of 22% to 26%,[35,36] have been reported in the literature at 1 to 3 years after abdominal sacral colpopexy.[20] In contrast, Lefranc and colleagues[31] reported no issues with constipation up to 10 years after sacral colpopexy, and patients participating in the CARE trial demonstrated a significant reduction in obstructive defecatory and other bowel symptoms 1 year after surgery regardless of concomitant posterior repair.[37]

Sexual activity after sacral colpopexy is also not sufficiently documented. Studies have generally indicated a low or improved rate of dyspareunia following abdominal sacral colpopexy.[20] Sexual function before and 1 year after abdominal sacral colpopexy was assessed in patients participating in the CARE trial.[38] This study showed a significant increase in the number of sexually active women after surgery and a significant decrease in the number of women avoiding sex because of a vaginal bulge. There was also a significant decrease in the number of women reporting intercourse limited by pain and pelvic symptoms, or fear of incontinence interfering with sexual activity. In addition, sacral colpopexy showed no impact on sexual desire.

Intra- and postoperative complications with abdominal sacral colpopexy have also been previously reviewed.[14,20] The most common complications are postoperative cystitis (median rate 10.9%), wound issues (median rate 4.6%), and hemorrhage or transfusion (median rate 4.4%). Commonly reported intraoperative events include cystotomy (median rate 3.1%), enterotomy or proctotomy (median rate 1.6%), and ureteral injury (median rate 1%). Deep venous thromboembolism or pulmonary embolism (3.3% median rate) and ileus (3.6% median rate) are other reported postoperative complications. Rare events include such things as nerve injury (femoral or obturator) and vertebral osteomyelitis. Mesh erosion is a postoperative complication well documented in the literature, but varies according to type of graft material used, concomitant procedures performed, and patient characteristics.[14,20] Nygaard and colleagues reported an overall mesh erosion rate of 3.4% and a total reoperation rate for mesh erosion of 3%. A recent study demonstrated a minor and major mesh erosion rate of 5.9% and 0.6%, respectively, after abdominal-vaginal sacral colpoperineopexy.[21]

There are currently three prospective studies comparing abdominal sacral colpopexy with vaginal colpopexy by bilateral or unilateral sacrospinous fixation.[39–41] Taking the results of these studies together, sacral colpopexy was shown to be superior to vaginal colpopexy, with a lower rate of recurrent vaginal vault prolapse, a better overall postoperative stage of prolapse, and less postoperative dyspareunia.[42] However, these studies also showed that abdominal sacral colpopexy has a longer operating time, a longer recovery period, and is more expensive than vaginal colpopexy.[42]

Laparoscopic sacral colpopexy/colpoperineopexy This approach was popularized in an attempt to improve pelvic visualization, operative morbidity, and postoperative functional results. All of the current data on laparoscopic sacral colpopexy are drawn from observational studies of various sizes, without any evidence from clinical trials and no systematic reviews of surgical outcomes.

A long-term study followed a cohort of 51 patients for 5 years after laparoscopic sacral colpopexy, and reported a 93% objective cure rate.[43] After 5 years, only three patients had recurrent vault prolapse and all went onto corrective surgery. Another group followed 103 patients who underwent laparoscopic sacral colpopexy, and showed that 92% had successful vault support, but nonvault prolapse recurrence occurred in 35% of these patients.[44] Of the patients followed, 79% stated their symptoms were cured or improved. Agarwala and colleagues[45] followed a group of patients who had either laparoscopic sacral colpopexy or cervicopexy. There was no prolapse recurrence and a subjective cure rate of 97% in all patients who underwent colpopexy. The most recent study performed by Claerhout and colleagues[46] followed 120 patients who had laparoscopic sacral colpopexy and 12 patients who had laparoscopic sacral cervicopexy. At the end of the follow-up period (mean 12.5 months), overall vault recurrence was 2%, anterior vaginal wall recurrence 3%, and posterior vaginal wall recurrence 18%. The reported subjective cure rate was 92%.

Bladder, bowel, and sexual function after laparoscopic sacral colpopexy are not well described in the literature. One study described an 86% improvement or no change in bladder symptoms after surgery.[44] Another study noted 2.8% of patients had postoperative stress urinary incontinence and 18% had de novo or persistent urge urinary incontinence; however, these symptoms were not differentiated between patients who did and did not have a concomitant sling procedure.[45] In the study performed by Claerhout and colleagues,[46] only five patients underwent midurethral sling; however, approximately half of patients with preoperative symptoms had persistence of stress incontinence (13/23 patients), urge incontinence (13/24 patients), and urgency (16/38 patients), and 5% to 7% had de novo urinary symptoms. Information from postoperative questionnaires have described a persistent obstructed defecation rate of 17% in one study,[43] with another study reporting more than half of patients with persistent constipation and 5% with de novo constipation following surgery.[46] Sexual function after laparoscopic sacral colpopexy has been reported, with de novo dyspareunia rates ranging between 9% and 23%.[43,46] Other studies have shown that approximately half of patients with preoperative dyspareunia or difficulty with intercourse improve after this procedure.[43,46]

A recent retrospective study assessed the complication rates in 402 laparoscopic sacral colpopexy cases.[47] This study compared patients who had a concomitant laparoscopic-assisted vaginal hysterectomy with those that had a previous hysterectomy. This group showed no significant difference in intra- or perioperative complications, as well as similar rates of mesh erosion between the two surgical groups. Overall complication rates for the entire cohort included 0.75% for hematoma, 2.2% for ileus or small bowel obstruction, 1.5% for bladder injury, 0.75% for bowel injury, and 0.25% for ureteric injury. After 1 year of follow-up, the overall mesh erosion rate was 1.2% and the overall mesh revision rate was also 1.2%.

There are two cohort studies that compare outcomes of laparoscopic sacral colpopexy with those of open sacral colpopexy.[48,49] Both studies showed that the laparoscopic approach was associated with significantly longer operative time, less intraoperative blood loss, and shorter hospital stay. Paraiso and colleagues[48] showed that both procedures had similar complication and reoperation rates for both recurrent prolapse and postoperative complications. Hsiao and colleagues[49] had no laparoscopic patients and only one laparotomy patient with recurrent apical prolapse. Three laparoscopic patients required repeat prolapse surgery (two anterior vaginal wall repairs and one posterior vaginal wall repair) and seven laparotomy patients required repeat surgery (four anterior vaginal wall repairs and three posterior vaginal wall repair), with similar patient numbers in each surgical group. Patients from neither group with polypropylene mesh placement had postoperative vaginal mesh erosion. This study also showed that the critical point in the learning curve with laparoscopic sacral colpopexy was 10 cases, after which the operative time significantly dropped and became comparable with the open sacral colpopexy.

In addition, a recent study by Su and colleagues[50] assessed pelvic floor quality of life outcomes in 29 patients after open sacral colpoperineopexy and 20 patients after laparoscopic sacral colpoperineopexy. There was a significant improvement in quality of life scores and POP-Q measurements at 6 months after surgery, with no significant differences between the 2 surgical groups.

Robotic-assisted laparoscopic sacral colpopexy/colpoperineopexy This procedure was devised to shorten the learning curve associated with traditional laparoscopic sacral colpopexy. The goal of using a robotic-assisted approach is to simplify the execution of laparoscopic maneuvers. The current body of literature on this approach is primarily limited to case series and cohort studies. A small series of 5 patients with an average follow-up of 4 months showed no recurrent prolapse in any vaginal compartment. Another small study of 12 patients and an average follow-up of 3.1 months reported a mean postoperative POP-Q stage of 0. Elliott and colleagues[51] followed 21 patients up until a year after surgery and reported a 95% apical cure rate. This study is the only one to report subjective outcomes with a surgical satisfaction rate of 100%. A recent study by Kramer and colleagues[52] followed 12 patients for an average of 25.2 months after robotic-assisted laparoscopic sacral colpopexy without any other concomitant procedure. This group had a significantly high reoperation rate (81%) for both prolapse and incontinence; however, only one patient had recurrent apical prolapse among those patients requiring repeat prolapse surgery. The largest series by Akl and colleagues[53] followed 80 patients and showed a recurrent prolapse rate of 3.7% (1 apical, 1 anterior, and 1 posterior). Finally, another retrospective study followed a cohort of 77 patients after robotic-assisted laparoscopic sacral colpoperineopexy.[54] This group showed only one patient with anatomic failure (stage II) and a 94% surgical satisfaction rate after 1 year of follow-up.

Postoperative bladder function has not been well investigated following robotic-assisted laparoscopic sacral colpopexy. Elliott and colleagues[51] noted that 9.5% of patients had significant postoperative urinary incontinence; however, type or de novo incontinence was not specified. Another study described resolution of preoperative urge urinary incontinence in 5 out of 6 patients (83%).[55] Kramer and colleagues[52] performed pre- and postoperative urodynamic studies on the first 7 patients in their series of robotic-assisted laparoscopic sacral colpopexy. None of these patients had a concomitant incontinence procedure at the time of sacral colpopexy. These investigators found that urodynamic parameters were not significantly changed by this procedure. In a cohort following robotic-assisted sacral colpoperineopexy, 5% required a postoperative midurethral sling procedure, 1% had persistent overactive bladder symptoms, and 19.5% had symptoms of de novo urge incontinence.[54] To date, there are no studies that describe bowel or sexual function relative to preoperative status following robotic-assisted laparoscopic sacral colpopexy.

Intra- and postoperative complications associated with robotic-assisted laparoscopic sacral colpopexy have been reported at very low rates.[51,52,55,56] The largest study to date reported a cystotomy rate of 1.2%, enterotomy rate of 1.2%, ureteric injury rate of 1.2%, postoperative ileus rate of 1.2%, and mesh erosion rate of 6%.[53] Complication rates for robotic-assisted sacral colpoperineopexy have been reported with a 5.2% cystotomy rate, 1.3% proctotomy rate, 6.5% postoperative ileus rate, and 9.1% suture or mesh erosion rate.

There is only one retrospective study comparing robotic-assisted sacral colpopexy with abdominal sacral colpopexy.[57] This group evaluated POP-Q scores at 6 weeks after surgery in 73 patients after robotic-assisted sacral colpopexy and 105 patients after an open sacral colpopexy. The robotic group had significantly higher POP-Q point C values (−9 vs −8), but all other anatomic measures were statistically similar. The robotic group had significantly longer operative time, less blood loss, and shorter hospital stay than those patients who underwent laparotomy. There were no significant differences for other secondary outcomes of intra- and postoperative complications, although the robotic group did show higher rates of postoperative fever. The results of these studies further substantiate the need for more comparative studies between different surgical approaches to sacral colpopexy, with longer follow-up and measured effects on bladder, bowel, and sexual function.

Other surgical considerations

Hysterectomy Many surgeons believe that a hysterectomy immediately before sacral colpopexy increases the risk of graft infection or erosion by exposing the graft material a vaginal incision. The impact of hysterectomy on graft erosion rates following sacral colpopexy is controversial within the literature. Two retrospective cohort studies showed no significant difference between postoperative mesh erosion rates in patients who did or did not have hysterectomy at the time of abdominal sacral colpopexy.[58,59] Another large retrospective cohort study also showed no difference in erosion rates when comparing patients who had laparoscopic sacral colpopexy with and without laparoscopic-assisted vaginal hysterectomy.[47]

On the other hand, a recent study showed a significantly increased risk of mesh erosion after sacral colpopexy and concomitant hysterectomy with an odds ratio of 4.9[60] Two other retrospective studies also showed significantly increased risk of mesh erosion in the hysterectomy groups.[61,62] Given these findings, some surgeons advocate performing a supracervical hysterectomy and subsequent sacral cervicopexy. The theoretical advantage of leaving the cervical stump is that it may act as a barrier to prevent ascending infection and graft erosion or prevent the issue of a vaginal incision having to heal over the graft. Until direct comparisons are studied in an appropriate fashion, controversy will remain.

Anterior/posterior colporrhaphy The need for concomitant anterior or posterior colporrhaphy at the time of sacral colpopexy is also a controversial issue among pelvic
floor surgeons. Early on, surgeons performing sacral colpopexy described the need
for concomitant anterior colporrhaphy.[5,6,63,64] As more surgeons extended graft
attachment and incorporated a retropubic urethropexy in conjunction with the sacral
colpopexy, the addition of a paravaginal defect repair also became more common to
help provide additional anterior wall support. Unfortunately there are no current
studies that directly compare sacral colpopexy with and without a separate anterior
vaginal wall repair. As such, proceeding with this additional procedure at the time of
sacral colpopexy is left to the discretion of the surgeon.

A traditional or site-specific posterior colporrhaphy may also be done at the time of
sacral colpopexy. Many surgeons advocate for this additional procedure,[8,39,41,64]
whereas others believe that suspending the vaginal apex with a separate posterior
vaginal graft is sufficient to correct posterior wall defects.[65] A recent study looked
at posterior wall measurements 1 year after abdominal sacral colpopexy without
posterior repair, and found an objective cure rate of 75% in this compartment.[66]
The investigators stated that the recurrence of posterior prolapse in their study was
comparable to other studies that performed sacral colpopexy with and without posterior colporrhaphies, indicating no true benefit of this additional procedure.[39,41,61] The
only comparative study in the literature to describe posterior measurements after
sacral colpopexy with and without site-specific posterior repair demonstrated that
the group with concomitant posterior repair had significantly better posterior measurements that persisted for 34 months after surgery.[67]

Sacral Cervicopexy/Hysteropexy

Uterine preservation in the face of uterovaginal prolapse was previously only considered if future fertility was a particular concern for the patient. Today, however, some
women are inclined to retain the cervix or the entire uterus in an attempt to prevent
a change in postoperative sexual function. Stoesser first described the abdominal
sacral cervicopexy procedure in 1955, using external oblique fascia to attach the
posterior cervix to the sacral promontory.[68] This study reported good surgical
outcomes although postoperative assessment was not explicitly defined. Arthure
and Savage described correction of uterovaginal prolapse in 1957 with direct attachment of the uterine fundus to the anterior sacrum using sutures.[3] Addison and
colleagues[69] then described sacral hysteropexy with the use of mersilene mesh attaching the posterior uterus to the anterior sacrum. This study described surgical
outcomes in only one patient, and showed no evidence of recurrent prolapse within
an undefined follow-up period. Other techniques of uterine fixation to the sacrum
have also been reported. Krause and colleagues[70] described a sacral suture hysteropexy whereby a permanent suture is run through the right uterosacral ligament
between the posterior cervix and sacrum. This procedure was performed in 81
patients, with a 95% objective cure rate and an 88% subjective cure rate. Cutner
and colleagues[71] described using a mersilene sling that is passed through the posterior cervix and both uterosacral ligaments, and then is anchored to the sacral promontory. This technique was performed in 8 patients, with no description of postoperative
anatomic outcomes.

Procedure

Other than graft placement, the sacral cervicopexy and hysteropexy use the same
surgical principles of the sacral colpopexy, and may be performed by laparotomy or
laparoscopy. In procedures whereby a cervical stump is retained, a subtotal

hysterectomy is first performed. The dissection and attachment of the anterior and posterior grafts are performed as in sacral colpopexy but with additional reinforcement sutures directly into the cervical stump. Sacral hysteropexy is commonly described with the use of a Y-shaped anterior graft (**Fig. 6**A) and a rectangular posterior graft (**Fig. 6**B) that are attached to the upper vagina and cervix. The arms of the anterior graft are passed bilaterally through though the right and left broad ligaments and then attached with the proximal portion of the posterior graft to the anterior longitudinal ligament overlying the sacrum. A rectangular or curvilinear anterior mesh that is passed only through the right broad ligament should be used in women who want to conceive post hysteropexy (**Fig. 7**). This approach may prevent lower uterine segment obstruction that can occur with placement of a Y-shaped anterior mesh.

Surgical outcomes
Abdominal sacral hysteropexy There are many studies reporting on outcomes following sacral hysteropexy; however, inconsistencies with regard to surgical

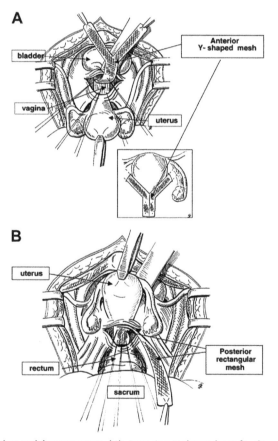

Fig. 6. Abdominal sacral hysteropexy. (*A*) Anterior Y-shaped graft placed along anterior vaginal wall and around uterine isthmus in sacral hysteropexy. (*B*) Posterior graft in sacral hysteropexy is rectangular and attached to posterior vaginal wall and posterior uterine isthmus. (*From* Costantini E, Mearini L, Bini V, et al. Uterus preservation in surgical correction of urogenital prolapse. Eur Urol 2005;48(4):642–9; with permission.)

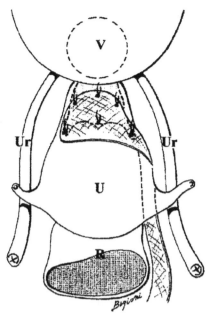

Fig. 7. Anterior curvilinear graft in sacral hysteropexy should be used in patients who want to conceive post-hysteropexy. Ur, ureter; U, uterus; R, rectum; V, bladder. (*From* Gadonneix P, Ercoli A, Salet-Lizee D, et al. Laparoscopic sacrocolpopexy with two separate meshes along the anterior and posterior vaginal walls for multicompartment pelvic organ prolapse. J Am Assoc Gynecol Laparosc 2004;11(1):29–35; with permission.)

approach, type of graft, and graft fixation make overall outcome analyses difficult to interpret. A small cohort study of 13 women after sacral hysteropexy using one piece of Y-shaped mesh wrapped posterior to anterior had only one recurrent stage I utero-vaginal prolapse.[72] This study showed an 88% improvement in prolapse symptoms, and 54% of patients believed the surgery had improved their overall quality of life. A larger study by Barranger and colleagues[73] followed 30 patients after sacral hystero-pexy using a 2-strap technique with an anterior Y-shaped graft. All patients also had a posterior colporrhaphy at the time of surgery. Only 6.5% of patients had recurrent uterovaginal prolapse attributed to cervical elongation. Another study followed 20 patients after sacral hysteropexy with only a single posterior mesh and concomitant posterior colporrhaphy.[74] The investigators reported only one patient with recurrent stage II prolapse that developed in the first month after surgery, and a significant improvement in postoperative questionnaire scores related to quality of life and prolapse symptoms.

Symptoms related to bladder, bowel, and sexual function after abdominal sacral hysteropexy have not been reported as primary outcomes related to this surgical procedure. Leron and Stanton[72] reported bladder symptoms both pre- and postoper-atively. In this study, no incontinence procedures were performed at the time of sacral hysteropexy and there was a significant reduction in reports of urgency, urge, and stress urinary incontinence. In another study where Burch urethropexies were per-formed in all patients, the rate of overall urinary incontinence went from 63% before surgery to 10% after surgery.[73] In the study by Demirci and colleagues[74] all patients had a Burch urethropexy, midurethral sling, or paravaginal defect repair. Before surgery, 65% had urodynamic stress incontinence and 25% had urge symptoms.

After sacral hysteropexy, only 5% had urodynamic stress incontinence and 15% had persistent urge symptoms. Defecatory dysfunction seems to be a symptom that is not significantly improved by sacral hysteropexy. Symptoms of constipation have been shown to be similar or worsened after surgery.[72,73] Sexual function seems to improve after sacral hysteropexy, with 89% to 95% of patients reporting improved or normal sexual function.[73,74] One study noted a 7% de novo dyspareunia rate.[73]

Complications associated with abdominal sacral hysteropexy seem to be comparable with those associated with sacral colpopexy. Barranger and colleagues[73] had a 7% rate for intraoperative complications and a 13% rate for minor postoperative complications. In this study, only one patient developed mesh erosion that was seen 2 years after surgery, and another patient developed a bowel obstruction secondary to occlusion by the mesh 4 years after surgery. In addition, postoperative pregnancy was assessed by one study that reported that 6 patients were interested in conceiving after surgery, with only 3 documented pregnancies occurring 3 to 6 years after the procedure.[73]

There are 2 studies that have compared abdominal sacral hysteropexy to other prolapse procedures. Costantini and colleagues[75] compared patients having abdominal sacral hysteropexy to those having abdominal sacral colpopexy. Abdominal sacral hysteropexy had shorter operative time, less blood loss, and shorter hospital stay. No patients in either group had recurrent cervical or vaginal vault prolapse, and there was no significant difference between objective (91% hysteropexy vs 92% colpopexy) and subjective cure rates (85% hysteropexy vs 82% colpopexy). Postoperative incontinence persisted in 18% of hysteropexy patients (7/20) and 35% of patients in the colpopexy group (4/22). Postoperative constipation persisted in 29% (4/14) of hysteropexy patients and 11% of colpopexy patients (2/18). There were no significant differences between surgical groups with regard to intra- or postoperative complications, although there were 3 patients with mesh erosion in the colpopexy group and none in the hysteropexy group. Roovers and colleagues[76] compared abdominal sacral hysteropexy to vaginal prolapse correction with a vaginal hysterectomy, uterosacral ligament vault suspension, and anterior and posterior colporrhaphy. One year after surgery, both groups had a 5% rate of stage II or greater recurrent uterine or vault prolapse. Recurrent cystocele (stage II or greater) occurred in 36% of the hysteropexy group and 39% of the vaginal group, and recurrent rectocele (stage II or greater) in 5% of the hysteropexy group and 15% of the vaginal group. The hysteropexy group, however, had significantly greater postoperative symptoms of prolapse, pelvic pain, overactive bladder, urinary incontinence, and obstructed voiding. In addition, 22% of hysteropexy patients required repeat pelvic surgery compared with only 2% in the vaginal group. There were no significant differences for intra- or postoperative complications between the 2 procedures. The investigators concluded that the vaginal approach with removal of the uterus was a preferable treatment for uterovaginal prolapse compared with abdominal sacral hysteropexy.

Laparoscopic sacral cervicopexy/hysteropexy Data on a laparoscopic approach to this procedure is even more limited, as many of the studies include sacral colpopexies, cervicopexies, and hysteropexies in the description of their surgical cohorts. The heterogeneity of these surgical procedures limits the validity of most published data. For patients with uterovaginal prolapse who desire minimally invasive repair, laparoscopic surgeons will often perform a supracervical hysterectomy followed by a sacral cervicopexy. This approach to hysterectomy is often considered technically easier and faster than a total laparoscopic hysterectomy, laparoscopic-assisted vaginal hysterectomy, or vaginal hysterectomy. Indeed, much of the literature cited as pertaining to laparoscopic sacral colpopexy is in fact based on evidence whereby the majority of patients actually underwent laparoscopic sacral cervicopexy.[77,78] One study followed a cohort of 40 patients after laparoscopic sacral cervicopexy using only a single posterior mesh.[79] There was a mean follow-up of approximately 8 months and all patients were cured of apical prolapse, with the cervix being higher than preoperative status and above the plane of the hymen. This group did not report postoperative outcomes for bladder, bowel, or sexual function. There were few complications reported, including one patient with an undetected rectal injury that later required bowel resection and colostomy. Only one patient developed postoperative mesh erosion.

There are several studies that have reported anatomic and functional outcomes wherein more than half of the patients underwent laparoscopic sacral hystero-pexy.[80–82] These results, however, are combined with the surgical outcomes of patients who underwent laparoscopic sacral colpopexy and cervicopexy, and are therefore difficult to interpret. There is only one study that followed a small cohort of 15 women who underwent laparoscopic sacral hysteropexy using a 2-strap technique with the anterior mesh being conformed to a V-shape.[83] All patients also had a concomitant Burch urethropexy. Patients were followed for a minimum of 2 years, and during this time no patients had objective or subjective evidence of recurrent uterine prolapse and no one required repeat surgery. Postoperative bladder and bowel symptoms were not reported, but 86% of patients with preoperative dyspareunia had complete resolution. There were no intraoperative complications and no postoperative mesh erosions. Three patients became pregnant after the surgery, with 2 carrying to term and delivering by cesarean section.

Uterosacral Colpopexy/Hysteropexy

Native tissue repair for prolapse makes use of structures and tissue found in the pelvis to reconstruct pelvic support. One of the most common structures used has been the uterosacral ligament. Its use in prolapse surgery was first described in 1927, and has been used in a variety of ways since.[84] In 1957 the McCall culdoplasty appeared in the literature and described plication of the uterosacral ligaments, incorporating both the posterior cul de sac peritoneum and posterior vaginal cuff.[85] Several variations of this technique, including the Mayo McCall modification, have since been introduced.[86] These variations differ in the number of sutures and points of fixation used, but all rely on the uterosacral ligament for the providing the foundation of support. In the late 1990s, Shull reported excellent anatomic results with the use of multiple attachment points along the ligament with fixation to both the anterior and posterior vaginal walls (**Fig. 8**). More recently, abdominal and laparoscopic approaches to prolapse correction using this ligament have been described.

From its name as a "ligament" to its anatomic description, the uterosacral ligament itself remains controversial. Its attachment to the cervix and upper vagina have been fairly reproducible in both gross dissections and magnetic resonance imaging (MRI) studies. Its attachment to the sacrum is more disputed. Some studies have shown attachments to the lateral sacrum ranging from S1 to S4, and to areas of the pelvic sidewall overlying the fascia of the levator ani, coccygeus, and obturator internus muscles. One MRI study showed attachment to the sacrum in only 7% of studies while 82% attached to the sacrospinous/coccygeus complex.[87] The composition of the structure is also debated. Dissection of fetal and adult cadavers has yielded relatively little organized connective tissue. Instead, varying amount of neural tissue, vascular channels, elastin, collagen, and fat have been found.[88] Despite the varied composition, the intermediate portion of the ligament has been recommended as the strongest and safest to use in vault suspension procedures.[89] Approach to this ligament can be

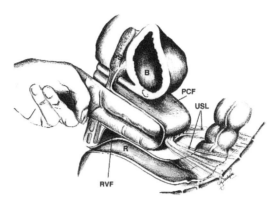

Fig. 8. Sagittal view of pubocervical fascia/vaginal muscularis and rectovaginal fascia/vaginal muscularis suspended to uterosacral ligaments. PCF, pubocervical fascia; RVF, rectovaginal fascia; USL, uterosacral ligament; PS, pubic symphysis; B, bladder; R, rectum. (*From* Shull BL, Bachofen C, Coates KW, et al. A transvaginal approach to repair of apical and other associated sites of pelvic organ prolapse with uterosacral ligaments. Am J Obstet Gynecol 2000;183(6):1365–73 [discussion: 73–4]; with permission.)

vaginal or abdominal, as it has been previously shown that there is no difference in the tensile strength of sutures placed vaginally or laparoscopically.[90] The proximity of other vital structures is a major concern when using this structure for apical support. One study using embalmed cadavers showed the average distance between the ligament and ureter ranged from 0.9 cm at the ligament's distal end to 4.1 cm at the ligament's proximal end.[89] These findings differ from those of another study using fresh cadavers, where the ureter was an average of 1.4 cm away from the ligament at both its distal and proximal ends.[91] Ureteric injury during vaginal uterosacral vault suspension has been documented in several studies, with one study reporting an 11% rate of ureteral compromise.[92] In other cadaver studies, sutures placed into the uterosacral ligament injured several other structures including the rectum, pelvic sidewall vessels, and neural structures such as the S3 sacral nerve and inferior hypogastric nerve plexus (**Fig. 9**).[91,93] All of these injuries have been reported as complications in the literature. One case series reported nerve injury in seven out of 182 cases in the distribution of S2 to S4.[94] In all of these cases, however, prompt suture removal or prolonged medical therapy led to complete symptom resolution.[94] These studies should remind the surgeon of the anatomy lying beneath the surface of the uterosacral ligaments and to be wary of deeply placed sutures. In general, placement of the distal sutures should be 1 cm posterior to the level of the ischial spine, with additional sutures placed more proximally to achieve higher apical support.

Procedure
Although primarily used in vaginal repairs, several case series and cohort studies document the use of the uterosacral ligament for vaginal vault suspension in abdominal surgery, both open and laparoscopic. The same general techniques should apply to both approaches and are performed in a similar manner to the vaginal approach. Uterosacral ligaments may be tagged during hysterectomy or identified by traction placed on the vaginal cuff if no uterus is present. The familiar tenting of the peritoneum extending back to the ischial spine area and lateral sacral boundaries is identified. The ureters are visualized and sutures are placed in the intermediate portion of the ligament. The suture location can be identified by use of a vaginal stent to outline the

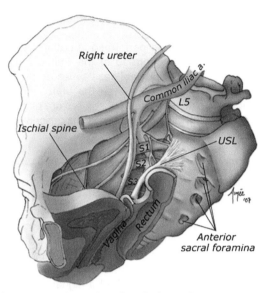

Fig. 9. Anatomy of the right pelvic sidewall with the peritoneum removed and the rectum opened is shown. Note the relationship of uterosacral ligament (USL) to the rectum, ureter, and other pelvic sidewall structures. First sacral nerve (S1), second sacral nerve (S2), third sacral nerve (S3), and fifth lumbar vertebrae (L5) are shown. (*From* Wieslander CK, Roshan-ravan SM, Wai CY, et al. Uterosacral ligament suspension sutures: Anatomic relationships in unembalmed female cadavers. Am J Obstet Gynecol 2007;197(6):672. e1–6; with permission.)

vaginal apex and then placing the uterosacral sutures at a corresponding level. It is recommended to suture away from the ureters to theoretically lesson the chance of ureteral injury. Anywhere from 1 to 3 sutures are placed on each side and then through the appropriate areas of the anterior and posterior vaginal wall where the muscularis is intact. Posterior sutures should not be passed through the rectovaginal septum as this is a 3 cm structure extending proximally from the perineal body, and attachment of the ligaments to this structure would significantly compromise vaginal length.[95] The sutures should direct the vaginal apex toward the S3 level of the sacrum without constricting the rectosigmoid. Suture selection varies by surgeon. Variations include the use of nonabsorbable sutures placed subepithelially,[96] absorbable sutures placed through full vaginal wall thickness,[97] or a combination of both. Current data do not prove one suture type to be superior over another. Based on ureteral location, relaxing incisions in the peritoneum between the ureter and the uterosacral ligament may be used. This action may prevent kinking of the ureter, although one cadaveric study showed no difference in pressures measured within the ureter before and after these relaxing incisions.[89] Transvesical or transurethral cystoscopy should be done before closing, to document ureteral integrity.

This repair can also be done through traditional or robotic-assisted laparoscopy. After appropriate port placement is achieved, the uterosacral ligaments are identified either at the time of hysterectomy or with strong traction provided by a vaginal stent. After identifying the ureters, sutures are placed below them at the appropriate level through the ligaments. Some surgeons use a rectal stent to help avoid placing these sutures into the rectum. The use of helical sutures through the uterosacral ligaments has been described or, as in the vaginal approach, anywhere from one to three individual sutures can be placed and tied bilaterally. As in the open approach, relaxing peritoneal incisions can be considered and ureteral integrity must be confirmed after sutures are tied.

Uterosacral hysteropexy can also be performed in patients who wish to maintain their uterus. The patient should be informed of the limited data available to help counsel her in this decision, although several case series do provide some outcome information. The procedure is done exactly as the uterosacral vault suspension, with the exception that the uterosacral ligament sutures are placed into the posterior cervix (**Fig. 10**). Single, helical, and multiple sutures are described, and relaxing peritoneal ureteral incisions remain an option.

Surgical outcomes

Limited data exist for the abdominal and laparoscopic approaches to uterosacral ligament vault suspension, and almost all are retrospective studies or case series. As with other studies that describe prolapse surgery, differences in outcome measures make direct comparisons between studies difficult. One retrospective series compared 79 patients who underwent abdominal uterosacral suspension with 34 patients who underwent sacral colpopexy.[98] After a follow-up of 12 months, there were no significant differences in outcomes or recurrence rates between the 2 groups, although it was noted that the sacral colpopexy group had a higher stage of prolapse before surgery than the uterosacral group.

Ostrzenski[99] reported on patients who had laparoscopic repair using uterosacral ligaments with (n = 11) and without (n = 16) concomitant paravaginal defect repair. No laxity was shown in 69% of patients who had no concomitant paravaginal repair, whereas no laxity was found in 91% of patients who did have a concomitant paravaginal repair. Seman and colleagues[100] reported no anatomic failures 8 months after surgery in a cohort of 47 patients undergoing laparoscopic uterosacral vault suspension. The largest cohort study to date that followed 113 patients after laparoscopic

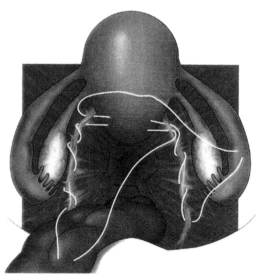

Fig. 10. Uterosacral hysteropexy with helical suture placed through each uterosacral ligament and posterior aspect of the cervix. (*From* Maher CF, Carey MP, Murray CJ. Laparoscopic suture hysteropexy for uterine prolapse. Obstet Gynecol 2001;97(6):1010–4; with permission.)

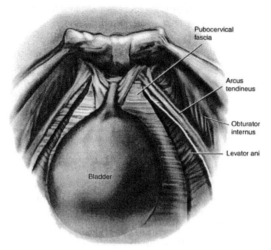

Fig. 11. Bilateral paravaginal defect as seen from the space of Retzius. (*From* Miklos JR, Kohli N. Laparoscopic paravaginal repair plus Burch colposuspension: review and descriptive technique. Urology 2000;56(6 Suppl 1):64–9; with permission.)

uterosacral vaginal vault suspension (mean follow-up 3.2 years), showed a stage II or greater failure rate of 12.8%.[101]

A recent retrospective cohort study examined uterosacral vault suspension done either laparoscopically or vaginally at the time of vaginal hysterectomy. Ninety-six patients in the vaginal group (mean follow-up 8.8 months) and 22 patients in the laparoscopic group (mean follow-up 10.8 months) were compared. Estimated blood loss was higher in the vaginal group, and ureteral compromise occurred in 4.2% of the

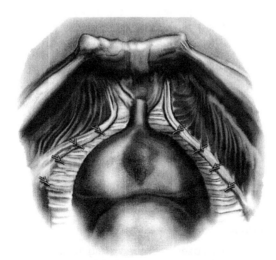

Fig. 12. Reapproximation of the lateral anterior vaginal wall to the obturator internus at the arcus tendineus fascia pelvis. (*From* Miklos JR, Kohli N. Laparoscopic paravaginal repair plus Burch colposuspension: review and descriptive technique. Urology 2000;56(6 Suppl 1):64–9; with permission.)

vaginal cases and none in the laparoscopic cases. Apical failure rates were not statistically significant between the 2 groups, but were noted in 6.3% of the vaginal group and 0% in the laparoscopic group.[102]

Other studies have combined abdominal uterosacral hysteropexy and uterosacral colpopexy within their surgical cohorts. One such multicenter nonrandomized, prospective study reported on patients with stage II or greater uterine (n = 42) or vaginal vault prolapse (n = 30, mean follow-up 46.1 weeks). This study reported no major complications, and statistically significant improvements in postoperative vaginal measurements and symptom scores for both groups.[103]

One study investigated 43 patients who underwent laparoscopic uterosacral hysteropexy (follow-up 12 months), with 16% requiring repeat surgery for uterine prolapse. Complications included uterine artery laceration (1 patient) and ureteral kinking (2 patients). Two women went on to deliver term infants by cesarean section.[104] Another study followed 23 patients (mean follow-up 15.9 months) that had uterosacral hysteropexy, and showed significant improvement in postoperative vault measurements with no reported failures.[105] In a study comparing 25 patients after laparoscopic uterosacral hysteropexy (mean follow-up 26 weeks) with 25 patients after total vaginal hysterectomy and a variety of vaginally approached vault suspension techniques (mean follow-up 46 weeks), blood loss and hospital stay were lower and shorter in the laparoscopic group. Postoperative vault measurements were significantly worse in the vaginal group than in the laparoscopic group. Furthermore, 3 patients required reoperation for apical prolapse in the vaginal group compared with none in the laparoscopic group. For short-term outcomes related to this procedure, this study suggests that there is a benefit to maintaining the uterus in situ.[106]

Other surgical considerations

One of the issues not addressed in any of the current studies is the discrepancy between the anterior and posterior vaginal walls at the time of hysterectomy. Most often, the anterior vaginal wall is shorter, and this needs to be considered when placing uterosacral sutures. If only the longer posterior wall is used to judge vaginal length and guide uterosacral ligament suture placement, excess tension may be placed on the anterior wall. If a hysterectomy was performed at an earlier date, the new apex may or may not be the same as the original cuff, and suture placement is generally easier as no open cuff is present to limit suture placement. Sutures should include only areas where the full thickness muscularis is intact on the anterior and posterior vaginal wall. Some experts advocate repair of other defects first so the new anterior or posterior wall can be included in the apical sutures, but currently there is no data to support one technique over the other.

Incontinence procedures at the time of uterosacral vault suspension are performed when indicated by patient complaint and objective demonstration of stress urinary incontinence. Unlike the sacral colpopexy procedure, there are no current studies to direct the surgeon as to whether incontinence procedures should be included in patients who do not complain of or demonstrate urodynamic stress incontinence.

Other Apical Suspensions

Abdominal colpopexy has also been described using the sacrospinous ligament. One case series described patients with anterior wall defects and stress incontinence who underwent abdominal paravaginal defect repair and Burch urethropexy with concomitant vaginal vault suspension to the sacrospinous ligament.[107] No repeat surgeries for vault prolapse were required in 55 patients with a mean follow-up of 23 months.

Abdominal hysteropexy using other pelvic ligaments remains controversial but has been described in the literature. Joshi[108] described transabdominal bilateral suspension of the uterus to the pectineal ligaments using Mersilene tape in 20 women. There were no reported complications, no recurrence of symptoms during the follow-up period (6–30 months), and seven patients conceived within the first 6 months after surgery. In contrast, O'Brien and Ibrahim[109] reported on nine postmenopausal patients who underwent laparoscopic round ligament ventrosuspension whereby the ligaments were fixated through the abdominal rectus sheath. Eight patients had recurrent prolapse within 3 months after surgery, and this technique has since been considered not suitable for patients with uterine prolapse.

ABDOMINAL ANTERIOR VAGINAL WALL SUPPORT

The occurrence of anterior vaginal wall prolapse has previously been described as a result of one or more defects in the pubocervical fascia (muscularis) that are midline, lateral or paravaginal, transverse or superior, or pubourethral.[110]

A historical abdominal approach to anterior vaginal wall prolapse was to correct the midline defect with a triangular colpectomy or wedge resection of the anterior vaginal wall. This technique was first proposed by Weinstein and Roberts in 1949,[111] and later by Schauffler[112] in 1951 and Macer[113] in 1978, as a means of correcting anterior vaginal wall prolapse after abdominal hysterectomy without having to proceed with a concomitant vaginal repair. In 2001, Lovatsis and Drutz[114] showed that there were significantly more anterior vaginal wall prolapse recurrences in patients who had Burch urethropexy with anterior wedge resection than in those who had Burch urethropexy alone (11% vs 4%). As such, this procedure is no longer considered a suitable abdominal procedure to correct anterior vaginal wall prolapse.

Lateral wall defects have been described in two-thirds of women presenting with anterior vaginal wall prolapse.[92,115] In 1912, White[116] noted that a complete cure for cystocele required reapproximation of the lateral vaginal fornices to the arcus tendineus. This approach to anterior vaginal wall repair was dismissed until Richardson and colleagues[110] reported results of abdominal paravaginal defect repair in 1976. Shull and Baden[117] later described this repair through a vaginal approach; however, many felt this was technically more difficult and would negatively impact pudendal and perineal innervation.[118] The abdominal paravaginal defect repair restores the normal attachment of the anterolateral vaginal sulcus to the pubococcygeus and obturator internus fascia at the level of the arcus tendineus fascia pelvis. This technique remains the only accepted abdominal approach to cystocele correction.

Procedure

This surgery can be done by laparotomy or laparoscopy. The surgical approach is left to the discretion of the surgeon and may be determined by concomitant procedures being done. For both surgical approaches, the patient is placed in the dorsal supine lithotomy position and is prepared both abdominally and vaginally. For laparotomy, a transverse or midline incision can be used, and is dependent on previous scars and other procedures being performed. Once all other procedures are completed, the peritoneum is left open and the transversalis fascia is separated from the superior ramus of the pubis so that the space of Retzius can be entered. The laparoscopic approach to paravaginal defect repair begins with port placement in a manner similar to that described for laparoscopic sacral colpopexy. Once in the peritoneal cavity, the bladder can be retrogradely filled to adequately visualize the bladder edge. The space of Retzius is entered through the parietal peritoneum 3 to 4 cm above the bladder reflection using electrocautery. This incision extends between the two medial-lateral umbilical ligaments and transects the urachus.

Once in the space of Retzius, both surgical approaches involve the same technical steps. The vagina and bladder are pulled medially to expose the lateral retropubic space that contains the obturator internus and levator muscles as well as the obturator neurovascular bundle. Gentle blunt dissection of the loose areolar tissue is then performed until the ischial spine is identified. The arcus tendineus fascia pelvis may be seen as a white band running from the symphysis pubis to the ischial spine over the pubococcygeus and obturator internus muscles (**Fig. 11**). The anterior vagina is elevated to its normal attachment point along the arcus tendineus. This position may improve visualization of the defect in the fascia. The veins along the vaginal wall occasionally may have to be sutured or clipped during dissection or repair to help maintain hemostasis.

Starting at the vaginal apex, a nonabsorbable suture is placed through the full thickness of the vagina while avoiding the vaginal epithelium, and then through the ipsilateral obturator internus fascia or arcus tendineus fascia pelvis, at the level of the ischial spine. This suture is tied down and an additional four to five sutures are passed in a similar fashion, at 1 cm intervals, with distal progression until the last stitch is passed through the pubourethral ligament, 1 to 2 cm proximal to the urethrovesical junction (**Fig. 12**). If the patient has stress urinary incontinence, the final distal suture may be replaced with a Burch urethropexy whereby two sutures are passed at the level of the bladder neck and urethra and anchored to the pectineal ligament; this is performed on both the right and left sides to correct bilateral defects. Bladder and ureteric integrity should be checked by cystoscopy once the defect is repaired, and the abdominal or laparoscopic incisions are closed in a standard fashion.

Surgical Outcomes

In studies that looked at abdominal paravaginal defect repair without any other concomitant reconstructive procedure, anatomic cure rates range from 95% to 97%, although the definition of "cure" differs among most studies.[110,115,117] Bruce and colleagues[119] compared anatomic rates between patients who had abdominal paravaginal defect repair with and without a rectus muscle sling, and found a higher recurrence of cystocele in the group that did not have a concomitant sling procedure (12% vs 4%). There are several other studies that report on anterior wall outcomes after this procedure; however, these studies also include patients with concomitant sacral colpopexy or hysteropexy, thereby confounding postoperative measurements.[120,121] One of the first reported studies on laparoscopic paravaginal defect repair reported a 93% cure rate based on objective and subjective data in a series of 28 patients who had no other concomitant procedures.[122] There was another larger study that reported the outcomes after laparoscopic paravaginal defect repair in 212 patients.[123] This study showed that only 1% of patients had postoperative failure at the site of paravaginal reattachment, although 20% of patients also had concomitant laparoscopic sacral colpopexy or hysteropexy.

Many studies have not done subgroup analyses on patients who have had paravaginal defect repairs in conjunction with various incontinence procedures. Richardson and colleagues[110] analyzed patients who only had abdominal paravaginal defect repairs, and found that 8% had persistent stress incontinence and none had postoperative urinary urgency. Bruce and colleagues[119] showed that the cure rate for stress incontinence was 72% in patients with abdominal paravaginal defect repair alone, compared with those that had the addition of a rectus muscle sling for whom the cure rate for stress incontinence was 85%. In a study by Shull and Baden[117] no concomitant Burch was performed, although the middle sutures within the paravaginal defect repair were anchored to the pectineal ligament bilaterally. Postoperatively, 3% of patients had persistent stress urinary incontinence.

Bowel and sexual function following abdominal paravaginal defect repair have not been described in the literature. Furthermore, intra- and postoperative complications reported in studies dealing with abdominal paravaginal defect repairs are difficult to interpret given the number of other procedures performed simultaneously.

There are no clinical trials that have directly compared abdominal to vaginal paravaginal defect repairs. Trials by Benson and colleagues[39] and Maher and colleagues[41] have both compared outcomes between abdominal sacral colpopexy and vaginal sacrospinous ligament fixation. In both studies, a paravaginal defect repair was added to the abdominal group when required. For the vaginal group, Maher and colleagues[124] performed only an anterior colporrhaphy when required, whereas Benson and colleagues performed an anterior colporrhaphy with or without vaginal paravaginal defect repair when required. When results of these trials were analyzed together, the abdominal sacral colpopexy with paravaginal defect repair with or without Burch urethropexy significantly reduced the risk of recurrent anterior vaginal wall prolapse when compared with sacrospinous ligament fixation with anterior colporrhaphy (relative risk 0.25; 95% confidence interval 0.09–0.85).

ABDOMINAL POSTERIOR VAGINAL WALL SUPPORT

No series with notable numbers of patients have reported on outcomes after enterocele repair alone. Most experts would agree that any culdoplasty surgery (Moschcowitz or Halban) should be performed in conjunction with an appropriate apical support procedure. Furthermore, there are sparse data available on abdominally approached rectocele repairs. Using an abdominal approach, 33 patients with rectocele and symptoms of obstructed defecation underwent an abdominal mesh rectopexy. Postoperative complications occurred in 16% of patients, ranging from abscess formation (n = 1) to urinary tract infection (n = 4). Evacuation proctography demonstrated rectoceles greater than 3 cm in 100% of patients preoperatively and in only 7% of patients postoperatively. Preoperative findings of enterocele (39% of patients) and intussusception (24% of patients) were eliminated in all patients postoperatively. In patients with normal colonic transit time preoperatively, 55% continued to have symptoms of obstructed defecation postoperatively despite adequate anatomic repair.[125]

A laparoscopic approach placing polyglactin mesh for rectocele repair in conjunction with other prolapse correction procedures was conducted in 20 patients.[126] One year after surgery, 80% reported relief of digital defecation and prolapse. In another study comparing 40 laparoscopic rectocele repairs with 40 transanal rectocele repairs (median follow-up 44 months), patients in the transanal group had significantly improved symptoms (63% vs 28%) but a higher dyspareunia rate (36% vs 22%).[127] There was also a significant decrease in mean resting anal pressure in the transanal group and, although it did not reach statistical significance, 13% of the transanal group compared with 3% of the laparoscopic group experienced a decline in anal continence. Over time, 56% of patients in both groups experienced a deterioration in bowel function.

SUMMARY

Abdominal correction of pelvic organ prolapse remains a viable option for patients and surgeons. The transition from open procedures to less invasive laparoscopic and robotic-assisted surgeries is evident in the literature. Long-term follow-up and appropriately designed studies will further help direct surgeons in deciding which approach to incorporate into their practice.

REFERENCES

1. Summers A, Winkel LA, Hussain HK, et al. The relationship between anterior and apical compartment support. Am J Obstet Gynecol 2006;194(5):1438–43.
2. Rooney K, Kenton K, Mueller ER, et al. Advanced anterior vaginal wall prolapse is highly correlated with apical prolapse. Am J Obstet Gynecol 2006;195(6): 1837–40.
3. Arthure HG, Savage D. Uterine prolapse and prolapse of the vaginal vault treated by sacral hysteropexy. J Obstet Gynaecol Br Emp 1957;64(3):355–60.
4. Huguier J, Scali P. [Posterior suspension of the genital axis on the lumbosacral disk in the treatment of uterine prolapse]. Presse Med 1958;66(35):781–4 [in French].
5. Lane FE. Repair of posthysterectomy vaginal-vault prolapse. Obstet Gynecol 1962;20:72–7.
6. Birnbaum SJ. Rational therapy for the prolapsed vagina. Am J Obstet Gynecol 1973;115(3):411–9.
7. Sutton GP, Addison WA, Livengood CH 3rd, et al. Life-threatening hemorrhage complicating sacral colpopexy. Am J Obstet Gynecol 1981;140(7):836–7.
8. Addison WA, Livengood CH 3rd, Sutton GP, et al. Abdominal sacral colpopexy with Mersilene mesh in the retroperitoneal position in the management of post-hysterectomy vaginal vault prolapse and enterocele. Am J Obstet Gynecol 1985;153(2):140–6.
9. Cundiff GW, Harris RL, Coates K, et al. Abdominal sacral colpoperineopexy: a new approach for correction of posterior compartment defects and perineal descent associated with vaginal vault prolapse. Am J Obstet Gynecol 1997; 177(6):1345–53 [discussion: 1353–5].
10. Latini JM, Brown JA, Kreder KJ. Abdominal sacral colpopexy using autologous fascia lata. J Urol 2004;171(3):1176–9.
11. FitzGerald MP, Edwards SR, Fenner D. Medium-term follow-up on use of freeze-dried, irradiated donor fascia for sacrocolpopexy and sling procedures. Int Urogynecol J Pelvic Floor Dysfunct 2004;15(4):238–42.
12. Flynn MK, Webster GD, Amundsen CL. Abdominal sacral colpopexy with allograft fascia lata: one-year outcomes. Am J Obstet Gynecol 2005;192(5): 1496–500.
13. Amid PK. Classification of biomaterials and their related complications in abdominal wall hernia surgery. Hernia 1997;1:15–21.
14. Nygaard IE, McCreery R, Brubaker L, et al. Abdominal sacrocolpopexy: a comprehensive review. Obstet Gynecol 2004;104(4):805–23.
15. Iglesia CB, Fenner DE, Brubaker L. The use of mesh in gynecologic surgery. Int Urogynecol J Pelvic Floor Dysfunct 1997;8(2):105–15.
16. Ridgeway B, Chen CC, Paraiso MF. The use of synthetic mesh in pelvic reconstructive surgery. Clin Obstet Gynecol 2008;51(1):136–52.
17. Culligan PJ, Blackwell L, Goldsmith LJ, et al. A randomized controlled trial comparing fascia lata and synthetic mesh for sacral colpopexy. Obstet Gynecol 2005;106(1):29–37.
18. Gregory WT, Otto LN, Bergstrom JO, et al. Surgical outcome of abdominal sacrocolpopexy with synthetic mesh versus abdominal sacrocolpopexy with cadaveric fascia lata. Int Urogynecol J Pelvic Floor Dysfunct 2005;16(5):369–74.

19. Boukerrou M, Orazi G, Nayama M, et al. [Promontofixation procedure: use of non-absorbable sutures or Tackers?]. J Gynecol Obstet Biol Reprod (Paris) 2003;32(6):524–8 [in French].
20. Beer M, Kuhn A. Surgical techniques for vault prolapse: a review of the literature. Eur J Obstet Gynecol Reprod Biol 2005;119(2):144–55.
21. Su KC, Mutone MF, Terry CL, et al. Abdominovaginal sacral colpoperineopexy: patient perceptions, anatomical outcomes, and graft erosions. Int Urogynecol J Pelvic Floor Dysfunct 2007;18(5):503–11.
22. Fitzgerald MP, Kulkarni N, Fenner D. Postoperative resolution of urinary retention in patients with advanced pelvic organ prolapse. Am J Obstet Gynecol 2000; 183(6):1361–3 [discussion: 1363–4].
23. Albo ME, Richter HE, Brubaker L, et al. Burch colposuspension versus fascial sling to reduce urinary stress incontinence. N Engl J Med 2007;356(21): 2143–55.
24. Ward KL, Hilton P. A prospective multicenter randomized trial of tension-free vaginal tape and colposuspension for primary urodynamic stress incontinence: two-year follow-up. Am J Obstet Gynecol 2004;190(2):324–31.
25. Liapis A, Bakas P, Creatsas G. Burch colposuspension and tension-free vaginal tape in the management of stress urinary incontinence in women. Eur Urol 2002; 41(4):469–73.
26. McGuire EJ. Urodynamic findings in patients after failure of stress incontinence operations. Prog Clin Biol Res 1981;78:351–60.
27. El-Barky E, El-Shazly A, El-Wahab OA, et al. Tension free vaginal tape versus Burch colposuspension for treatment of female stress urinary incontinence. Int Urol Nephrol 2005;37(2):277–81.
28. Silva WA. Treatment of stress urinary incontinence—midurethral slings: top-down, bottom-up, "outside-in," or "inside-out". Clin Obstet Gynecol 2007; 50(2):362–75.
29. Porena M, Costantini E, Frea B, et al. Tension-free vaginal tape versus transobturator tape as surgery for stress urinary incontinence: results of a multicentre randomised trial. Eur Urol 2007;52(5):1481–90.
30. Brubaker L, Nygaard I, Richter HE, et al. Two-year outcomes after sacrocolpopexy with and without Burch to prevent stress urinary incontinence. Obstet Gynecol 2008;112(1):49–55.
31. Lefranc JP, Atallah D, Camatte S, et al. Longterm followup of posthysterectomy vaginal vault prolapse abdominal repair: a report of 85 cases. J Am Coll Surg 2002;195(3):352–8.
32. Burgio KL, Nygaard IE, Richter HE, et al. Bladder symptoms 1 year after abdominal sacrocolpopexy with and without Burch colposuspension in women without preoperative stress incontinence symptoms. Am J Obstet Gynecol 2007;197(6): 647.e641–6.
33. Baessler K, Schuessler B. Abdominal sacrocolpopexy and anatomy and function of the posterior compartment. Obstet Gynecol 2001;97(5 Pt 1):678–84.
34. Fox SD, Stanton SL. Vault prolapse and rectocele: assessment of repair using sacrocolpopexy with mesh interposition. BJOG 2000;107(11):1371–5.
35. Geomini PM, Brolmann HA, van Binsbergen NJ, et al. Vaginal vault suspension by abdominal sacral colpopexy for prolapse: a follow up study of 40 patients. Eur J Obstet Gynecol Reprod Biol 2001;94(2):234–8.
36. Virtanen H, Hirvonen T, Makinen J, et al. Outcome of thirty patients who underwent repair of posthysterectomy prolapse of the vaginal vault with abdominal sacral colpopexy. J Am Coll Surg 1994;178(3):283–7.

37. Bradley CS, Nygaard IE, Brown MB, et al. Bowel symptoms in women 1 year after sacrocolpopexy. Am J Obstet Gynecol 2007;197(6):642.e641–8.

38. Handa VL, Zyczynski HM, Brubaker L, et al. Sexual function before and after sacrocolpopexy for pelvic organ prolapse. Am J Obstet Gynecol 2007;197(6):629.e621–6.

39. Benson JT, Lucente V, McClellan E. Vaginal versus abdominal reconstructive surgery for the treatment of pelvic support defects: a prospective randomized study with long-term outcome evaluation. Am J Obstet Gynecol 1996;175(6):1418–21 [discussion: 1421–2].

40. Lo T, Wang A. Abdominal colposacropexy and sacrospinous ligament suspension for severe uterovaginal prolapse: a comparison. J Gynecol Surg 1998;14(2):59–64.

41. Maher CF, Qatawneh AM, Dwyer PL, et al. Abdominal sacral colpopexy or vaginal sacrospinous colpopexy for vaginal vault prolapse: a prospective randomized study. Am J Obstet Gynecol 2004;190(1):20–6.

42. Maher C, Baessler K, Glazener CM, et al. Surgical management of pelvic organ prolapse in women: a short version Cochrane review. Neurourol Urodyn 2008;27(1):3–12.

43. Ross JW, Preston M. Laparoscopic sacrocolpopexy for severe vaginal vault prolapse: five-year outcome. J Minim Invasive Gynecol 2005;12(3):221–6.

44. Higgs PJ, Chua HL, Smith AR. Long term review of laparoscopic sacrocolpopexy. BJOG 2005;112(8):1134–8.

45. Agarwala N, Hasiak N, Shade M. Laparoscopic sacral colpopexy with Gynemesh as graft material—experience and results. J Minim Invasive Gynecol 2007;14(5):577–83.

46. Claerhout F, De Ridder D, Roovers JP, et al. Medium-term anatomic and functional results of laparoscopic sacrocolpopexy beyond the learning curve. Eur Urol 2009;55:1459–68.

47. Stepanian AA, Miklos JR, Moore RD, et al. Risk of mesh extrusion and other mesh-related complications after laparoscopic sacral colpopexy with or without concurrent laparoscopic-assisted vaginal hysterectomy: experience of 402 patients. J Minim Invasive Gynecol 2008;15(2):188–96.

48. Paraiso MF, Walters MD, Rackley RR, et al. Laparoscopic and abdominal sacral colpopexies: a comparative cohort study. Am J Obstet Gynecol 2005;192(5):1752–8.

49. Hsiao KC, Latchamsetty K, Govier FE, et al. Comparison of laparoscopic and abdominal sacrocolpopexy for the treatment of vaginal vault prolapse. J Endourol 2007;21(8):926–30.

50. Su KC, Terry CL, Hale DS. Abdominovaginal sacral colpoperineopexy: a quality of life assessment. J Pelvic Med Surg 2007;14(4):181–90.

51. Elliott DS, Krambeck AE, Chow GK. Long-term results of robotic assisted laparoscopic sacrocolpopexy for the treatment of high grade vaginal vault prolapse. J Urol 2006;176(2):655–9.

52. Kramer BA, Whelan CM, Powell TM, et al. Robot-assisted laparoscopic sacrocolpopexy as management for pelvic organ prolapse. J Endourol 2009;23(4):655–8.

53. Akl MN, Long J, Giles DL, et al. Robotic-assisted sacrocolpopexy: technique and learning curve. Surg Endosc 2009. January 27, 2009. [epub ahead of print].

54. Shariati A, Maceda JS, Hale DS. Da Vinci assisted laparoscopic sacral colpopexy: surgical technique on a cohort of 77 patients. J Pelvic Med Surg 2008;14(3):163–71.

55. Daneshgari F, Kefer JC, Moore C, et al. Robotic abdominal sacrocolpopexy/sacrouteropexy repair of advanced female pelvic organ prolapse (POP): utilizing POP-quantification-based staging and outcomes. BJU Int 2007; 100(4):875–9.

56. Dimarco DS, Chow GK, Gettman MT, et al. Robotic-assisted laparoscopic sacrocolpopexy for treatment of vaginal vault prolapse. J Urol 2004;63:373–6.

57. Geller EJ, Siddiqui NY, Wu JM, et al. Short-term outcomes of robotic sacrocolpopexy compared with abdominal sacrocolpopexy. Obstet Gynecol 2008;112(6): 1201–6.

58. Wu JM, Wells EC, Hundley AF, et al. Mesh erosion in abdominal sacral colpopexy with and without concomitant hysterectomy. Am J Obstet Gynecol 2006; 194(5):1418–22.

59. Brizzolara S, Pillai-Allen A. Risk of mesh erosion with sacral colpopexy and concurrent hysterectomy. Obstet Gynecol 2003;102(2):306–10.

60. Cundiff GW, Varner E, Visco AG, et al. Risk factors for mesh/suture erosion following sacral colpopexy. Am J Obstet Gynecol 2008;199(6):688.e681–5.

61. Culligan PJ, Murphy M, Blackwell L, et al. Long-term success of abdominal sacral colpopexy using synthetic mesh. Am J Obstet Gynecol 2002;187(6): 1473–80 [discussion: 1481–2].

62. Imparato E, Aspesi G, Rovetta E, et al. Surgical management and prevention of vaginal vault prolapse. Surg Gynecol Obstet 1992;175(3):233–7.

63. Arthure HG. Vault-suspension. Proc R Soc Med 1949;42(6):388–90.

64. Feldman GB, Birnbaum SJ. Sacral colpopexy for vaginal vault prolapse. Obstet Gynecol 1979;53(3):399–401.

65. Snyder TE, Krantz KE. Abdominal-retroperitoneal sacral colpopexy for the correction of vaginal prolapse. Obstet Gynecol 1991;77(6):944–9.

66. Guiahi M, Kenton K, Brubaker L. Sacrocolpopexy without concomitant posterior repair improves posterior compartment defects. Int Urogynecol J Pelvic Floor Dysfunct 2008;19(9):1267–70.

67. Yau JL, Rahn DD, McIntire DD, et al. The natural history of posterior vaginal wall support after abdominal sacrocolpopexy with and without posterior colporrhaphy. Am J Obstet Gynecol 2007;196(5):e45–7.

68. Stoesser FG. Construction of a sacrocervical ligament for uterine suspension. Surg Gynecol Obstet 1955;101(5):638–41.

69. Addison WA, Timmons MC. Abdominal approach to vaginal eversion. Clin Obstet Gynecol 1993;36(4):995–1004.

70. Krause HG, Goh JT, Sloane K, et al. Laparoscopic sacral suture hysteropexy for uterine prolapse. Int Urogynecol J Pelvic Floor Dysfunct 2006;17(4):378–81.

71. Cutner A, Kearney R, Vashisht A. Laparoscopic uterine sling suspension: a new technique of uterine suspension in women desiring surgical management of uterine prolapse with uterine conservation. BJOG 2007;114(9):1159–62.

72. Leron E, Stanton SL. Sacrohysteropexy with synthetic mesh for the management of uterovaginal prolapse. BJOG 2001;108(6):629–33.

73. Barranger E, Fritel X, Pigne A. Abdominal sacrohysteropexy in young women with uterovaginal prolapse: long-term follow-up. Am J Obstet Gynecol 2003; 189(5):1245–50.

74. Demirci F, Ozdemir I, Somunkiran A, et al. Abdominal sacrohysteropexy in young women with uterovaginal prolapse: results of 20 cases. J Reprod Med 2006; 51(7):539–43.

75. Costantini E, Mearini L, Bini V, et al. Uterus preservation in surgical correction of urogenital prolapse. Eur Urol 2005;48(4):642–9.

76. Roovers JP, van der Vaart CH, van der Bom JG, et al. A randomised controlled trial comparing abdominal and vaginal prolapse surgery: effects on urogenital function. BJOG 2004;111(1):50–6.

77. Cosson M, Rajabally R, Bogaert E, et al. Laparoscopic sacrocolpopexy, hysterectomy, and Burch colposuspension: feasibility and short-term complications of 77 procedures. JSLS 2002;6(2):115–9.

78. Rivoire C, Botchorishvili R, Canis M, et al. Complete laparoscopic treatment of genital prolapse with meshes including vaginal promontofixation and anterior repair: a series of 138 patients. J Minim Invasive Gynecol 2007;14(6):712–8.

79. Rosenblatt PL, Chelmow D, Ferzandi TR. Laparoscopic sacrocervicopexy for the treatment of uterine prolapse: a retrospective case series report. J Minim Invasive Gynecol 2008;15(3):268–72.

80. Gadonneix P, Ercoli A, Salet-Lizee D, et al. Laparoscopic sacrocolpopexy with two separate meshes along the anterior and posterior vaginal walls for multicompartment pelvic organ prolapse. J Am Assoc Gynecol Laparosc 2004;11(1): 29–35.

81. Rozet F, Mandron E, Arroyo C, et al. Laparoscopic sacral colpopexy approach for genito-urinary prolapse: experience with 363 cases. Eur Urol 2005;47(2): 230–6.

82. Antiphon P, Elard S, Benyoussef A, et al. Laparoscopic promontory sacral colpopexy: is the posterior, recto-vaginal, mesh mandatory? Eur Urol 2004;45(5): 655–61.

83. Seracchioli R, Hourcabie JA, Vianello F, et al. Laparoscopic treatment of pelvic floor defects in women of reproductive age. J Am Assoc Gynecol Laparosc 2004;11(3):332–5.

84. Miller N. A new method of correcting complete inversion of the vagina: with or without complete prolapse; report of two cases. Surg Gynecol Obstet 1927; 44:550–5.

85. McCall ML. Posterior culdeplasty; surgical correction of enterocele during vaginal hysterectomy; a preliminary report. Obstet Gynecol 1957;10(6):595–602.

86. Lee RA, Symmonds RE. Surgical repair of posthysterectomy vault prolapse. Am J Obstet Gynecol 1972;112(7):953–6.

87. Umek WH, Morgan DM, Ashton-Miller JA, et al. Quantitative analysis of uterosacral ligament origin and insertion points by magnetic resonance imaging. Obstet Gynecol 2004;103(3):447–51.

88. Ramanah R, Parratte B, Arbez-Gindre F, et al. The uterosacral complex: ligament or neurovascular pathway? Anatomical and histological study of fetuses and adults. Int Urogynecol J Pelvic Floor Dysfunct 2008;19(11):1565–70.

89. Buller JL, Thompson JR, Cundiff GW, et al. Uterosacral ligament: description of anatomic relationships to optimize surgical safety. Obstet Gynecol 2001;97(6): 873–9.

90. Culligan PJ, Miklos JR, Murphy M, et al. The tensile strength of uterosacral ligament sutures: a comparison of vaginal and laparoscopic techniques. Obstet Gynecol 2003;101(3):500–3.

91. Wieslander CK, Roshanravan SM, Wai CY, et al. Uterosacral ligament suspension sutures: Anatomic relationships in unembalmed female cadavers. Am J Obstet Gynecol 2007;197(6):672.e671–6.

92. Barber MD, Visco AG, Weidner AC, et al. Bilateral uterosacral ligament vaginal vault suspension with site-specific endopelvic fascia defect repair for treatment of pelvic organ prolapse. Am J Obstet Gynecol 2000;183(6):1402–10 [discussion: 1410–1].

93. Collins SA, Downie SA, Olson TR, et al. Nerve injury during uterosacral ligament fixation: a cadaver study. Int Urogynecol J Pelvic Floor Dysfunct 2009. January 27, 2009. [epub ahead of print].

94. Flynn MK, Weidner AC, Amundsen CL. Sensory nerve injury after uterosacral ligament suspension. Am J Obstet Gynecol 2006;195(6):1869–72.

95. DeLancey JO. Structural anatomy of the posterior pelvic compartment as it relates to rectocele. Am J Obstet Gynecol 1999;180(4):815–23.

96. Shull BL, Bachofen C, Coates KW, et al. A transvaginal approach to repair of apical and other associated sites of pelvic organ prolapse with uterosacral ligaments. Am J Obstet Gynecol 2000;183(6):1365–73 [discussion: 1373–4].

97. Silva WA, Pauls RN, Segal JL, et al. Uterosacral ligament vault suspension: five-year outcomes. Obstet Gynecol 2006;108(2):255–63.

98. Bai SW, Kwon HS, Chung DJ. Abdominal high uterosacral colpopexy and abdominal sacral colpopexy with mesh for pelvic organ prolapse. Int J Gynaecol Obstet 2006;92(2):147–8.

99. Ostrzenski A. Laparoscopic colposuspension for total vaginal prolapse. Int J Gynaecol Obstet 1996;55(2):147–52.

100. Seman EI, Cook JR, O'Shea RT. Two-year experience with laparoscopic pelvic floor repair. J Am Assoc Gynecol Laparosc 2003;10(1):38–45.

101. Lin LL, Phelps JY, Liu CY. Laparoscopic vaginal vault suspension using uterosacral ligaments: a review of 133 cases. J Minim Invasive Gynecol 2005;12(3):216–20.

102. Rardin CR, Erekson EA, Sung VW, et al. Uterosacral colpopexy at the time of vaginal hysterectomy: comparison of laparoscopic and vaginal approaches. J Reprod Med 2009;54(5):273–80.

103. Schwartz M, Abbott KR, Glazerman L, et al. Positive symptom improvement with laparoscopic uterosacral ligament repair for uterine or vaginal vault prolapse: interim results from an active multicenter trial. J Minim Invasive Gynecol 2007; 14(5):570–6.

104. Maher CF, Carey MP, Murray CJ. Laparoscopic suture hysteropexy for uterine prolapse. Obstet Gynecol 2001;97(6):1010–4.

105. Medina C, Takacs P. Laparoscopic uterosacral uterine suspension: a minimally invasive technique for treating pelvic organ prolapse. J Minim Invasive Gynecol 2006;13(5):472–5.

106. Diwan A, Rardin CR, Strohsnitter WC, et al. Laparoscopic uterosacral ligament uterine suspension compared with vaginal hysterectomy with vaginal vault suspension for uterovaginal prolapse. Int Urogynecol J Pelvic Floor Dysfunct 2006;17(1):79–83.

107. Hale DS, Rogers RM Jr. Abdominal sacrospinous ligament colposuspension. Obstet Gynecol 1999;94(6):1039–41.

108. Joshi VM. A new technique of uterine suspension to pectineal ligaments in the management of uterovaginal prolapse. Obstet Gynecol 1993;81(5 (Pt 1)):790–3.

109. O'Brien PM, Ibrahim J. Failure of laparoscopic uterine suspension to provide a lasting cure for uterovaginal prolapse. Br J Obstet Gynaecol 1994;101(8): 707–8.

110. Richardson AC, Lyon JB, Williams NL. A new look at pelvic relaxation. Am J Obstet Gynecol 1976;126(5):568–73.

111. Weinstein M, Roberts M. Simultaneous repair of cystocele and high rectal prolapse during total hysterectomy. West J Surg Obstet Gynecol 1949;57(1): 34–7.

112. Schauffler GC. The management of cystocele during abdominal hysterectomy. Urol Cutaneous Rev 1951;55(5):269–70.

113. Macer GA. Transabdominal repair of cystocele, a 20 year experience, compared with the traditional vaginal approach. Am J Obstet Gynecol 1978; 131(2):203–7.

114. Lovatsis D, Drutz HP. Is transabdominal repair of mild to moderate cystocele necessary for correction of prolapse during a modified Burch procedure? Int Urogynecol J Pelvic Floor Dysfunct 2001;12(3):193–8.

115. Richardson AC, Edmonds PB, Williams NL. Treatment of stress urinary incontinence due to paravaginal fascial defect. Obstet Gynecol 1981;57(3):357–62.

116. White GR. An anatomical operation for the cure of cystocele. Am J Obstet Gynecol 1912;65:286–90.

117. Shull BL, Baden WF. A six-year experience with paravaginal defect repair for stress urinary incontinence. Am J Obstet Gynecol 1989;160(6):1432–9 [discussion: 1439–40].

118. Benson JT, McClellan E. The effect of vaginal dissection on the pudendal nerve. Obstet Gynecol 1993;82(3):387–9.

119. Bruce RG, El-Galley RE, Galloway NT. Paravaginal defect repair in the treatment of female stress urinary incontinence and cystocele. Urology 1999;54(4): 647–51.

120. Demirci F, Ozdemir I, Somunkiran A, et al. Abdominal paravaginal defect repair in the treatment of paravaginal defect and urodynamic stress incontinence. J Obstet Gynaecol 2007;27(6):601–4.

121. Scotti RJ, Garely AD, Greston WM, et al. Paravaginal repair of lateral vaginal wall defects by fixation to the ischial periosteum and obturator membrane. Am J Obstet Gynecol 1998;179(6 Pt 1):1436–45.

122. Ostrzenski A. Genuine stress urinary incontinence in women. New laparoscopic paravaginal reconstruction. J Reprod Med 1998;43(6):477–82.

123. Behnia-Willison F, Seman EI, Cook JR, et al. Laparoscopic paravaginal repair of anterior compartment prolapse. J Minim Invasive Gynecol 2007;14(4):475–80.

124. Maher C, Baessler K. Surgical management of anterior vaginal wall prolapse: an evidencebased literature review. Int Urogynecol J Pelvic Floor Dysfunct 2006; 17(2):195–201.

125. Oom DM, Gosselink MP, van Wijk JJ, et al. Rectocele repair by anterolateral rectopexy: long-term functional outcome. Colorectal Dis 2008;10(9):925–30.

126. Lyons TL, Winer WK. Laparoscopic rectocele repair using polyglactin mesh. J Am Assoc Gynecol Laparosc 1997;4(3):381–4.

127. Thornton MJ, Lam A, King DW. Laparoscopic or transanal repair of rectocele? A retrospective matched cohort study. Dis Colon Rectum 2005;48(4):792–8.

Use of Mesh and Materials in Pelvic Floor Surgery

Miles Murphy, MD, MSPH[a,b,c,*]

KEYWORDS

• Mesh • Graft • Prolapse • Incontinence • Pelvic floor surgery

Grafts have been used in reconstructive pelvic surgery for more than 100 years, but the turn of the 20th century brought a new wave of controversial, packaged graft procedures that has significantly changed the practice of urogynecology. Early graft procedures primarily used the patient's own tissues to aid in repair. Treatment of stress urinary incontinence (SUI) using these "autologous" grafts varied from use of the patient's own gracilis muscle in 1907,[1] to the round ligament,[2] and the rectus fascia.[3] Use of biologic grafts eventually expanded to the repair of pelvic organ prolapse (POP) defects,[4] but as will be shown in this article, the recent trend in graft use has been toward synthetic materials.

The annual direct cost of POP surgery in the United States is estimated at more than $1 billion.[5] Evidence suggests that a fair amount of this expense can be attributed to failed primary surgery. One retrospective study showed that over a 10-year period more than one in four women will develop a recurrence of her prolapse.[6] A prospective study showed that within 5 years, 13% of women will undergo reoperation for failed surgery for prolapse and incontinence.[7] Values such as these have driven practitioners to seek more durable techniques for repair of these complex defects.

One field that pelvic surgeons have looked to for help in guiding these innovations is that of general surgery. The widespread use of grafts in abdominal hernia repair preceded that of reconstructive pelvic surgery. The results of early randomized clinical trials of traditional suture-based versus synthetic mesh repairs of inguinal hernia showed superior success rates with mesh, and more recent long-term follow-up of these trials have shown a persistence of the decreased risk of recurrence with

[a] Department of Obstetrics/Gynecology & Reproductive Sciences, 3500 N. Broad St., Temple University School of Medicine, Philadelphia, PA 19140, USA
[b] Division of Urogynecology, Department of Obstetrics and Gynecology, 1200 Old York Road, Abington Memorial Hospital, Abington, PA 19001, USA
[c] Institute for Female Pelvic Medicine and Reconstructive Surgery, 1010 Horsham Road, Suite 205, North Wales, PA 18104, USA
* Corresponding author. Institute for Female Pelvic Medicine and Reconstructive Surgery, 1010 Horsham Road - Suite 205, North Wales, PA 18104.
E-mail address: milesmurphy@comcast.net

Obstet Gynecol Clin N Am 36 (2009) 615–635
doi:10.1016/j.ogc.2009.08.007
0889-8545/09/$ – see front matter © 2009 Elsevier Inc. All rights reserved.

obgyn.theclinics.com

mesh repair.[8] But the functional requirements of a vaginal repair are often drastically different from an abdominal hernia repair. The need for optimal urinary, defecatory, and sexual function requires that a repair be more than just durable.

Nonetheless, recent surveys of professional subspecialty societies have shown widespread adoption of at least some form of graft repair by their surgeons. As early as 2002, a survey of practice patterns of the International Urogynecological Association showed that more surgeons were using a synthetic midurethral sling as their procedure of choice for SUI than were using a suture-based colposuspension.[9] More recent surveys of the American Urogynecologic Society have shown that nearly half of respondents used minimally invasive transobturator devices for cystocele repair[10] and nearly all use synthetic mesh for at least some of their reconstructive procedures for SUI and/or POP.[11]

Despite this near universal use of some form of graft-based repair among this subspecialist organization, great controversy exists over the use of materials in pelvic floor surgery. This controversy is particularly acute in regard to synthetic mesh grafts, especially when packaged with delivery-system kits produced by medical device manufacturers. This issue came to a head in October 2008 when the Center for Devices and Radiological Health, a division of the US Food and Drug Administration (FDA), issued public health notifications to both the general public and health care practitioners regarding the complications that can be associated with the transvaginal placement of surgical mesh in repair of POP and SUI.[12,13]

This article will attempt to get to the root of the complex issues regarding the use of mesh and materials in pelvic floor dysfunction. We examine the various types of grafts available for use and the outcomes of the case series and comparative studies of graft repairs used in the treatment of SUI and POP.

TYPES OF MESH AND MATERIALS
Biologic

Grafts used in pelvic reconstructive surgery can be divided into two basic types: biologic and synthetic. Subtypes of these two divisions can be found in **Table 1**.

Biologic grafts can be autologous, heterologous, or xenogenic. Autologous grafts are harvested from and then implanted in the same patient. The most commonly known examples of this type of graft are the fascia lata and rectus fascia grafts that are harvested from women with SUI and fashioned into suburethral slings. Because these grafts come from the patient herself there is very little risk of a foreign body reaction or transmission of infection. However, autologous grafts may produce morbidity at the harvest site and procurement of the graft adds operative time and

Table 1	
Types of grafts used in vaginal reconstructive surgery	
Biologics	Autologous graft: rectus sheath, fascia lata, vaginal mucosa
	Allograft: cadaveric fascia lata, cadaveric dura mater, cadaveric dermis (these tissues may have been freeze-dried, solvent dehydrated, or irradiated)
	Xenograft: porcine dermis, porcine small intestine submucosa, bovine pericardium, fetal bovine dermis (these tissues may or may not have been cross-linked)
Synthetics	Absorbable: polyglycolic acid, polyglactin, hybrid: polyglactin/polypropylene
	Non-absorbable: polyester, polytetrafluorethylene (PTFE), polypropylene, polyethylene, and nylon (often categorized by pore size and mono- or multifilament construction)

the potential for increased blood loss to the reconstructive procedure. Heterologous grafts (aka allografts) are materials harvested from a human donor other than the patient herself. Allografts are usually harvested from cadavers and processed with solvent dehydration or freeze-drying. Because morbidity from the harvest site is not a concern with cadaveric material, larger pieces of allograft have been used to repair POP. One of the more common procedures using these materials is the abdominal sacral colpopexy.

The other type of biologic graft is a xenograft. These are materials that are harvested from other species and processed for use in humans. Because of the risk of rejection and infection, these products are usually processed into acellular collagen scaffolds. In some of these grafts the collagen is cross-linked to minimize degradation by host collagenases. The most common forms of xenografts used in pelvic reconstruction are porcine and bovine derivatives.

Synthetic

Synthetic grafts have traditionally been categorized by a classification system first described by Amid and colleagues[14] in regard to abdominal hernia repair (**Table 2**). Synthetic implants can be made from knitted single-fiber filaments (monofilament materials) or they can be braided with monofilament yarns, further woven as multifilament fibers in different ways and pore sizes.

Multiple factors influence the suitability of mesh for human use: the degree of inflammatory reaction is related to its chemical composition and the amount of material used, flexibility of the mesh can affect organ function, and strength can be related to the durability of the repair. One of the critical categories in the Amid system is pore size of the mesh, which has been related to infectious risk and fibroblast infiltration. Bacteria, which can measure as little as or less than 1 micron in size, easily enter into synthetic meshes. However, larger pore sizes are required to allow passage of

Table 2 Classification of synthetic grafts				
Type	**Pore Size Macro > 75 μm, Micro < 75 μm**	**Component**	**Fiber Type**	**Trade Name**
Type I	Macroporous and monofilamentous	Polypropylene	Monofilament Monofilament Monofilament Monofilament	Prolene (Ethicon) Marlex (Bard) Atrium (Atrium) Gynemesh (Gynecare)
Type II	Microporous (<10 μm) and multifilamentous	Expanded PTFE	Multifilament	Gore-Tex-DualMesh (WL Gore)
Type III	Macroporous Patch with multifilament or Microporous elements	Woven polyethylene (Dacron) PTFE Woven polypropylene Perforated PTFE Polyglactin 910	Multifilament Multifilament Multifilament Multifilament Multifilament	Merselene (Ethicon) Teflon Surgipro Mycro Mesh Vicryl (Ethicon)
Type IV	Submicro <1 μm	Polypropylene sheet	Monofilament	Cellguard

Abbreviation: PTFE, polytetrafluorethylene.

leukocytes (9–15 μm in size) and macrophages (16–20 μm in size). In general, knitted materials have greater porosity than woven materials.[15] Interstices between multifilament fibers is also important, in that those with interstices of less than 10 μm may theoretically allow passage of bacteria but not the cells from the host's microbial defense system. Pore sizes larger than 75 μm can allow for rapid ingrowth of fibroblasts (50 μm) and vascular elements necessary to anchor the implant within the native tissue.[16]

The other major characteristic that affects the natural history of implanted mesh is its absorbability. Most of the materials listed in the Amid classification system are permanent, nonabsorbable materials such as polypropylene, polytetrafluoroethylene, and polyethylene. However, absorbable meshes made out of materials such as polyglactin 910 do exist. There are also hybrid meshes that include nonabsorbable materials like polypropylene either knitted with fibers of absorbable polyglactin or poliglecaprone 25 or coated with hydrophilic porcine collagen.

GRAFT USE IN RECONSTRUCTIVE PELVIC SURGERY
Urinary Incontinence

Biologic grafts
The Kelly plication was the predominant surgical procedure performed for SUI in women during the first half of the 20th century. This was overwhelming replaced by retropubic urethropexies in the 1950s, as the popularity of the Burch and Marshall-Marchetti-Kranz (MMK) procedures spread across North America. These suture-based procedures (especially the latter two) are still performed today, but the introduction of the tension-free vaginal tape (TVT) procedure in the late 1990s greatly reduced the frequency with which suture-based surgeries were done. Before the TVT, sling surgeries were generally reserved for patients with hypermobility of the bladder neck combined with incompetence of the proximal urethral closure mechanism (commonly referred to as intrinsic sphincter deficiency or ISD).

Although the concept of suburethral support was originally introduced in 1907, it was not until its reintroduction in 1978 by McGuire and Lytton that it gained increased clinical use.[17] Since this initial description a number of different techniques for securement and sling materials have been used, but the performance of the traditional pubovaginal sling has had only minor modifications since 1978.[18] A 6.0 to 8.0 × 1.0 to 1.5-cm portion of the rectus fascia is harvested through a Pfannenstiel incision and secured at the ends with suture. An inverted U or midline incision is centered over the proximal urethra, and the endopelvic fascia is sharply perforated lateral and distal to the bladder neck thus entering into the retropubic position. The sling sutures are passed from the vaginal to the abdominal incision lateral to the rectus muscle and then tied across the midline over the rectus fascia with the least amount of tension required to prevent urethral motion.

Early series of 67 women undergoing autologous fascial slings revealed very good results with a cure rate of 82% and another 9% improved at a mean follow-up of 3.5 years.[19] Most of the failures were felt to be the result of urge incontinence. A later, much larger series of almost 250 women noted similar cure rates with favorable responses to the short form of the Urinary Distress Inventory (UDI-6), a validated, condition-specific quality of life instrument.[18] In this series there was a less than 1% incisional hernia rate and no sling erosions.

Despite these good results, in an attempt to minimize the invasiveness of the procedure and to limit harvest-site morbidity, many surgeons moved toward allogeneic grafts for their suburethral slings. One early series of 16 women undergoing sling surgery using allogeneic human cadaver fascia lata showed acceptable short-term results.[20] They reported an objective success rate of 79% at follow-up ranging from 6 to 12 months. The mean duration of postoperative bladder drainage was 29 days.

Longer-term follow-up in other similar series, however, showed less favorable results. Failure was noted in 52% of patients, with recurrent SUI symptoms occurring from 2 weeks to 24 months (median 3 months) after the procedure.[21] Results are not significantly better when bone anchors are used to anchor the sling into the posterior aspect of the pubic bone. One study showed recurrent SUI in 37.6% of patients at 10.6 months of follow-up using freeze-dried fascia[22] and another using nonfrozen solvent-dehydrated fascia showed recurrent SUI in 37.0% of patients at 24 months.[23] Furthermore, there appears to be a relatively high erosion rate with cadaveric fascia. Within as little as 45 days, one study showed a 23% vaginal erosion rate.[24]

Fitzgerald and colleagues[25] theorize recurrent SUI in patients treated with freeze-dried irradiated fascia *allograft* sling may be the result of material failure. They note that on reoperation, the graft was either grossly degenerated (6%) or completely absent (14%) in up to 20% of patients. On the other hand, this same group of investigators note in a smaller series of patients with *autologous* rectus fascia slings, that these slings remain viable. There appears to be proliferation of fibroblasts, neovascularization, and remodeling of the graft with no evidence of an inflammatory reaction or graft degeneration.[26]

Synthetic grafts

Following the rebirth of suburethral autologous sling surgery for the treatment of SUI in the 1970s, a number of synthetic slings were also investigated. One of the first nonbiologic materials used for SUI was woven polyethylene (Mersilene),[27] but this multifilamentous material was, in some cases, associated with significant complications such as delayed transection of the urethra.[28] Other synthetic materials used in procedures for SUI that did not ultimately prove ideal for vaginal use included the "Teflon tape suspension,"[29] and the "Marlex"[30] and the "Silastic"[31] sling operations.

In the 1980s a number of surgeons started using polytetrafluoroethylene (Gore-Tex) for their slings. Short-term objective and subjective cure rates were good at 85%, but even at this 3-month postoperative evaluation, complications such as urinary retention and wound seromas were noted.[32] Longer follow-up studies showed that voiding difficulties often required prolonged catheterization and/or sling revision; in some cases, even sling removal did not relieve these patients' urinary retention.[33] One study of patients who were at least 1 year out from surgery showed postoperative wound complications in 40% and noted that 22% of the grafts were eventually removed.[34] In a 1997 review of the use of mesh in gynecologic surgery, Iglesia and colleagues[35] concluded that "The ideal synthetic mesh material for pelvic surgery, one that induces minimal foreign-body reaction with minimal risk of infection, rejection and erosion, has yet to be developed."

It was around this time that surgical device manufacturers began partnering with surgeons to create and market prepackaged slings. Several different materials were used in an attempt to avoid the complications associated with other synthetic slings. One of the first was a woven polyester sling treated with pressure-injected bovine collagen (ProteGen, Boston Scientific, Natick, MA), which was recalled in January 1999. One multicenter study reported on 34 patients who had undergone removal of the polyester slings within the 2 previous years.[36] The average patient presented within 8 months of original sling placement. Of the 34 women, 17 (50%) had vaginal erosion only, 7 (20%) had isolated urethral erosion, and 6 (17%) had urethrovaginal fistula. Another polyester mesh sling, this one coated with silicone (American Medical Systems, Minnetonka, MN) was noted to have similar problems in a premarket, multicenter trial.[37] Ten of 31 (32%) required a second surgical procedure at an average of 6 months (range 68 to 343 days) postoperatively. Eight (26%) had vaginal extrusion of the mesh, one required sling lysis, and one required sling removal because of infection. This product was subsequently not marketed in the United States. It is not entirely clear why these devices had such high erosion rates, but one study of polyester and polypropylene meshes removed for erosion showed bacterial contamination in all cases.[38] Most cultures demonstrated multimicrobial growth, but when only one bacterium was found, it was *Proteus mirabilis* in 25% of cases. However, bacterial quantifications varied greatly and because quantification was often low, the authors concluded that the role of bacterial contamination in mesh erosion "is not yet clear."

In 1996, a landmark paper was published out of Sweden describing an ambulatory surgical procedure for SUI.[39] Ulmsten and colleagues had been working for a number of years on a surgical procedure they called intravaginal slingplasty.[40] They experimented with different sling materials including polytetrafluoroethylene and polyethylene before settling on a macroporous, monofilament polypropylene mesh. This procedure differed from previous sling procedures in three key ways: first, the sling was placed via a vaginal route rather than the traditional abdominal approach; second, the sling was covered by a plastic sheath to theoretically prevent contamination before placement; and third, the sling was placed at the level of the midurethra, loosely positioned, with the sling arms not fixed to a static structure. This procedure came to be known as the tension-free vaginal tape (TVT).[41]

TVT came to be one of the most studied surgical procedures for female SUI. Long-term follow-up of TVT at 7[42] and 11[43] years showed very little decline in efficacy over time with a 90% objective and 77% subjective cure rate (with another 20% subjectively improved) at greater than 10 years out from surgery. Furthermore, the troublesome complication of infection and/or erosion seen with other synthetic slings was not a significant issue with this technique and material. These findings published by the creators of this procedure proved to be highly reproducible by other investigators.[44,45]

Despite the impressive safety and efficacy of the TVT, it is not without potential complications. Although the most common complication of this "blind" procedure, bladder perforation, does not produce significant adverse sequelae as long as it is recognized and corrected intraoperatively; the much less common complications of bowel[46] and major vessel injury can be catastrophic. Concern over these potential complications spurred the development of similar midurethral tension-free slings that were placed through the obturator space instead of the retropubic space. These "transobturator" slings can be passed from under the urethra, through the obturator foramen, and out through skin incisions at the thigh folds (the so called "inside-out" technique) or from the skin incisions in toward the midurethra (the "outside-in" technique), significantly decreasing the risk of bladder perforation and essentially eliminating the risk of bowel injury. Initial series of these procedures reported similar efficacy outcomes to the retropubic TVT.[47,48] Most of these transobturator slings used mesh similar to or the same as TVT, but one used a polypropylene graft prepared through a heat-welding process with smaller pore size than the TVT and was shown to carry an erosion risk as high as 13%.[49]

Comparative studies

Despite a plethora of comparative data on sling materials and placement techniques, there is still no definitive consensus as to the ideal anti–stress incontinence procedure. However, the studies discussed in the following paragraphs should help to guide surgeons in their decision-making process.

Comparisons of autograft and allograft pubovaginal slings show, for the most part, similar outcomes. In a retrospective review of pubovaginal slings performed with either autologous fascia or freeze-dried cadaveric fascia lata, Wright and colleagues[50] found similar improvements in a symptom scoring system between the two groups at a mean follow-up of approximately 1 year. There were no complications related to the cadaveric origin of the allograft and its use significantly shortened operative time and hospital stay. Another retrospective review comparing these types of grafts showed a small number of early failures with the cadaveric fascia, but the overall success rates were ultimately comparable and operative time and postoperative pain were decreased in the cadaveric group.[51] However, a recent long-term comparison of autologous fascia lata to solvent dehydrated fascia lata showed urodynamic stress incontinence in 41.7% of the allograft patients at 2 years compared with 0% of the autograft patients,[52] suggesting that long-term follow-up may reveal differences in biologic grafts that may not be seen during a standard postoperative observation period. Although donor antigens associated with allografts may play a role in host incorporation, the exact significance of this antigenicity is unknown.[53]

Human use is the ultimate test of the worth of a material in pelvic reconstruction, but laboratory evaluation of sling properties can be of value as well. Using a rabbit model, Dora and colleagues[54] looked at time-dependent variations in the biomechanical properties of cadaveric fascia, porcine dermis and small intestine mucosa, polypropylene mesh, and autologous fascia. They noted a rapid loss of tensile strength in the cadaveric and porcine allografts. There was no loss of strength with the autologous fascia, but it did show a 50% decrease in its surface area. The synthetic mesh did not have a decrease in tensile strength or a significant decrease in surface area when compared with the other sling types. Human trials seem to validate this model in that most comparative studies of the autologous pubovaginal sling and TVT show similar success rates,[55–57] but those comparing TVT and autologous sling to xenografts show poorer outcomes with the latter.[58,59] In some of these studies there were higher rates of voiding dysfunction with pubovaginal sling than TVT; in others no difference was seen.

TVT has also been compared with a number of suture-based repairs. A randomized trial of TVT and endopelvic fascia plication with permanent suture in women with POP and occult SUI showed significantly higher subjective and objective continence rates in the TVT arm.[60] Paraiso and colleagues[61] showed higher objective and subjective cure rates with TVT at 1 to 2 years postoperatively in a randomized trial of TVT and laparoscopic Burch colposuspension. In their long-term (4–8 years) follow-up of these subjects, the dryness rates were 10% higher in the TVT arm, but this difference was no longer statistically significant.[62] A similar randomized trial was conducted in the United Kingdom, but in it TVT was compared with open colposuspension. Short-term results showed no significant difference in cure at 6 months between groups (66% of TVT and 57% of colposuspension group).[63] The overall complication rate was comparable between groups, but the TVT arm had more intraoperative complications (mostly bladder perforations) whereas the colposuspension arm had more postoperative complications. Over a 6-month period, TVT was less costly than colposuspension.[64] Operative time and time to resumption of normal voiding were shorter in the TVT arms of both the US laparoscopic and UK open colposuspension trials. At 2-year follow-up there was a statistically significant difference in objective cure favoring TVT.[65] By 5 years out, nearly two thirds of the study population had been lost to follow-up and there was no difference in cure between arms in this reduced population, but vault and posterior vaginal wall prolapse was seen more commonly after colposuspension. On the other hand, three late TVT erosions were detected.[66]

TVT also fairs well when compared with other retropubic midurethral slings. In two studies of TVT and the "top-down" suprapubic arc sling (SPARC), TVT appeared to perform as well or better than the SPARC. In a large retrospective study, TVT had higher objective and subjective cure rates.[67] In a smaller prospective randomized trial, the TVT arm had a higher cure rate and a lower rate of bladder perforation. Neither of these differences was statistically significant, but with only 31 patients in each arm, very large differences would have been needed to reach statistical significance.[68] When compared with another "bottom-up" midurethral sling, the difference in outcomes was more clear. The intravaginal slingplasty (IVS) (Tyco Healthcare, Mansfield, MA) is made from polypropylene as is TVT, but the IVS uses multifilament threads with small pores unlike TVT, which is a knitted macroporous monofilament mesh. In a large randomized trial of these two slings, both were effective for stress incontinence, but 9% of the women treated with the IVS required removal of the tape for vaginal erosion/infection as compared with 0% of the TVT group ($P < .01$) after 2 years of follow-up.[69] In a subanalysis of another comparative trial, delayed erosions of the IVS sling were noted at up to 34 months of follow-up.[70]

There have been many comparative studies of retropubic and obturator midurethral slings. In 2007, Sung and colleagues[71] performed a very informative systematic review and meta-analysis on this topic. They felt that there was insufficient evidence to determine if one approach leads to better objective outcomes. They did note a higher rate of complication with the retropubic approach but this was mostly composed of bladder perforations, which may be of little clinical significance. Since then, a number of other investigations have been conducted that for the most part confirm these findings. One multicenter, randomized trial of an "outside-in" obturator sling with 18-month follow-up showed that it was not inferior to TVT and had a lower bladder perforation rate.[72] Another trial of an "inside-out" obturator sling showed comparable short-term objective and subjective cure, but a higher rate of complication with the obturator.[73] This was because they included postoperative groin pain as a complication. Their 1-year follow-up study showed persistent equivalence in regard to success and they noted an equal complication rate between groups.[74]

Where the differences in outcomes may exist becomes more evident when one looks at different subtypes of incontinence and pelvic function. The conventional wisdom suggests that obturator slings may have the potential for having a negative impact on sexual function but more forgiving for people with voiding dysfunction in addition to stress incontinence. One study did show a decreased risk of urethrolysis and need for postoperative anticholinergic medications following obturator slings,[75] although others have not shown a difference in voiding symptoms.[76] Likewise, there does not appear to be a difference in sexual function either.[77]

Where there does appear to be an emerging difference in outcomes is in patients with severe SUI, what is often referred to as intrinsic sphincter deficiency. Although the International Continence Society has not provided an agreed upon definition for this condition, many practitioners use the following urodynamic parameters to make this diagnosis: a leak point pressure (LPP) of 60 or less or a maximum urethral closure pressure (MUCP) of 20 cm or less of water pressure. In a randomized trial of patients meeting these criteria, Schierlitz and colleagues[78] found a 6-month failure rate of 21% of TVT versus a 45% failure rate in the transobturator arm ($P = .004$). Other nonrandomized trials have found similar differences in outcomes with even less stringent urodynamic parameters such as an MUCP of 40.[79,80] Even factors such as the degree of stressful activity that is required to cause incontinence (minor versus major strains) has been shown to affect outcomes in these two types of midurethral slings.[81]

Pelvic Organ Prolapse

Abdominal surgery

The techniques for using grafts in abdominal prolapse repair has been covered extensively in the article by Douglass Hale, MD elsewhere in this issue, so this section will mostly focus on putative issues related to abdominal versus vaginal use of grafts and the types of grafts used in these repairs. By far, the most commonly performed grafted abdominal procedure for prolapse is the sacral colpopexy. This technique was first described by Lane in 1962,[82] in which a graft was used to bridge the gap from vaginal cuff to the sacrum. Early case series of this procedure describe the use of polyethylene terephthalate (Mersilene),[83] polyethylene (Marlex),[84] and polytetrafluoroethylene (Gore-Tex)[85] synthetic mesh for reconstruction. This procedure was noted to be highly effective, and when there were failures they were generally attributed to separation of the graft from the vagina and not as a failure of the graft material itself.[86]

The first large series of sacral colpopexy using a polypropylene graft was published in 1990.[87] Since then a comprehensive review of sacral colpopexy has suggested that vaginal erosion rate of polypropylene appears to be lower than with other synthetic grafts.[88] This systematic review included erosion data from more than 2000 patients and noted erosions in less than 1% of polypropylene and in greater than 3% of polyethylene graft procedures. Although rare, two cases of sacral osteomyelitis have also been reported with the use of polyethylene mesh.[89]

A number of biologic grafts have also been used for abdominal sacral colpopexy including rectus fascia,[90] lyophilized cerebral dura mater allograft, and cadaveric fascia lata.[24,91] The goal of using a biologic graft can vary, but certainly one would hope to be at least as effective at preventing recurrent prolapse while minimizing the risks of untoward effects of using a permanent, synthetic mesh such as vaginal erosion. Some series suggest that these goals may not be reached. One investigation of cadaveric fascia lata showed an early erosion rate of 27%[24] and another reported a 43% failure rate at 1 year.[21] Unlike synthetic graft, which showed intact mesh at reoperation that had separated from the vagina, reoperation on the donor fascia repairs showed graft between the sacrum and vagina in only 19% of cases.

As we see with suburethral slings, a number of factors seem to influence the rate of graft erosion. Like surgery for SUI, the type of graft material used is certainly an important factor when repairing prolapse. As with suburethral sling surgery, polytetrafluoroethylene (Gore-Tex) and silicone-coated polyester meshes tend to lead to unacceptably high erosion rates. One retrospective chart review of 92 patients over a 6-year period, found a 9% erosion rate with Gore-Tex and a 19% rate with silicone-coated mesh as compared with no erosions with polypropylene or fascia grafts.[92] A similar erosion rate (24%) was found in another retrospective study of abdominal and laparoscopic sacral colpopexy with silicone-coated polyester mesh as compared with a 0% rate with uncoated polypropylene at a mean follow-up of 12 months.[93] Only one of these erosions was successfully managed transvaginally, the remainder required abdominal exploration.

Another factor of interest is whether or not the vaginal cavity is entered during abdominal repair. In an attempt to fully correct the posterior fascial defects often associated with perineal descent, Cundiff and colleagues[94] modified the traditional sacral colpopexy by dissecting the full length of the rectovaginal space and, if necessary, attaching the posterior mesh directly to the perineal body. In patients with distal detachment of the posterior fascia from the perineal body or in cases in which it appears that the posterior vaginal fascia is severely attenuated, this group used a combined abdominal and vaginal colpoperineopexy. In a retrospective review of purely abdominal versus combined vaginal-abdominal sacral colpoperineopexy, they noted a higher rate of and shorter time to mesh erosion when suture or mesh placement was performed transvaginally.[95] Likewise, there is some concern regarding hysterectomy with entry into the vaginal lumen at the time of sacral colpopexy for utero-vaginal prolapse. Here the literature provides conflicting evidence, with some studies showing a higher rate of mesh erosion[96,97] whereas others show no increased risk as compared with colpopexy for vaginal vault prolapse.[98,99] One interesting note, in the latter studies showing no difference only polypropylene mesh was used, whereas in the others, a variety of other synthetic grafts were used.

Vaginal surgery

The variety of grafted transvaginal prolapse surgeries is more diverse than abdominal surgery. The abdominal sacral colpopexy is designed to treat apical defects and is most commonly performed with anterior and posterior grafts, whereas transvaginal operations are more likely to address individual compartment defects. The introduction of biologic grafts into transvaginal reconstruction demonstrates this. One of the more common uses of transvaginal biologic graft is for repair of a rectocele. Suture-based posterior compartment defect repairs tend to use plication of rectovaginal "fascia" or of the levator musculature, and are historically associated with the risk of de novo dyspareunia.[100] In 2002, Miklos and colleagues[101] published two case reports of patients with postoperative dyspareunia following levatorplasty who were subsequently treated with release and reconstruction of the rectovaginal septum with a dermal allograft. This treatment corrected their rectocele and their dyspareunia. The authors followed-up this case report with a series of 43 women with advanced posterior wall prolapse who underwent dermal graft augmentation of site-specific rectocele repair.[102] They reported a 93% cure rate with no complications at an average of more than 1 year of follow-up. However, a prospective study of rectocele repair using a porcine dermal xenograft showed a 41% failure rate at 3-year follow-up.[103]

Biologic grafts have also been used to treat isolated anterior compartment defects as well. Chung and colleagues[104] have reported on the combined repair of stress incontinence and central cystocele using a single piece of cadaveric dermal graft. At 2 years of follow-up, only 2 (11%) of 18 patients had a recurrence of their cystocele. One patient developed an acute infection and the autolysed graft was removed and she subsequently underwent a successful repair with an autologous graft. Vaginal paravaginal defect repairs with dermal allograft have not fared as well, with failure rates as high as 41% at 18 months[105] and greater than 50% at long-term follow-up.[106] There were no graft erosions or rejection at a mean follow-up of 52 months.

As with slings, the safety of many biologic grafts is attractive to some, but questions over repair durability have led others to investigate the use of synthetic grafts for vaginal prolapse repair. Whereas some of these studies have been with absorbable or hybrid mesh,[107] most have looked at the use of permanent grafts (most commonly polypropylene mesh). One early observational study of recurrent cystoceles showed excellent cure rates with polypropylene (Marlex) mesh but also a high rate (25%) of vaginal mesh exposures.[108] One series of anterior and posterior compartment repairs with polypropylene mesh also showed very good anatomic results but an unacceptably high rate of postoperative dyspareunia.[109] In both series, the operations involved augmentation of traditional colporrhaphy with the mesh.

Other investigators have sought new techniques for the transvaginal repair of prolapse with synthetic monofilament mesh. A group of French gynecologists, inspired by the tension-free concept first demonstrated with midurethral slings, developed a technique and procedure that they termed the Tension-free Vaginal Mesh (TVM)[110] and initiated a prospective multicenter study. Instead of augmenting a traditional repair, the procedure involves placing bodies of mesh in the vesico-vaginal and/or recto-vaginal space (in essentially the same space as the abdominal sacral colpopexy but accessed through a transvaginal incision) that are held in place by attached arms of mesh that traverse the obturator and/or ischio-rectal fossae, and associated muscles and connective tissues, instead of being sutured in place. Early results showed low failure rates but an erosion rate of 12.3%, and it was suggested that avoidance of T-colpotomy and concomitant hysterectomy could drastically reduce this rate of erosion.[111] After instituting these guidelines, a short-term series showed a low failure (4.7%) and erosion (4.7%) rate.[112]

An independent group of Nordic gynecologists also embarked on a prospective, multicenter study of this technique. Using a standardized protocol, 25 centers enrolled 248 women in this series starting in October of 2005. Early perioperative data showed a 4.4% rate of serious complications; one was an intraoperative hemorrhage and the rest were visceral injuries.[113] Short-term (2-month) outcomes from this group showed an anatomic cure in 87% of the anterior, 91% of the posterior, and 88% of the total repairs and no severe adverse events attributed to the polypropylene mesh.[114] One-year data showed only a small drop in anatomic cure rates, improvement in domain-specific quality of life instruments, and repeat surgical intervention because of mesh exposure in only 2.8% of cases.[115] Another 1-year series showed an even lower rate of mesh-related complications.[116]

Despite these relatively low rates of adverse events in large series with this emerging technique, other case reports and case series of adverse events have given many pause for concern. These events include postoperative vesicovaginal fistula,[117] hematoma,[118] mesh exposures, and chronic pain.[119] All of these reports involved monofilament, macroporous polypropylene mesh, but the rate at which these complications occur outside of large series is unknown because of a lack of a denominator in these case reports. However, other tension-free prolapse repairs appear to have more definable device-related adverse event rates. Although initial reports on the efficacy of an apical suspension procedure known as the posterior intravaginal slingplasty (IVS) were encouraging,[120] larger longer-term series were more concerning. As with its related anti-incontinence sling procedure, this operation involves placement of a multifilament polypropylene tape. This posterior IVS is placed in a transgluteal fashion to reinforce the atrophied uterosacral ligaments. Two series with a combined patient population of more than 200 women showed a 17% erosion rate necessitating a high reoperation rate.[121,122]

Comparative studies

Comparative studies (especially randomized controlled trials) involving graft-based prolapse repairs are scarce, but most of the investigations that have been published were conducted in the past few years. Hopefully, this represents a trend toward higher-quality research in pelvic reconstructive surgery. In this section, comparisons of graft studies involving abdominal versus other abdominal, abdominal versus vaginal, and vaginal versus other vaginal repairs will be examined.

One of the only trials comparing abdominal sacral colpopexy performed with a synthetic graft versus a biologic graft was published in 2005.[123] In this study, 100 women were randomized to either polypropylene or solvent-dehydrated cadaveric fascia lata. By 1 year out from surgery, significant differences were seen between groups in regard to prolapse stage, anterior and apical compartment support, and objective failure, all favoring the synthetic graft. Although a lack of subjective outcomes were a limitation of this study, the difference in objective failure (32% versus 9%, $P < .01$) was significant. A smaller, nonrandomized trial of synthetic versus biologic graft, however, showed no significant difference.[124] This study compared synthetic mesh to a porcine xenograft in abdominal sacral colpopexy. The objective success was based on a mean follow-up of only 7 months, but long-term (2–4 years) subjective outcomes were comparable between groups.

In regard to suture-based versus graft-based transabdominal reconstruction for prolapse, one interesting study looked at a comparison of three techniques: abdominosacral colpopexy with mesh and hysterectomy, abdominosacral uteropexy with mesh, and abdominal uterosacrocardinal colpopexy and hysterectomy (no mesh). Although hysterectomy has traditionally been considered an important part of the surgical correction of uterovaginal prolapse, the authors of this study concluded that the use of mesh, rather than removal of the uterus, was associated with higher success rates for correction of pelvic organ prolapse.[125]

When comparing abdominal versus vaginal reconstruction, all of the available studies involving grafts look at grafted abdominal versus suture-based vaginal repairs. One of the first was a randomized comparison of colposacral suspension with synthetic mesh versus transvaginal bilateral sacrospinous ligament suture suspension.[126] In this trial, the vaginal approach was less effective and reoperation was needed twice as often as compared with the grafted abdominal group. Although some studies have supported these findings,[127,128] others have found more equivocal outcomes between groups.[129,130] But even if all these studies showed a difference between groups, could one know if the difference was because of the route taken for repair or to the use (or lack) of graft? Until well-designed comparative studies of abdominal versus vaginal graft repairs are performed, it will be difficult to truly know the answer to that question.

With the exception of one study of absorbable mesh,[131] most of the comparative transvaginal graft studies looking at isolated posterior compartment repair have investigated the use of biologic grafts. The only randomized trial involved three arms: posterior colporrhaphy, sutured site-specific repair, and site-specific repair augmented with porcine small intestine submucosa (Fortagen).[132] Not only was the grafted repair not superior to the suture-based repairs, it was actually inferior in regard to anatomic outcomes at 1 year. One nonrandomized comparative study failed to show a difference in anatomic outcomes with porcine dermal graft,[133] but another showed superior results on a domain-specific sexual function questionnaire when compared with site-specific rectocele repair.[134]

Randomized trials of biologic grafts used in the transvaginal repair of anterior compartment defects have also shown varied results when compared with suture-based repairs. One study showed that augmentation of anterior colporrhaphy with porcine dermis helped prevent the recurrence of cystocele,[135] whereas another suggested that solvent-dehydrated fascia lata did not.[136] The two randomized trials of absorbable synthetic (polyglactin) mesh used in the repair of anterior compartment defects also showed conflicting results, with one showing no difference as compared with traditional and ultralateral colporrhaphy[137] and the other showing a significant decrease in the risk of recurrence with mesh augmentation.[131]

The results of a number of recent randomized trials investigating the use of nonabsorbable polypropylene mesh in the transvaginal repair of anterior compartment defects have been much more consistent. Although there may be trade-offs with regard to the risk of mesh erosion and de novo SUI, three trials in the past 3 years have shown a decreased risk of recurrence associated with permanent mesh in the anterior compartment. The first, a study by Hiltunen and colleagues,[138] showed that recurrence (defined as stage II or greater prolapse at points Aa or Ba of the pelvic organ prolapse quantification (POP-Q) system) at 12-month follow-up was seen in 38.5% of the anterior colporrhaphy alone group as compared with 6.7% of the group with the same repair augmented with mesh ($P < .001$). A higher rate of postoperative stress incontinence, however, occurred in the mesh group (23% versus 10%, $P = .02$). Sivaslioglu and colleagues[139] compared transvaginal paravaginal defect repair to transobturator cystocele repair with a macroporous, monofilament polypropylene mesh. They found a 91% anatomic cure rate in the mesh group as compared with 72% cure in the suture-based repair ($P < .01$). Nguyen and Burchette[140] compared traditional colporrhaphy to repair with a commercially available transobturator polypropylene mesh "kit" (Perigee) in 76 women. One-year outcomes showed anatomic success in 55% versus 87% and de novo dyspareunia in 16% versus 9% of the two groups, all in favor of the mesh repair. Vaginal mesh erosion rates in these three studies ranged from 5% to 17%.

SUMMARY

A recent editorial in the *International Urogynecology Journal,*[141] published by a group of experts in the field suggested that calling midurethral synthetic mesh slings anything less than a gold standard procedure would poorly reflect the reality of the surgical management of SUI today, and yet this procedure falls within the category of procedures noted in the recent Public Health Notification by the FDA. Likewise, two recent publications by leading groups in North America[142] and Europe[143] have indicated that surgical repair of vaginal prolapse may be more efficacious than traditional surgical repair without mesh, but this type of surgery also falls within the FDA warning.

However, there are reasons that the controversy over the use of mesh and materials in pelvic floor surgery exist. Although the use of grafts has the potential to improve the quality of life of many patients, it also carries with it unique risks. It is obviously impossible to develop a mesh erosion if a graft isn't used in a repair. Many graft materials are permanent and yet very few studies of grafted reconstruction extend more than 2 to 4 years. Continued research of graft use in pelvic reconstructive surgery is needed and patients need to be made aware that there are unique risks associated with graft use. Ultimately, it comes down to the fact that each individual patient has a unique set of clinical needs, expectations, and level of risk tolerance and it is incumbent on each reconstructive surgeon to discuss these issues and the known and potentially unknown risks and benefits of various actions or inactions when managing their pelvic floor dysfunction.

REFERENCES

1. Wall LL. Urinary stress incontinence. In: Rock JA, Thompson JD, editors. TeLindes operative gynecology. 8th edition. Philadelphia: Lippincott Williams & Wilkins; 1997. p. 1087–134.
2. Barns HH. Round ligament sling operation for stress incontinence. J Obstet Gynaecol Br Emp 1950;57(3):404–7.
3. Aldridge AH. Transplantation of fascia for relief of urinary stress incontinence. Am J Obstet Gynecol 1942;44:398.
4. Austin RC, Damstra EF. New fascia plastic repair of enterocele. Surg Gynecol Obstet 1955;101(3):297–304.

5. Subak LL, Waetjen LE, van den Eeden S, et al. Cost of pelvic organ prolapse surgery in the United States. Obstet Gynecol 2001;98(4):646–51.

6. Fialkow MF, Newton KM, Weiss NS. Incidence of recurrent pelvic organ prolapse 10 years following primary surgical management: a retrospective cohort study. Int Urogynecol J Pelvic Floor Dysfunct 2008;19:1483–7.

7. Clark AL, Gregory T, Smith VJ, et al. Epidemiologic evaluation for surgically treated pelvic organ prolapse and urinary incontinence. Am J Obstet Gynecol 2003;189(5):1261–7.

8. van Veen RN, Wijsmuller AR, Vrijland WW, et al. Long-term follow-up of a randomized clinical trial of non-mesh versus mesh repair of primary inguinal hernia. Br J Surg 2007;94:506–10.

9. Davila GW, Ghoniem GM, Kapoor DS, et al. Pelvic floor dysfunction management practice patterns: a survey of members of the International Urogynecological Association. Int Urogynecol J Pelvic Floor Dysfunct 2002;13(5):319–25.

10. Shippey S, Gutman RE, Quiroz LH, et al. Contemporary approaches to cystocele repair: a survey of AUGS members. J Reprod Med 2008;53(11):8326.

11. Pulliam SJ, Ferzandi TR, Hota LS, et al. Use of synthetic mesh in pelvic reconstructive surgery: a survey of attitudes and practice patterns of urogynecologists. Int Urogynecol J Pelvic Floor Dysfunct 2007;18:1405–8.

12. Information on surgical mesh for pelvic organ prolapse and stress urinary incontinence. Available at: www.fda.gov/cdrh/consumer/surgicalmesh-popsui.html. Accessed August 11, 2009.

13. FDA Public Health Notification. Serious complications associated with transvaginal placement of surgical mesh in repair of pelvic organ prolapse and stress urinary incontinence. Available at: www.fda.gov/cdrh/safety/102008-surgical mesh.html. Accessed August 11, 2009.

14. Amid PK, Shulman AG, Lichtenstein IL, et al. Biomaterials for abdominal hernia surgery and principles of their application. Langenbecks Arch Chir 1994;379(3):168–71.

15. Chu CC, Welch L. Characterization of morphologic and mechanical properties of surgical mesh fabrics. J Biomed Mater Res 1985;19(8):903–16.

16. Deprest J, Zheng F, Konstantinovic M, et al. The biology behind fascial defects and the use of implants in pelvic organ prolapse repair. Int Urogynecol J Pelvic Floor Dysfunct 2006;17:S16–25.

17. McGuire EJ, Lytton B. Pubovaginal sling procedure for stress urinary incontinence. J Urol 1978;119:82.

18. Morgan TO, Westney L, McGuire EJ. Pubovaginal sling: 4-year outcome analysis and quality of life assessment. J Urol 2000;163:1845–8.

19. Blaivas JG, Jacobs BZ. Pubovaginal fascial sling for the treatment of complicated stress urinary incontinence. J Urol 1991;145(6):1214–8.

20. Handa VL, Jensen JK, Germain MM, et al. Banked human fascia lata for the suburethral sling procedure: a preliminary report. Obstet Gynecol 1996;88(6):1045–9.

21. Fitzgerald MP, Edwards SR, Fenner D. Medium-term follow-up on use of freeze-dried, irradiated donor fascia for sacrocolpopexy and sling procedures. Int Urogynecol J Pelvic Floor Dysfunct 2004;15(4):238–42.

22. Carbone JM, Kavaler E, Hu JC, et al. Pubovaginal sling using cadaveric fascia and bone anchors: disappointing early results. J Urol 2001;165:1605–11.

23. Nazemi TM, Rapp DE, Govier FE, et al. Cadaveric fascial sling with bone anchors: minimum of 24 months of follow-up. Urology 2008;71(5):834–8.

24. Kammerer-Doak DN, Rogers RG, Bellar B. Vaginal erosion of cadaveric fascia lata following abdominal sacrocolpopexy and suburethral sling urethropexy. Int Urogynecol J Pelvic Floor Dysfunct 2002;13(2):106–9.
25. Fitzgerald MP, Mollenhauer J, Brubaker L. Failure of allograft suburethal slings. BJU Int 1999;84(7):785–8.
26. Fitzgerald MP, Mollenhauer J, Brubaker L. The fate of rectus fascia suburethral slings. Am J Obstet Gynecol 2000;183(4):964–6.
27. Nichols DH. The Mersilene mesh gauze-hammock for severe urinary stress incontinence. Obstet Gynecol 1973;41(1):88–93.
28. Melnick I, Lee RE. Delayed transection of urethra by mersilene tape. Urology 1976;8(6):580–1.
29. Cato RJ, Murray AG. Teflon tape suspension for the control of stress incontinence. Br J Urol 1981;53(4):364–7.
30. Morgan JE, Farrow GA, Stewart FE. The Marlex sling operation for the treatment of recurrent stress urinary incontinence. Am J Obstet Gynecol 1985;151(2):224–6.
31. Stanton SL, Brindley GS, Holmes DM. Silastic sling for urethral sphincter incompetence in women. Br J Obstet Gynaecol 1985;92(7):747–50.
32. Horbach NS, Blanco JS, Ostergard DR, et al. A suburethral sling procedure with polytetrafluoroethylene for the treatment of genuine stress incontinence in patients with low urethral closure pressure. Obstet Gynecol 1988;71(4):648–52.
33. Weinberger MW, Ostergard DR. Postoperative catheterization, urinary retention, and permanent voiding dysfunction after polytetrafluoroethylene suburethral sling placement. Obstet Gynecol 1996;87(1):50–4.
34. Weinberger MW, Ostergard DR. Long-term clinical and urodynamic evaluation of the polytetrafluoroethylene suburethral sling for the treatment of genuine stress incontinence. Obstet Gynecol 1995;86(1):92–6.
35. Iglesia CB, Fenner DE, Brubaker L. The use of mesh in gynecologic surgery. Int Urogynecol J Pelvic Floor Dysfunct 1997;8(2):105–15.
36. Kobashi KC, Dmochowski R, Mee SL, et al. Erosion of woven polyester pubovaginal sling. J Urol 1999;162:2070–2.
37. Govier FE, Kobashi KC, Kuznetsov DD, et al. Complications of transvaginal silicone-coated polyester synthetic mesh sling. Urology 2005;66(4):741–5.
38. Boulanger L, Boukerrou M, Rubod C, et al. Bacteriological analysis of meshes removed for complications after surgical management of urinary incontinence or pelvic organ prolapse. Int Urogynecol J Pelvic Floor Dysfunct 2008;19(6):827–31.
39. Ulmsten U, Henriksson L, Johnson P, et al. An ambulatory surgical procedure under local anesthesia for treatment of female urinary incontinence. Int Urogynecol J Pelvic Floor Dysfunct 1996;7:81–6.
40. Ulmsten U, Petros P. Intravaginal slingplasty (IVS): an ambulatory surgical procedure for treatment of female urinary incontinence. Scand J Urol & Nephrology 1995;29(1):75–82.
41. Ulmsten U, Falconer C, Johnson P, et al. A multicenter study of tension-free vaginal tape (TVT) for surgical treatment of stress urinary incontinence. Int Urogynecol J Pelvic Floor Dysfunct 1998;9:210–3.
42. Nilson CG, Falconer C, Rezapour M. Seven-year follow-up of the tension-free vaginal tape procedure for treatment of urinary incontinence. Obstet Gynecol 2004;104(6):1259–62.
43. Nilson CG, Palva K, Rezapour M, et al. Eleven years prospective follow-up of the tension-free vaginal tape procedure for treatment of urinary incontinence. Int Urogynecol J Pelvic Floor Dysfunct 2008;19:1043–7.

44. Mescia M, Pifarotti P, Gernasconi F, et al. Tension-free vaginal tape: analysis of outcome and complications in 404 stress incontinent women. Int Urogynecol J Pelvic Floor Dysfunct 2001;12:24–7.

45. Levin I, Groutz A, Pauzner D, et al. Surgical complications and medium-term outcome results of tension-free vaginal tape: a prospective study of 313 consecutive patients. Neurourol Urodyn 2004;23:7–9.

46. Gruber DD, Wiersma DS, Dunn JS, et al. Cecal perforation complicating placement of a transvaginal tension-free vaginal tape. Int Urogynecol J Pelvic Floor Dysfunct 2007;18(6):671–3.

47. de Leval J. Novel surgical technique for the treatment of female stress urinary incontinence: transobturator vaginal tape inside-out. Eur Urol 2003;44(6):724–30.

48. Davila GW, Johnson JD, Serels S. Multicenter experience with the Monarc transobturator sling system to treat stress urinary incontinence. Int Urogynecol J Pelvic Floor Dysfunct 2006;17(5):460–5.

49. Yamada BS, Govier FE, Stefanovic KB, et al. High rate of vaginal erosions associated with the Mentor ObTape. J Urol 2006;176:651–4.

50. Wright EJ, Iselin CE, Carr LK, et al. Pubovaginal sling using cadaveric allograft fascia for the treatment of intrinsic sphincter deficiency. J Urol 1998;160:759–62.

51. Brown SL, Govier FE. Cadaveric versus autologous fascia lata for the pubovaginal sling: surgical outcome and patient satisfaction. J Urol 2000;164:1633–7.

52. McBride AW, Ellerkman RM, Bent AE, et al. Comparison of long-term outcomes of autologous fascia lata slings with suspend Tutoplast fascia lata allograft slings for stress incontinence. Am J Obstet Gynecol 2005;192:1677–81.

53. Fitzgerald MP, Mollenhauer J, Brubaker L. The antigenicity of fascia lata allografts. BJU Int 2000;86(7):826–8.

54. Dora CD, Dimarco DS, Zobitz ME, et al. Time dependent variations in biomechanical properties of cadaveric fascia, porcine dermis, porcine small intestine submucosa, polypropylene mesh and autologous fascia in the rabbit model: implications for sling surgery. J Urol 2004;171:1970–3.

55. Wadie BS, Edwan A, Nabeeh AM. Autologous fascial sling vs polypropylene tape at short-term follow-up: a prospective randomized study. J Urol 2005;174:990–3.

56. Sharifiaghdas F, Mortazavi N. Tension-free vaginal tape and autologous rectus fascia pubovaginal sling for the treatment of urinary stress incontinence: a medium-term follow-up. Med Princ Pract 2008;17(3):209–14.

57. Jeon MJ, Jung HJ, Chung SM, et al. Comparison of the treatment outcome of pubovaginal sling, tension-free vaginal tape, and transobturator tape for stress urinary incontinence with intrinsic sphincter deficiency. Am J Obstet Gynecol 2008;199:76, e1–4.

58. Morgan DM, Dunn RL, Fenner DE, et al. Comparative analysis of urinary incontinence severity after autologous fascia pubovaginal sling, pubovaginal sling and tension-free vaginal tape. J Urol 2007;177:604–9.

59. Shippey SH, Green IC, Quiroz LH, et al. Midurethral sling outcomes: tension-free vaginal tape versus Pelvilace. Int Urogynecol J Pelvic Floor Dysfunct 2008;19(9):1199–204.

60. Meschia M, Pifarotti P, Spennacchio M, et al. A randomized comparison of tension-free vaginal tape and endopelvic fascia plication in women with genital prolapse and occult stress urinary incontinence. Am J Obstet Gynecol 2004;190:609–13.

61. Paraiso MF, Walters MD, Karram MM, et al. Laparoscopic Burch colposuspension versus tension-free vaginal tape: a randomized trial. Obstet Gynecol 2004;104(6):1249–58.

62. Jelovsek JE, Barber MD, Karram MM, et al. Randomized trial of laparoscopic Burch colposuspension versus tension-free vaginal tape: long-term follow-up. BJOG 2008;115(2):219–25.

63. Ward K, Hilton P. Prospective multicentre randomised trial of tension-free vaginal tape and colposuspension as a primary treatment for stress incontinence. BMJ 2002;325:7355.

64. Manca A, Sculpher MJ, Ward K, et al. A cost-utility analysis of tension-free vaginal tape versus colposuspension for primary urodynamic stress incontinence. BJOG 2003;110(3):255–62.

65. Ward KL, Hilton P. A prospective multicenter randomized trial of tension-free vaginal tape and colposuspension as a primary treatment for stress incontinence: two-year follow-up. Am J Obstet Gynecol 2004;190:324–31.

66. Ward KL, Hilton P. Tension-free vaginal tape versus colposuspension for primary urodynamic stress incontinence: 5-year follow up. BJOG 2008; 115(2):226–33.

67. Ghandi S, Abramov Y, Kwon C, et al. TVT versus SPARC: comparison of outcomes for two midurethral tape procedures. Int Urogynecol J Pelvic Floor Dysfunct 2006;17(2):125–30.

68. Tseng LH, Wang AC, Lin YH, et al. Randomized comparison of the suprapubic arc sling procedure vs tension-free vaginal taping for stress incontinent women. Int Urogynecol J Pelvic Floor Dysfunct 2005;16(3):230–5.

69. Meschia M, Pifarotti P, Bernasconi F, et al. Tension-free vaginal tape (TVT) and intravaginal slingplasty (IVS) for stress urinary incontinence: a multicenter randomized trial. Am J Obstet Gynecol 2006;195:1338–42.

70. Balakrishnan S, Lim YN, Barry C, et al. Sling distress: a subanalysis of the IVS tapes from the SUSPEND trial. Aust N Z J Obstet Gynaecol 2007;47(6):496–8.

71. Sung VW, Schleinitz MD, Rardin CR, et al. Comparison of retropubic vs transobturator approach to midurethral slings: a systematic review and meta-analysis. Am J Obstet Gynecol 2007;197(1):3–11.

72. Barber MD, Kleeman S, Karram MM, et al. Transobturator compared with tension-free vaginal tape for the treatment of stress urinary incontinence. Obstet Gynecol 2008;111(3):611–21.

73. Laurikainen E, Valpas A, Kivela A, et al. Retropubic compared with transobturator tape placement in treatment of urinary incontinence. Obstet Gynecol 2007; 109(1):4–11.

74. Rinne K, Laurikainen E, Kivela A, et al. A randomized trial comparing TVT with TVT-O: 12-month results. Int Urogynecol J Pelvic Floor Dysfunct 2008;19(8): 1049–54.

75. Barber MD, Gustilo-Ashby AM, Chen CCG, et al. Perioperative complications and adverse events of the MONARC transobturator tape, compared with the tension-free vaginal tape. Am J Obstet Gynecol 2006;195:1820–5.

76. Ballert KN, Kanofsky JA, Nitti VW. Effect of tension-free vaginal tape and TVT-obturator on lower urinary tract symptoms other than stress urinary incontinence. Int Urogynecol J Pelvic Floor Dysfunct 2008;19:335–40.

77. Murphy M, van Raalte J, Mercurio E, et al. Incontinence-related quality of life and sexual function following the tension-free vaginal tape versus the "inside-out" tension-free vaginal tape obturator. Int Urogynecol J Pelvic Floor Dysfunct 2008;19(4):481–7.

78. Schierlitz L, Dwyer PL, Rosamilia A, et al. Effectiveness of tension-free vaginal tape compared with transoburator tape in women with stress urinary incontinence and intrinsic sphincter deficiency. Obstet Gynecol 2008;112(6):1253–61.

79. Miller JJ, Botros SM, Akl MN, et al. Is transobturator tape as effective as tension-free vaginal tape in patients with borderline maximum urethral closure pressure? Am J Obstet Gynecol 2006;195:1799–804.

80. Guerette NL, Bena JF, Davila GW. Transobturator slings for stress incontinence: using urodynamic parameters to predict outcomes. Int Urogynecol J Pelvic Floor Dysfunct 2008;19(1):97–102.

81. Araco F, Gravante G, Sorge R, et al. TVT-O vs TVT: a randomized trial in patients with different degrees of urinary stress incontinence. Int Urogynecol J Pelvic Floor Dysfunct 2008;19:917–26.

82. Lane FE. Repair of posthysterectomy vaginal-vault prolapse. Obstet Gynecol 1962;20:72–7.

83. Addison WA, Livengood CH 3rd, Sutton GP, et al. Abdominal sacral colpopexy with Mersilene mesh in the retroperitoneal position in the management of posthysterectomy vaginal vault prolapse and enterocele. Am J Obstet Gynecol 1985;153(2):140–6.

84. Drutz HP, Cha LS. Massive genital and vaginal vault prolapse treated by abdominal sacropexy with use of Marlex mesh: review of the literature. Am J Obstet Gynecol 1987;156(2):387–92.

85. van Lindert AC, Groenendijk AG, Scholten PC, et al. Surgical support and suspension of genital prolapse, including preservation of the uterus, using the Gore-Tex soft tissue patch (a preliminary report). Eur J Obstet Gynecol Reprod Biol 1993;50(2):133–9.

86. Addison WA, Timmons MC, Wall LL, et al. Failed abdominal sacral colpopexy: observations and recommendations. Obstet Gynecol 1989;74:480–3.

87. Baker KR, Beresford JM, Campbell C. Colposacropexy with Prolene mesh. Surg Gynecol Obstet 1990;171:51–4.

88. Nygaard IE, McCreery R, Brubaker L, et al. Abdominal sacrocolpopexy: a comprehensive review. Obstet Gynecol 2004;104(4):805–23.

89. Weidner AC, Cundiff GW, Harris RL, et al. Sacral osteomyelitis: an unusual complication of abdominal sacral colpopexy. Obstet Gynecol 1997;90(4):689–91.

90. Maloney JC, Dunton CJ, Smith K. Repair of vaginal vault prolapse with abdominal sacropexy. J Reprod Med 1990;35(1):6–10.

91. Virtanen H, Hirvonen T, Makinen J, et al. Outcome of thirty patients who underwent repair of posthysterectomy prolapse of the vaginal vault with abdominal sacral colpopexy. J Am Coll Surg 1994;178(3):283–7.

92. Begley JS, Kupferman SP, Kuznetsov DD, et al. Incidence and management of abdominal Sacrocolpopexy mesh erosions. Am J Obstet Gynecol 2005;192:1956–62.

93. Govier FE, Kobashi KC, Kozlowski PM, et al. High complication rate identified in Sacrocolpopexy patients attributed to silicone mesh. Urology 2005;65(6):1099–103.

94. Cundiff GW, Harris RL, Coates K, et al. Abdominal sacral colpoperineopexy: a new approach for correction of posterior compartment defects and perineal descent associated with vaginal vault prolapse. Am J Obstet Gynecol 1997;177(6):1345–53.

95. Visco AG, Weidner AC, Barber MD, et al. Vaginal mesh erosion after abdominal sacral colpopexy. Am J Obstet Gynecol 2001;184(3):297–302.

96. Culligan PJ, Murphy M, Blackwell L, et al. Long-term success of abdominal sacral colpopexy using synthetic mesh. Am J Obstet Gynecol 2002;187(6):1473–80.

97. Wu JM, Wells EC, Hundley AF, et al. Mesh erosion in abdominal sacral colpopexy with and without concomitant hysterectomy. Am J Obstet Gynecol 2006;194:1418–22.

98. Marinkovic SP. Will hysterectomy at the time of Sacrocolpopexy increase the rate of polypropylene mesh erosion? Int Urogynecol J Pelvic Floor Dysfunct 2008;19: 199–203.

99. Brizzolara S, Pillai-Allen A. Risk of mesh erosion with sacral colpopexy and concurrent hysterectomy. Obstet Gynecol 2003;102(2):306–10.

100. Kahn MA, Stanton SL. Posterior colporrhaphy: its effects on bowel and sexual function. Br J Obstet Gynaecol 1997;104:82–6.

101. Miklos JR, Kohli N, Moore R. Levatorplasty release and reconstruction of rectovaginal septum using allogenic dermal graft. Int Urogynecol J Pelvic Floor Dysfunct 2002;13(1):44–6.

102. Kohli N, Miklos JR. Dermal graft-augmented rectocele repair. Int Urogynecol J Pelvic Floor Dysfunct 2003;14(2):146–9.

103. Altman D, Zetterstrom J, Mellgren A, et al. A three-year prospective assessment of rectocele repair using porcine xenograft. Obstet Gynecol 2006;107(1):59–65.

104. Chung SY, Franks M, Smith CP, et al. Technique of combined pubovaginal sling and cystocele repair using a single piece of cadaveric dermal graft. Urology 2002;59(4):538–41.

105. Clemons JL, Myers DL, Aguilar VC, et al. Vaginal paravaginal repair with an Alloderm graft. Am J Obstet Gynecol 2003;189(6):1612–8.

106. Ward RM, Sung VW, Clemons JL, et al. Vaginal paravaginal repair with an Alloderm graft: long-term outcomes. Am J Obstet Gynecol 2007;197(6):670, e1–5.

107. YN Lim, Rane A, Muller R. An ambispective observational study in the safety and efficacy of posterior colporrhaphy with composite vicryl-prolene mesh. Int Urogynecol J Pelvic Floor Dysfunct 2005;16:126–31.

108. Julian TM. The efficacy of Marlex mesh in the repair of severe, recurrent vaginal prolapse of the anterior midvaginal wall. Am J Obstet Gynecol 1996;175(6): 1472–5.

109. Milani R, Salvatore S, Soligo M, et al. Functional and anatomical outcome of anterior and posterior vaginal prolapse repair with prolene mesh. BJOG 2005; 112(1):107–11.

110. Debodinance P, Berrocal J, Clave H, et al. Changing attitudes on the surgical treatment of urogenital prolapse: birth of the tension-free vaginal mesh. J Gynecol Obstet Biol Reprod (Paris) 2004;33(7):577–88.

111. Collinet P, Belot F, Debodinance P, et al. Transvaginal mesh technique for pelvic organ prolapse repair: mesh exposure management and risk factors. Int Urogynecol J Pelvic Floor Dysfunct 2006;17:315–20.

112. Fatton B, Amblard J, Debodinance P, et al. Transvaginal repair of genital prolapse: preliminary results of a new tension-free vaginal mesh (Prolift TM technique)—a case series multicentric study. Int Urogynecol J Pelvic Floor Dysfunct 2007;18:743–52.

113. Altman D, Falconer C. Perioperative morbidity using transvaginal mesh in pelvic organ prolapse repair. Obstet Gynecol 2007;109(2):303–8.

114. Altman D, Vayrynen T, Engh ME, et al. Short-term outcome after transvaginal mesh repair of pelvic organ prolapse. Int Urogynecol J Pelvic Floor Dysfunct 2008;19:787–95.

115. Elmer C, Altman D, Engh ME, et al. Trocar-guided transvaginal mesh repair of pelvic organ prolapse. Obstet Gynecol 2009;113(1):117–26.
116. van Raalte HM, Lucente VR, Molden SM, et al. One-year anatomic and quality of life outcomes after the Prolift procedure for treatment of posthysterectomy prolapse. Am J Obstet Gynecol 2008;199:694, e1–6.
117. Yamada BS, Govier FE, Stefanovic KB, et al. Vesicovaginal fistula and mesh erosion after Perigee (transobturator polypropylene mesh anterior repair). Urology 2006;68(5):1121, e5–7.
118. LaSala CA, Schimpf MO. Occurrence of postoperative hematomas after prolapse repair using a mesh augmentation system. Obstet Gynecol 2007;109:569–72.
119. Marguiles RU, Lewicky-Gaupp C, Fenner DE, et al. Complication requiring reoperation following vaginal mesh kit procedures for prolapse. Am J Obstet Gynecol 2008;199:687, e1–4.
120. Farnsworth BN. Posterior intravaginal slingplasty infracoccygeal sacropexy_ for severe posthysterectomy vaginal vault prolapse—a preliminary report on efficacy and safety. Int Urogynecol J Pelvic Floor Dysfunct 2002;13(1):4–8.
121. Hefni M, Yousri N, El-Toukhy T, et al. Morbidity associated with posterior intravaginal slingplasty for uterovaginal and vault prolapse. Arch Gynecol Obstet 2007;276(5):499–504.
122. Luck AM, Steele AC, Leong GC, et al. Short-term efficacy and complications of posterior intravaginal slingplasty. Int Urogynecol J Pelvic Floor Dysfunct 2008; 19(6):795–9.
123. Culligan PJ, Blackwell L, Goldsmith LJ, et al. A randomized controlled trial comparing fascia lata and synthetic mesh for sacral colpopexy. Obstet Gynecol 2005;106(1):29–37.
124. Altman D, Anzen B, Brismar S, et al. Long-term outcome of abdominal sacrocolpopexy using xenograft compared with synthetic mesh. Urology 2006;67(4):719–24.
125. Jeon MJ, Jung HJ, Choi HJ, et al. Is hysterectomy or the use of graft necessary for the reconstructive surgery for uterine prolapse? Int Urogynecol J Pelvic Floor Dysfunct 2008;19:351–5.
126. Benson JT, Lucente V, McClellan E. Vaginal versus abdominal reconstructive surgery for the treatment of pelvic support defects: a prospective randomized study with long-term outcome evaluation. Am J Obstet Gynecol 1996;175(6):1418–21.
127. Lo TS, Wang AC. Abdominal colposacropexy and sacrospinous ligament suspension for severe uterovaginal prolapse: a comparison. J Gynecol Surg 1998;14:59–64.
128. Sze EH, Meranus J, Kohli N, et al. Vaginal configuration on MRI after abdominal Sacrocolpopexy and sacrospinous ligament suspension. Int Urogynecol J Pelvic Floor Dysfunct 2001;12(6):375–9.
129. Roovers JP, van der Vaart CH, van der Born JG, et al. A randomized controlled trial comparing abdominal and vaginal prolapse surgery: effects on urogenital function. BJOG 2004;111(1):50–6.
130. Maher CF, Qatawneh AM, Dwyer PL, et al. Abdominal sacral colpopexy or vaginal sacrospinous colpopexy for vaginal vault prolapse: a prospective randomized study. Am J Obstet Gynecol 2004;190:20–6.
131. Sand PK, Koduri S, Lobel RW, et al. Prospective randomized trial of polyglactin 910 mesh to prevent recurrence of cystoceles and rectoceles. Am J Obstet Gynecol 2001;184:1357–62.
132. Paraiso MF, Barber MD, Muir TW, et al. Rectocele repair: a randomized trial of three surgical techniques including graft augmentation. Am J Obstet Gynecol 2006;195:1762–71.

133. Altman D, Mellgren A, Blomgren B, et al. Clinical and histological safety assessment of rectocele repair using collagen mesh. Acta Obstet Gynecol Scand 2004;83:995–1000.
134. Novi JM, Bradley CS, Mahmoud NN, et al. Sexual function in women after rectocele repair with acellular porcine dermis graft vs site-specific rectovaginal fascia repair. Int Urogynecol J Pelvic Floor Dysfunct 2007;18:1163–9.
135. Meschia M, Pifarotti P, Bernasconi F, et al. Porcine skin collagen implants to prevent anterior vaginal wall prolapse recurrence: a multicenter, randomized study. J Urol 2007;177:192–5.
136. Gandhi S, Goldberg RP, Kwon C, et al. A prospective randomized trial using solvent dehydrated fascia lata for the prevention of recurrent anterior vaginal wall prolapse. Am J Obstet Gynecol 2005;192:1649–54.
137. Weber AM, Walters MD, Piedmonte MR, et al. Anterior colporrhaphy: a randomized trial of three surgical techniques. Am J Obstet Gynecol 2001;185: 1299–304.
138. Hiltunen R, Nieminen K, Takala T, et al. Low-weight polypropylene mesh for anterior vaginal wall prolapse: a randomized controlled trial. Obstet Gynecol 2007;110:455–62.
139. Sivaslioglu AA, Unlubilgin E, Dolen I. A randomized comparison of polypropylene mesh surgery with site-specific surgery in the treatment of cystocele. Int Urogynecol J Pelvic Floor Dysfunct 2008;19:467–71.
140. Nguyen JN, Burchette RJ. Outcome after anterior vaginal prolapse repair. Obstet Gynecol 2008;111(4):891–8.
141. Serati M, Salvatore S, Uccella S, et al. Surgical treatment for female stress urinary incontinence: what it the gold-standard procedure? Int Urogynecol J Pelvic Floor Dysfunct 2009;20:619–21.
142. Murphy M. Society of Gynecologic Surgeons Systematic Review Group. Clinical practice guidelines on vaginal graft use from the Society of Gynecologic Surgeons. Obstet Gynecol 2008;112(5):1123–30.
143. National Institute for Health and Clinical Excellence—surgical repair of vaginal wall prolapse using mesh. Available at: www.nice.org.uk/guidance/index.jsp. Accessed August 11, 2009.

Obliterative Vaginal Surgery for Pelvic Organ Prolapse

Thomas L. Wheeler II, MD, MSPH[a],*, Kimberly A. Gerten, MD[b],
Jeffrey B. Garris, MD, MS[a]

KEYWORDS

- Obliterative surgery • Colpocleisis • Older women
- Management • Pelvic organ prolapse

Estimates for surgeries performed for female pelvic organ prolapse in the United States exceed more than 500,000 surgical procedures per year.[1] Considering that only 10% to 20% of women with prolapse are currently believed to seek medical attention and that the number of American women greater than age 50 is projected to increase by more than 70% over the next 30 years, the number of surgeries performed for prolapse is expected to dramatically increase.[2–4] Although restorative reconstructive surgical procedures may be indicated for those patients with prolapse who desire to maintain sexual function, many other patients with prolapse may be medically compromised or have other reasons why postoperative coital function is not desired. For those patients, whether elderly or of younger age, with no desire to preserve postoperative coital function, an obliterative surgical procedure to repair pelvic organ prolapse has many advantages and should be considered.

Typically, obliterative procedures are less invasive, require shorter operative times, and have less surgical risks over traditional vaginal reconstructive procedures.[5,6] Various techniques have been described for performing obliterative surgery. These obliterative procedures can be generally divided into partial or total colpocleisis. Either procedure can be performed with or without levator myorrhaphy and high perineorrhaphy. When pelvic anatomy limits or prevents more traditional techniques of colpocleisis, a constricting anterior and posterior colporrhaphy with levator myorrhaphy and high perineorraphy is an option.

The pelvic reconstructive surgeon who performs these procedures should have comfort in preoperative discussion with the patient of the risks and benefits associated with the procedure, the surgical skills needed to perform the procedure, and

---

[a] Division of Female Pelvic Medicine and Reconstructive Pelvic Surgery, University of South Carolina, Greenville Campus, 480 West Faris Road, Greenville, SC 29608, USA
[b] Park Nicollet Urogynecology and Reconstructive Pelvic Surgery, 6490 Excelsior Boulevard, Suite E111, St. Louis Park, MN 55426, USA
* Corresponding author.
E-mail address: twheeler@ghs.org (T.L. Wheeler II).

Obstet Gynecol Clin N Am 36 (2009) 637–658
doi:10.1016/j.ogc.2009.08.003
0889-8545/09/$ – see front matter © 2009 Elsevier Inc. All rights reserved.

obgyn.theclinics.com

the experience to recognize and address any complications as a result of the procedure. With this in mind, appropriate patient selection for obliterative operations should
be of utmost consideration. Colpocleisis procedures should not be the sole surgery
offered for prolapse, but rather a part of the pelvic surgeon's armamentarium for treatment of severe pelvic organ prolapse and associated conditions.

HISTORY

Despite a rapidly increasing incidence and need for improved surgical correction of
female pelvic organ prolapse, advancements in the detailed understanding and treatment of prolapse have been comparatively slow. From the time of ancient cultures,
women have endured severe pelvic organ prolapse. Through the years treatment
has included vaginal packing, crude pessaries, exercises, instillation of caustic materials, and hanging the prolapsed patient upside down for an extended period of time.
Early attempts at surgical management entailed amputation of the prolapsed
segments or closure of the vaginal introitus.[7]

Perhaps the earliest idea to surgically obliterate severe prolapse should be credited
to Gerardin[8] who in 1823 suggested, but never performed, the method of suturing
surgically denuded anterior and posterior vaginal walls together. With advancements
in anesthesia and general surgical techniques, it was during the mid-nineteenth
century that Neugebauer[9] performed the first known surgical procedure for correction
of prolapse. Neugebauer obliterated the vagina by denuding 6 × 3 cm anterior and
posterior areas near the introitus and sutured them together. Later in 1877, LeFort[10]
published a modification of Neugebauer's 1867 technique; he denuded longer and
narrower areas of vaginal epithelium at the time of initial surgery and then returned
to the operating room 8 days later to perform a secondary colpoperineoplasty.
Although today this partial colpocleisis technique is typically referred to as a "LeFort
colpocleisis," a less common eponym is the Neugebauer-LeFort procedure.

It was not until the early twentieth century that further understanding of prolapse led
to Edebohls[11,12] first published report of a total colpocleisis with levator myorraphy
following hysterectomy, which he called a panhysterectomy. Edenbohls results of
1901 soon were followed by several case series that noted comparable results with
the partial colpocleisis-type procedures.[13] To make the colpocleisis procedures
more universally acceptable, many of the surgical modifications were subsequently
directed at reducing the postoperative risk of recurrent prolapse or decreasing the
incidence of urinary incontinence.[14] Further modifications, such as those by Wyatt,[15]
were directed at reducing prolapse recurrence by creating a wider vaginal septum and
by other surgeons who addressed postoperative urinary incontinence by either
sparing the distal vagina near the urethra or supporting the bladder neck with a high
perineorraphy.[7,15–19] In 1937, Goodall and Power[20] documented efforts at reducing
postoperative urinary incontinence and preserving sexual function by creating a triangular septum higher in the vagina. During the late twentieth and twenty-first centuries,
understanding of pelvic organ prolapse has rapidly increased, including a better
understanding of improvement in pelvic floor symptoms with obliterative surgery
and patient satisfaction.

PATIENT SELECTION AND PERIOPERATIVE MANAGEMENT

The ideal candidate for colpocleisis is an older, sexually inactive patient who has
medical comorbidities that make an efficient and relatively noninvasive procedure to
treat advanced pelvic organ prolapse attractive. Advanced age, however, is not
a requirement. Before surgical intervention, she has either declined conservative

treatment (pessary use) or had unsatisfactory results. The patient (and potentially her spouse or partner) needs to be counseled that penetrative intercourse is not possible after colpocleisis. Candidates should also be counseled that reported satisfaction rates are greater than 85% and regret rates are less than 11%.[6,19,21–29]

Urinary Incontinence

An important consideration when evaluating potential candidates for an obliterative procedure is postoperative urinary incontinence. Urinary incontinence is associated with significant impairment of quality of life. Historically, the occurrence of postoperative urinary incontinence, up to 25%,[14] was the biggest deterrent against the performance of the procedure. De novo stress incontinence has been attributed to distal vaginal dissection with scarring and resultant downward traction on the urethra, and to unmasking of occult stress urinary incontinence by reducing the prolapse, which previously had "kinked" the bladder neck. To minimize this problem, contemporary colpocleisis techniques avoid distal dissections that predispose to downward traction on the urethra and include incontinence procedures for appropriately selected patients.[14,25–31]

The decision to perform an incontinence procedure in these patients is difficult and should be individualized. Patients should be preoperatively evaluated for urinary incontinence and bladder function because the morbidity of postoperative stress incontinence against the possibility of urinary retention must be considered. There are mixed results on the impact of colpocleisis on bladder emptying,[14,31] but it does not seem to commonly occur.[32] If no voiding dysfunction is suspected, candidates should be evaluated at least with simple cystometrics with reduction of the prolapse and measurement of a postvoid residual. Otherwise, urodynamic evaluation is warranted. Of note, the role of complex urodynamics is debatable because urodynamics have not been shown to be ultrasensitive in distinguishing whether poor bladder emptying is caused by severe prolapse or detrusor motor impairment.

In addition to bladder testing, the surgeon must also judge the patient's ability to perform self-catheterization, because decreased manual dexterity is common in these patients. All patients, whether or not an incontinence procedure is performed, should be counseled on the possible need for prolonged bladder drainage with indwelling Foley or intermittent catheterization.

Management of the Geriatric Patient

Advanced age alone is not a contraindication to any type of pelvic floor surgery, including colpocleisis. Increasing age is associated with more complications and mortality especially past age 80, where mortality with urogynecologic surgery is 2.8 out of 1000.[5] In general, however, surgery is well tolerated by the older woman, although complications are not as well tolerated. In women 80 years and older, fewer complications occur with obliterative surgery than with reconstructive surgery, making it an attractive surgical approach.[5] Regardless, surgeons who perform colpocleisis need to be adept at surgical care of the geriatric patient. **Table 1** summarizes some important considerations.

Preoperative Management

Aging is associated with several physiologic changes. In addition to open communication with the anesthesiologist regarding the optimal method of anesthesia, cardiac, pulmonary, nutritional, cognitive, and functional statuses may need to be assessed preoperatively. The goal is to minimize risk factors for the occurrence of complications.

Table 1 Perioperative considerations for the older woman		
Issue	**Background**	**Clinical Recommendation**
Deep venous thrombosis/ thromboembolic events	Older patients have 20%–40% risk of deep venous thrombosis because of advanced age (>60 y) and length of surgery	Perioperative use of sequential pneumatic compression devices and selective use of heparin prophylaxis, early ambulation
Cardiovascular	Perioperative myocardial infarction associated with 50% mortality rate	Perioperative β-blocker use in the high- and moderate-risk patient
Pulmonary	Increased perioperative morbidity and mortality rates with development of pneumonia	Pulmonary toilet with deep cough, incentive spirometry, early ambulation
Neuropathies	Neurologic injuries caused by nerve compression and ischemia as a result of patient positioning	Careful patient positioning with attention to the peroneal, femoral, ulnar, and sciatic nerves with padded stir-ups, avoid hyperflexion or extension of the lower extremities
Hypothermia	Decreased immunologic response, prolonged wound healing, increased perioperative cardiac events	Intraoperative forced warm air blanket use, warmed intravenous fluids
Infectious disease	Clean contaminated procedures: mixed flora of the vagina	Perioperative dose of first-generation cephalosporin
Pharmacology	Decreased pharmacologic metabolic rates in older patients. Risk of oversedation and delirium	Avoidance of polypharmacy, sedatives, and anticholinergic medications
Delirium	Abrupt change in cognition or consciousness, postsurgical prevalence estimate 37%, at risk for long-term cognitive deficiencies and increased mortality, underdiagnosis	Avoid merperidine and anticholinergic agents including promethazine, minimize hospital stay, allow a companion to stay at bedside, maintain circadian pattern
Urinary tract infection	Pelvic floor surgery postoperative rates up to 44%	Screen if new-onset bladder or voiding symptoms

From Gerten KA, Markland AD, Lloyd LK, et al. Prolapse and incontinence surgery in older women. J Urol 2008;179:2111–8; with permission.

Organ system functional reserve begins to decline after age 60. Cardiac changes include increased vessel and ventricular wall thickness, resulting in more dependence on diastolic filling and stroke volume to maintain cardiac output. Sympathetic response slows causing decreased heart rate and contractility.[33] The combination of these cardiovascular changes makes attention to perioperative fluid management paramount to avoid fluid overload.

Antihypertensives should be given the day of surgery and restarted immediately after surgery, because the risk of severe hypertension greatly outweighs the risk posed to giving medicine before anesthesia induction. Consultation with an internist or cardiologist should be considered for patients on multiple classes of antihypertensive medications or with a history of cardiac compromise.

Respiratory performance declines steadily after age 30 including decreases in vital capacity, respiratory compliance, and maximum voluntary ventilation. In advanced age, cough effort is less vigorous and mucociliary clearance is reduced further increasing the risk of respiratory complication.[33] Early ambulation and aggressive incentive spirometry use are encouraged.

Renal mass, blood flow, and filtration decline with age. Creatinine levels remain stable, however, because of decreased protein catabolism. Renin activity decreases and atrial naturiuretic peptide increases, causing potential impairment of the secretion of water and sodium loads.

Poor functional status, as shown by decreased activities of daily living, is predictive of pulmonary complications and should prompt a rigorous preoperative assessment.[33] Baseline dementia increases the incidence of acute postoperative delirium and adverse outcomes. A basic check of cognitive function should be performed in older surgical candidates and, if cognitive processes are impaired, consultation with an internist, geriatrician, neurologist, or other individual skilled in dementia management should be considered perioperatively to reduce the risk of postoperative delirium.

Poor nutrition inhibits wound healing, and a serum albumin may be checked to assess preoperative nutritional status.[33] A history of alcohol abuse should be elicited, and smoking should be stopped.

Recommended preoperative laboratories and testing in the older woman (>65 years) include hematocrit, blood urea nitrogen, creatinine, and electrocardiogram. Women aged 75 and older should also have a chest radiograph and blood glucose measurement. Other laboratories and testing should be ordered on an individualized basis. Additional tests based on age alone have not been shown to decrease morbidity and add economic burden.[34]

Perioperative Management

Perioperative and postoperative care are tailored for a speedy recovery and avoidance of a decline in functional status. No benefit has been demonstrated favoring one type of anesthesia in the older patient undergoing surgery.[35,36] General, regional, or local anesthesia technique should be tailored to the patient's needs and desires and anesthesiologist and surgeon preference and training.

Appropriate antibiotic prophylaxis should be administered perioperatively addressing the mixed flora of the vaginal environment.[37] Appropriate patient positioning should be ensured to lessen the occurrence of peripheral nerve injuries.

Postoperative Considerations

Postoperative delirium may be seen in up to 10% of older surgical patients and is often misdiagnosed leading to longer hospital stays, nursing home admissions, and morbidity. Delirium occurrence is reduced by improving orientation, decreasing sensory overload or deprivation, and providing reassurance. Prompt disposition to the home environment reduces the incidence of delirium.

Adequate pain control must be ensured, along with avoidance of common drug-drug interactions in this population. Oxidative drug metabolism decreases with age, and the effects of medications must be monitored. Medications to avoid in the older patient include meperidine and promethazine. Atelectasis is a common postoperative occurrence; incentive spirometry should be initiated immediately after surgery with turning, coughing, and deep breathing to prevent increased respiratory compromise and vigorous ambulation. Prophylaxis should also be used against deep venous thrombosis, infection, and constipation.[33]

Concurrent Hysterectomy

In general, hysterectomy should be reserved for pathologic indications or if a total colpocleisis is planned. The main benefit of routine hysterectomy is the prevention of endometrial or cervical cancer, in addition to the rare event of pyometra after partial colpocleisis secondary to blocked lateral channels.[38] Pyometra can be managed initially with attempted radiologically guided drainage as opposed to hysterectomy.[39] The main argument against routine hysterectomy is that the advantages of less operative time and a less invasive technique with partial colpocleisis are compromised. Two observational studies showed longer operating times, with one of these studies showing increased blood loss and longer hospital stay.[22,31] If hysterectomy is not performed, Papanicolaou smear, if indicated, and endometrial assessment with ultrasound or sampling should be considered.

Perineorrhaphy and Levator Myorrhaphy

The rationale behind performing this concurrent procedure is to narrow the introitus and create a platform whereby less gravitational tension is placed on the colpocleisis procedure. In theory, this platform may reduce the risk of anatomic failure and downward tension on the urethra, a proposed etiology of postoperative stress incontinence. This procedure is encouraged, especially for candidates who are physically active, but its necessity has not been proved.

TECHNIQUES
Partial Colpocleisis

A partial colpocleisis (ie, LeFort) should be considered for those patients with vaginal vault prolapse or uterovaginal prolapse who are viable candidates for an obliterative procedure. The procedure is begun by placing the patient in lithotomy position, and the bladder preferably drained. The vaginal cuff or cervix is grasped and exteriorized through the vaginal introitus. A marking pen is used to outline rectangular areas for incision on both the anterior and posterior vaginal walls (**Fig. 1**). With vaginal vault prolapse, the rectangular areas are begun cephalad approximately 1 cm distal to the vaginal cuff, longitudinally extend posteriorly to 2 cm proximal to the hymenal ring, and anteriorly to 2 cm proximal to the urethrovesical junction. When the cervix is present, the anterior rectangular area should extend longitudinally from approximately 0.5 cm distal from the cervicovaginal junction to 2 cm proximal to the urethrovescial junction. With both vaginal vault prolapse and uterovaginal prolapse, the lateral aspects of the vaginal wall rectangles should extend to encompass any cystocele or rectocele defect present.

To assist in dissection, the marked areas may be first injected with saline, anesthetic agent, or vasoconstrictor of choice into the subepithelial layer. The rectangular epithelial layers can then be completely excised by sharp dissection. The surgeon should make an effort to minimize blood loss and dissect in an avascular plane while trying to maintain the underlying musculoconnective tissue overlying the bladder and rectum (**Fig. 2**).

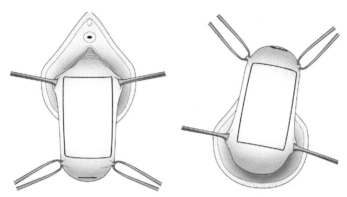

Fig. 1. Partial colpocleisis. Rectangular portions of the anterior and posterior vaginal walls are demarcated. A 2-cm space between the rectangles is left to allow for creation of drainage tunnels. Care is taken to be distal to the urethrovesical junction. (*From* Wheeler TL, Richter HE. Oblitertive procedures. In: Bent AE, Cundiff GW, Swift SE, editors. Ostergard's urogynecology and pelvic floor dysfunction. 6th edition. Philadelphia: Lippincott Williams and Wilkins; 2008. p. 514–20; with permission.)

If there is a cystocele or rectocele found to be so severe as to compromise the surgeon's field of visualization or is noted to have minimal central musculoconnective tissue for plication of the anterior wall to the posterior wall, the surgeon may first choose to reduce the defect by minimally plicating the musculoconnective tissue of the cystocele or rectocele before completing the colpocleisis. An enterocele, if noted, is not typically entered or separately repaired.

The newly created vaginal epithelial edges of the anterior vaginal wall are then sewn to the posterior vaginal wall with two opposing running delayed absorbable sutures

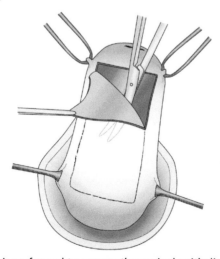

Fig. 2. Sharp dissection is performed to remove the vaginal epithelium leaving musculoconnective tissue on the bladder and rectum. (*From* Wheeler TL, Richter HE. Oblitertive procedures. In: Bent AE, Cundiff GW, Swift SE, editors. Ostergard's urogynecology and pelvic floor dysfunction. 6th edition. Philadelphia: Lippincott Williams and Wilkins; 2008. p. 514–20; with permission.)

(**Fig. 3**). During the sewing of the lateral vaginal edges together, the connective tissue overlying the bladder is plicated, proximally to distally, to the connective tissue overlying the rectum with delayed absorbable sutures in simple interrupted fashion (**Fig. 4**). Concurrent sewing of the lateral epithelial edges of the anterior and posterior vaginal walls together creates the lateral tunnels allowing for any possible future drainage.

The partial colpocleisis procedure is usually completed by tying the opposing anterior and posterior running epithelial sutures together with final resultant vaginal depth of approximately 3 to 4 cm (**Fig. 5**). An additional high perineorraphy or intoital modification may be performed if desired. Cystoscopy may then be performed to ensure ureteral patency.

Total Colpocleisis (Colpectomy)

For those patients with vaginal vault prolapse following hysterectomy and who desire obliterative procedure, a total colpocleisis can be performed. The procedure is begun by placing the patient in lithotomy position, and the bladder preferably drained. The subepthelial layer may first be injected with saline, local anesthesia, or vasoconstrictor to assist in sharp dissection. The vaginal epithelium is then completely excised en bloc. Dissection typically begins distally and progresses proximally with circumferential incision near the hymenal ring on the posterior vaginal wall (**Figs. 6** and **7**) and 2 cm proximal to the urethrovesical junction on the anterior vaginal wall. As in the partial colpocleisis, efforts should be made to minimize bleeding and maximize the remaining underlying musculoconnective tissue. Once denuded, the vaginal tube is obliterated with sequential purse string or interrupted delayed absorbable sutures (**Fig. 8**). The exposed vaginal epithelium is subsequently closed with absorbable suture. Concomitant perineorraphy, introital modification, or levatorpasty may be performed. Cystoscopy may then be performed to ensure ureteral patency.

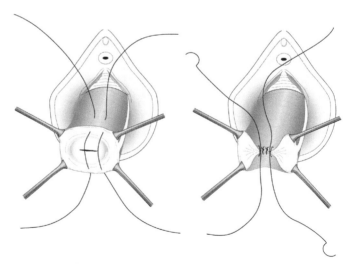

Fig. 3. Two delayed absorbable sutures are used to start the locking closure. The closure starts over the midline of the cervix or cuff and is run in opposite directions. (*From* Wheeler TL, Richter HE. Oblitertive procedures. In: Bent AE, Cundiff GW, Swift SE, editors. Ostergard's urogynecology and pelvic floor dysfunction. 6th edition. Philadelphia: Lippincott Williams and Wilkins; 2008. p. 514–20; with permission.)

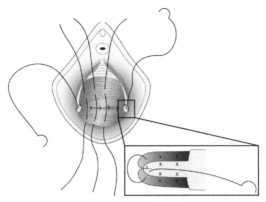

Fig. 4. Three or four absorbable sutures are sagittally placed in the musculoconnective tissue underlying the bladder and brought to that overlying the rectum to approximate the middle portions of the rectangles. (*Inset*) The locking closure is continued to create the lateral drainage channels. The x's represent appropriate needle placement paying attention to stay near the epithelial edge. (*From* Wheeler TL, Richter HE. Oblitertive procedures. In: Bent AE, Cundiff GW, Swift SE, editors. Ostergard's urogynecology and pelvic floor dysfunction. 6th edition. Philadelphia: Lippincott Williams and Wilkins; 2008. p. 514–20; with permission.)

Incontinence Procedure

When performing partial or total colpocleisis, the surgeon should be mindful to avoid plication near the urethrovesical junction to prevent traction on the bladder neck. The risk of postoperative stress urinary incontinence following an obliterative procedure has been reported to be greater than 25%.[14] Dissection and plication of periurethral

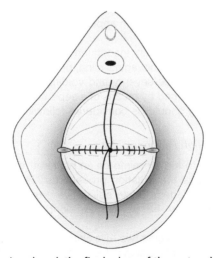

Fig. 5. After the prolapse is reduced, the final edges of the rectangles are closed either with a separate suture or from continuation of the running stitch. The lateral drainage channels are shown. (*From* Wheeler TL, Richter HE. Oblitertive procedures. In: Bent AE, Cundiff GW, Swift SE, editors. Ostergard's urogynecology and pelvic floor dysfunction. 6th edition. Philadelphia: Lippincott Williams and Wilkins; 2008. p. 514–20; with permission.)

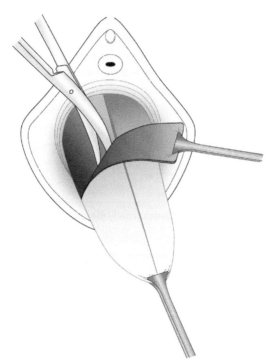

Fig. 6. Total colpocleisis. The prolapse is divided into four quadrants. A circumferential incision at the base of the prolapse starts the dissection. (*From* Wheeler TL, Richter HE. Obliterative procedures. In: Bent AE, Cundiff GW, Swift SE, editors. Ostergard's urogynecology and pelvic floor dysfunction. 6th edition. Philadelphia: Lippincott Williams and Wilkins; 2008. p. 514–20; with permission.)

connective tissue should typically remain approximately 2 cm proximal to the bladder neck.

At the time of colpocleisis, a urinary incontinence procedure may be performed. A Kelly plication-type procedure, pubovaginal sling, or midurethral sling may be considered as directed by incontinence severity and voiding function. These incontinence procedures are usually performed by means of a separate midline suburethral vaginal incision. Cystourethroscopy should be considered following the procedure.

Levator Myorraphy and High Perineorraphy

The surgeon may choose to further reinforce an obliterative procedure by modifying the vaginal introitus. Introital modification procedures are recommended when the genital hiatus is notably widened. These adjunctive procedures, levator myorraphy and high perineorraphy, may be performed along with either partial or total colpocleisis.

The procedure is begun by placing two Allis clamps at the 4- and 8-o'clock position of the hymenal ring. A horizontal incision is made in the vaginal epithelium from clamp to clamp. The incision is then extended cephalad from the clamps bilaterally to the distal edge of the mid colpocleisis to create a triangular-shaped wedge. The wedge is dissected in the rectovaginal space and then excised (**Fig. 9**). Dissection through this incision is further extended laterally to free the vaginal wall from the underlying

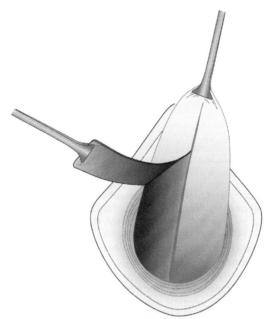

Fig. 7. The entire overlying vaginal epithelium is removed a quadrant at a time, leaving as much connective tissue as possible on the bladder and rectum. (*From* Wheeler TL, Richter HE. Oblitertive procedures. In: Bent AE, Cundiff GW, Swift SE, editors. Ostergard's urogynecology and pelvic floor dysfunction. 6th edition. Philadelphia: Lippincott Williams and Wilkins; 2008. p. 514–20; with permission.)

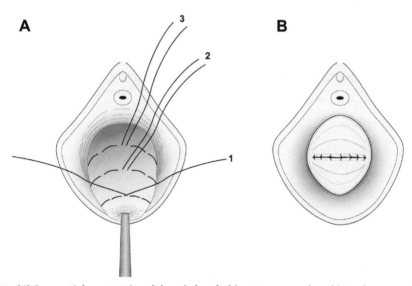

Fig. 8. (*A*) Sequential purse-string delayed absorbable sutures are placed into the connective tissue. The prolapse is reduced and the purse-string sutures are tied in the order shown (here 1 through 3). (*B*) The vaginal epithelium is then closed. (*From* Wheeler TL, Richter HE. Oblitertive procedures. In: Bent AE, Cundiff GW, Swift SE, editors. Ostergard's urogynecology and pelvic floor dysfunction. 6th edition. Philadelphia: Lippincott Williams and Wilkins; 2008. p. 514–20; with permission.)

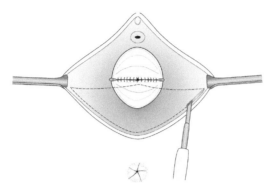

Fig. 9. Levator myorrhaphy and high perineorrhaphy. Two Allis clamps are placed opposite each other at the level of the hymenal ring or slightly distal to that at approximately 4 and 8 o'clock. A horizontal incision is made between the clamps. (*From* Wheeler TL, Richter HE. Oblitertive procedures. In: Bent AE, Cundiff GW, Swift SE, editors. Ostergard's urogynecology and pelvic floor dysfunction. 6th edition. Philadelphia: Lippincott Williams and Wilkins; 2008. p. 514–20; with permission.)

fascia of the puborectalis muscle, bulbocavernosus muscle, and perineal membrane (**Figs. 10** and **11**). The puborectalis muscle is plicated, contralaterally across the midline, posterior to the vaginal wall (**Fig. 12**). The bulbocavernosus muscles are also plicated across the midline in the same fashion (**Fig. 13**). The perineal body is then approximated (**Fig. 14**). Finally, the vaginal introital epithelium is approximated with absorbable running suture leaving the resultant genital hiatus about 1 to 2 cm in length (**Fig. 15**).

Constricting Colporrhaphy

It is not uncommon for a patient considered for an obliterative procedure to be found with minimal apical descensus, anterior wall prolapse, or posterior wall prolapse as to make colpocleisis technically infeasible. For these patients a constricting colporrhaphy with concurrent levator myorrhaphy and high perineorrhaphy should be

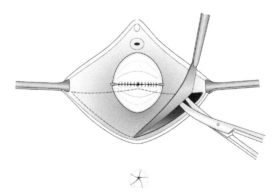

Fig. 10. This incision is then carried cephalad to the distal edge of the colpocleisis to dissect free the wedge to be removed (*hash marks*). (*From* Wheeler TL, Richter HE. Oblitertive procedures. In: Bent AE, Cundiff GW, Swift SE, editors. Ostergard's urogynecology and pelvic floor dysfunction. 6th edition. Philadelphia: Lippincott Williams and Wilkins; 2008. p. 514–20; with permission.)

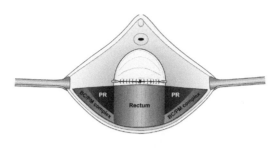

Fig. 11. The vaginal wall is freed from the fascia of the puborectalis (PR) and bulbocavernous muscles and from whatever perineal membrane is present. (*From* Wheeler TL, Richter HE. Oblitertive procedures. In: Bent AE, Cundiff GW, Swift SE, editors. Ostergard's urogynecology and pelvic floor dysfunction. 6th edition. Philadelphia: Lippincott Williams and Wilkins; 2008. p. 514–20; with permission.)

considered. The goal for successful constricting colporrhaphies is to narrow the vaginal tube to close the defect.

A recommended technique is to begin the procedure by outlining the entire defect on the vaginal epithelium with a marking pen. The subepithelium of the demarcated area is injected with saline anesthesia or vessel constrictor of choice. The infiltrated epithelium overlying the defect is dissected free of the underlying musculoconnective tissue and then excised. Dissection of the remaining epithelium is continued laterally to locate and expose underlying paravaginal connective tissue. The paravaginal connective tissue and vaginal epithelium are plicated across the midline with delayed absorbable suture thereby reducing vaginal tube diameter.

When performing the constricting colporrhaphy on the posterior vaginal wall a levator myorrhaphy and high perineorrhaphy should be performed as previously described. An enterocele, if noted, is not typically repaired separately. During

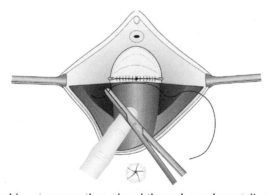

Fig. 12. Nonabsorbable sutures are then placed through a puborectalis muscle or its fascial covering approximately 3-cm posterior to its attachment to the pubic rami and then brought across to the same area of the contralateral muscle. (*From* Wheeler TL, Richter HE. Oblitertive procedures. In: Bent AE, Cundiff GW, Swift SE, editors. Ostergard's urogynecology and pelvic floor dysfunction. 6th edition. Philadelphia: Lippincott Williams and Wilkins; 2008. p. 514–20; with permission.)

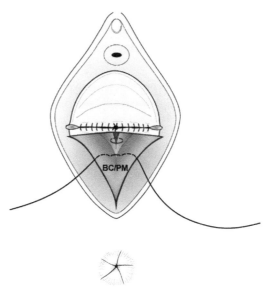

Fig. 13. The bulbocavernous muscles, which are not dissected from the perineal membrane, are plicated across the midline (BC/PM complex). (*From* Wheeler TL, Richter HE. Oblitertive procedures. In: Bent AE, Cundiff GW, Swift SE, editors. Ostergard's urogynecology and pelvic floor dysfunction. 6th edition. Philadelphia: Lippincott Williams and Wilkins; 2008. p. 514–20; with permission.)

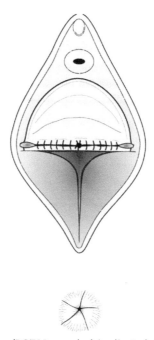

Fig. 14. The perineal membrane (BC/PM complex) is plicated. (*From* Wheeler TL, Richter HE. Oblitertive procedures. In: Bent AE, Cundiff GW, Swift SE, editors. Ostergard's urogynecology and pelvic floor dysfunction. 6th edition. Philadelphia: Lippincott Williams and Wilkins; 2008. p. 514–20; with permission.)

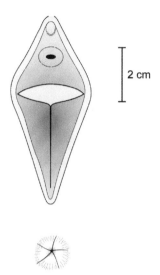

2 cm

Fig. 15. Closure of the vaginal wall, down to the introitus, is completed with the running absorbable suture. The genital hiatus should be approximately 2 cm. (*From* Wheeler TL, Richter HE. Oblitertive procedures. In: Bent AE, Cundiff GW, Swift SE, editors. Ostergard's urogynecology and pelvic floor dysfunction. 6th edition. Philadelphia: Lippincott Williams and Wilkins; 2008. p. 514–20; with permission.)

dissection of the posterior vaginal wall defect, exposure and plication of the perileva- tor and perirectal connective tissues are needed to complete the procedure. Plication is performed across the midline with delayed absorbable suture; however, care should be taken during the posterior plication as to allow for the levator myorrhaphy and high perineorraphy procedures that follow.

In addition to the techniques described previously, Conill's colpocleisis, Doderlein's cross-bar colporrhaphy, Labhardt's high perineoplasty, and their modifications have been described.[25] Two out of 39 had mesh exposures that were subsequently trimmed.[28] In patients undergoing concurrent tension-free vaginal tape, Agarwala and coworkers[28] interposed excess mesh strips from tension-free vaginal tape in the partial colpocleisis repair.

RESULTS

An anatomic success rate of 100% for colpocleisis was first reported by Edebohls[11] in 1901 for a series of four patients who underwent total colpocleisis. Since then, case series reports for total colpocleisis have ranged between 89% and 100% success with most close to or at 100%.[13,22–24,31,40–47] Likewise, anatomic success rates for partial colpocleisis are based on case series starting with Wyatt's[15] report of 83% success on eight patients in 1912 and range between 75% and 100%.[15–19,28,32,48–56] Case series reporting both techniques report anatomic success between 90% and 100%.[14,26,30,57–59] The inherent outcome bias associated with case series reports limits comparison of the techniques.

Recurrence, satisfaction, and incontinence after colpocleisis for published results since 1992 are listed in **Table 2**. Reports of satisfaction are high (86%–100%) and regret low (0%–13%) after colpocleisis. Following partial colpocleisis, Ubachs and coworkers[19] reported a 10.7% regret rate and Wheeler and colleagues[21] reported 9.3%; none cited regret over the loss of sexual function. For total colpocleisis,

Table 2
Results after obliterative vaginal prolapse surgery reported since 1992

Author Year	N	Duration of Follow-up	Recurrence, %	Incontinence	Colpocleisis-Related Complications	Satisfaction
Abbasy 2009	38	3 mo	97	POPDI and UDI improved; 13% SUI rate and 32% UUI rate postoperatively; urinary retention resolved in 0/11	None intraoperatively; 1 CHF; 1 N/V; 1 de novo elevated PVR	
van Huisseling 2009[a]	30	6 mo	3	Continence rates improved	1 hemorrhage; 1 dehiscence	No regret; most were satisfied and considered the result very good
Fitzgerald 2008	152	12 mo	93 POP-Q stage ≤2	All pelvic symptom scores and related bother, including UI, improved; 14% bothersome SUI and 15% UUI at 1 y	OR time longer for total versus partial colpocleisis (121 versus 94 min); 1 cystotomy; 1 ureteral kinking; AEs were uncommon for 1 y after surgery	95% satisfaction
Murphy 2008	45	17 mo	7	Significant improvements on UDI-6 and IIQ-7; no difference from reconstructive surgery	Colpocleisis had a longer OR time than reconstructive surgery with trocar-inserted mesh (156 versus 105 min)	High satisfaction on the Surgical Satisfaction Questionnaire; no difference from reconstructive surgery
Argawala 2007	39	24 mo	5	All had TVT with excess strips placed in the prolapse repair; 35 had improved SUI; no voiding postoperative difficulties	1 h mean OR time; 1 reoperation for POP; 2 interposed mesh exposures requiring local excision	95% satisfied with prolapse repair

Sung 2007	1181				Obliterative had fewer complications than reconstructive (17 versus 25%)
Hullfish 2007	46	33 mo	2/46	Improvements in IIQ and UDI	4 UTI; 5 urinaryincontinence; 1postoperative bleed; 1 A Fib; 1 chest pain; 1 rectal prolapse	95% satisfaction; patient goal attainment high
Barber 2006	30	12 mo		Significant improvements PFDI and PFIQ; no difference from reconstructive surgery	Colpocleisis had a shorter OR time than reconstructive surgery (150 versus 180 min); 2 transfusions; 1 cystotomy; 1 pulmonary	87% somewhat to very much better; 90% would choose obliterative surgery again
Wheeler 2005	32	28mo	7	Significant improvements on UDI-6 and IIQ-7 for both patients who did have and did not have an incontinence procedure		9.3% regret rate; 86% satisfied
Glavind 2005	42	46 mo	0	11/29 incontinent	1 postoperative bleed	90% satisfied
Fitzgerald 2003	64	12 wk	3	18/21 continent after sling; 8/30 new onset SUI	2 vaginal hematomas	
Harmanli 2003	41	28.7 mo	0	53.1% cure of SUI; 22.2% new-onset SUI	1 vesical injury; 4 late rectal bleeding	High satisfaction and no regret

(continued on next page)

Table 2
(continued)

Author/Year	N	Duration of Follow-up	Recurrence, %	Incontinence	Colpocleisis-Related Complications	Satisfaction
Von Pechmann 2003	92	12 mo (24 mo for telephone survey)	2	6/46 (13%) recurrent SUI; no new-onset SUI	4 ureteral occlusion; 1 proctotomy; 2 rectal prolapse; 2 laparotomies with TVH; 20 transfusions	90.3% (56/62) satisfaction; 12.9 (8/62) regret over loss of coital ability
Hoffman 2003	54	22 mo	0	22/33 improvement in bladder or bowel symptoms; 2 new-onset mixed UI; 4 new-onset SUI	1 CVA; 1 pulmonary edema; 1 A-fib	
Moore 2003	30	19.1 mo	10	94% cure of SUI with TVT	1 TVT release (continence maintained); 1 myocardial infarction	No regret
Cespedes 2001	38	24 mo	0	3 persistent SUI	1 urethrolysis after sling	100% satisfaction; no regret
DeLancey 1997	33	8 mo (35 mo for telephone survey)	1	100% cure SUI; no new-onset SUI; 2 cured, 1 improved, and 3 no change out of 8 with preoperative UUI	2 CHF; 1 pneumonia	1/22 remorse over loss of sexual function
Denehy 1995	21	25 mo	5		1 arrhythmia; 3 UTI	
Ahranjani 1992	38	30/38 patients followed long term	0		2 transfusions; 30% minor complication rate (11 respiratory; 2 cardiac; 5 urinary)	

Abbreviations: AE, adverse event; A-Fib, atrial fibrillation, CHF, congestive heart failure; CVA, cerebro vascular accident; IIQ, incontinence impact questionnaire, N/V, nausea/vomiting; OR, operating room; PFDI, pelvic floor distress inventory; PFIQ, pelvic floor impact questionnaire; POP, pelvic organ prolapse; POPDI, pelvic organ prolapse distress inventory; POP-Q, pelvic organ prolapse quantification; PVR, post void residual; SUI, stress urinary incontinence; TVH, tension-free vaginal tape; UDI, urinary distress inventory; UI, urinary incontinence; UTI, urinary tract infection; UUI, urge urinary incontinence.
[a] Modification of the Labhardt's high perineoplasty.

Harmanli and colleagues[23] had no reports of regret. As far as losing sexual function after total colpocleisis, Von Pechmann[22] reported that 12.9% were at least somewhat regretful, whereas DeLancey and Morley[24] reported that 1 patient out of 33 had remorse.

Changes in pelvic floor symptoms have been evaluated after obliterative surgery with concurrent incontinence procedures when indicated. Validated, symptom-specific quality of life questionnaires have shown improvements in the bother and impact of prolapse, coloanal, and urinary symptoms.[6,21,26,27,29,32] General quality of life also improves.[6,26]

There are relatively few studies comparing obliterative with reconstructive because of the heterogeneity between groups that can lead to selection bias. Two studies have shown shorter operative times with obliterative surgery (approximately 150 minutes).[6,26] One study found that trocar-guided mesh insertion took less time than colpocleisis (105 versus 156 minutes).[60]

SUMMARY

Obliterative vaginal surgery is an appropriate option for elderly women who do not desire vaginal intercourse and have failed or do not desire nonsurgical management of pelvic organ prolapse. Although increasing age does impose more risk with surgery, older women do tolerate obliterative surgery, especially when consideration is given to their age-related physiologic changes and risk of delirium. Overall, obliterative surgery has high success rates and improvement in pelvic floor symptoms.

REFERENCES

1. Handa VL, Garret E, Hendrix S, et al. Progression and remission of pelvic organ prolapse: a longitudinal study of menopausal women. Am J Obstet Gynecol 2004; 190:27–32.
2. Daneshgari F, Moore C. Epidemiology of pelvic organ prolapse. In: Raz S, Rodriguez LV, editors. Female Urology, 3rd edition. Philadelphia: Saunders Elsevier; 2008. p. 527.
3. Boyles SH, Weber AM, Meyn L. Procedures for pelvic organ prolapse in the United States, 1979–97. Am J Obstet Gynecol 2003;188:108–15.
4. Olsen AL, Smith VJ, Bergstrom JO, et al. Epidemiology of surgically managed pelvic organ prolapse and urinary incontinence. Obstet Gynecol 1997;89:501–6.
5. Sung VW, Weitzen S, Sokol ER, et al. Effect of patient age on increasing morbidity and mortality following urogynecologic surgery. Am J Obstet Gynecol 2006;194: 1411–7.
6. Barber MD, Admundsen CL, Paraiso FR, et al. Quality of life after surgery for genital prolapse in elderly women: obliterative and reconstructive surgery. Int Urogynecol J Pelvic Floor Dysfunct 2007;18:799–806.
7. Adair FL, DaSef L. The Le Fort colpocleisis. Am J Obstet Gynecol 1936;32: 218–26.
8. Geradin R. Memoire presente a la societe medicale de Metz en 1823. Arch Gen de Med 1825;8:1825 [in French].
9. Neugebauer JA. Einige worte uber die mediane vaginalnaht als mittel zur beseit-gung des gebarmuttervorfalls. Zentralbl Gynecol 1881;5:3–8 [in German].
10. LeFort L. Nouveau procede pour la guerison du prolapsus uterin. Bull Gen Ther 1877;92:337–46 [in French].
11. Edebohls GM. In: Panhysterokolpectomy: a new prolapsus operation, vol. 60. New York: Med red; 1901. p. 561–4.

12. Edebohls GM. Panhysterokolpectomy: a new prolapsus operation. Trans Am Gynecol Soc 1901;26:150–62.

13. Hayden RC, Levinson JM. Total vaginectomy, vaginal hysterectomy, and colpocleisis for advanced procidentia. Obstet Gynecol 1960;16:564–6.

14. Fitzgerald MP. Colpocleisis and urinary incontinence. Am J Obstet Gynecol 2003; 189:1241–4.

15. Wyatt J. Le Fort's operation for prolapse, with an account of eight cases. J Obstet Gynaecol Br Emp 1912;22:266–9.

16. Mazer C, Israel SL. The LeFort colpocleisis: an analysis of 43 operations. Am J Obstet Gynecol 1948;56:944–9.

17. Falk H, Kaufman S. Partial colpocleisis: the Le Fort procedure (analysis of 100 cases). Obstet Gynecol 1955;5:617.

18. Hanson GE, Keettel WC. The Neugebauer Le Fort operation (a review of 288 colpocleisis). Obstet Gynecol 1969;34:352–7.

19. Ubachs JM, van Sante TJ, Schellekens LA. Partial colpocleisis by a modification of LeFort's operation. Obstet Gynecol 1973;42:415–20.

20. Goodall JR, Power RMH. A modification of the Le Fort operation for increasing its scope. Am J Obstet Gynecol 1937;34:968–76.

21. Wheeler TL, Richter HE, Varner RE, et al. Regret, satisfaction and symptom improvement: analysis of the impact of partial colpocleisis for the management of severe pelvic organ prolapse. Am J Obstet Gynecol 2005;193:2067–70.

22. Von Pechmann WS, Mutone M, Fyffe J, et al. Total colpocleisis with high levator plication for the treatment of advanced pelvic organ prolapse. Am J Obstet Gynecol 2003;189:121–6.

23. Harmanli OH, Dandolu V, Chatwani AJ, et al. Total colpocleisis for severe pelvic organ prolapse. J Reprod Med 2003;48:703–6.

24. DeLancey JO, Morley GW. Total colpocleisis for vaginal eversion. Am J Obstet Gynecol 1997;176:1228–32 [discussion: 1232–5].

25. van Huisseling JCM. A modification of Labhardt's high perineoplasty for treatment of pelvic organ prolapse in the very old. Int Urogynecol J Pelvic Floor Dysfunct 2009;20:185–91.

26. Fitzgerald MP, Richter HE, Bradley CS, et al. Pelvic support, pelvic symptoms, and patient satisfaction after colpocleisis. Int Urogynecol J Pelvic Floor Dysfunct 2008;19:1603–9.

27. Murphy M, Sternschuss G, Haff R, et al. Quality of life and surgical satisfaction after vaginal reconstructive vs obliterative surgery for the treatment of advanced pelvic organ prolapse. Am J Obstet Gynecol 2008;198:573.e1–7.

28. Agarwala N, Hasiak N, Shade M. Graft interposition colpocleisis, perineorrhaphy, and tension-free sling for pelvic organ prolapse and stress urinary incontinence in elderly patients. J Minim Invasive Gynecol 2007;14(6):740–5.

29. Hullfish KL, Bovbjerg VE, Steers WD. Colpocleisis for pelvic organ prolapse: patient goals, quality of life, and satisfaction. Obstet Gynecol 2007;110(2): 341–5.

30. Moore RD, Miklos JR. Colpocleisis and tension-free vaginal tape sling for severe uterine and vaginal prolapse and stress urinary incontinence under local anesthesia. J Am Assoc Gynecol Laparosc 2003;10:276–80.

31. Hoffman MS, Cardosi RJ, Lockhart J, et al. Vaginectomy with pelvic herniorrhaphy for prolapse. Am J Obstet Gynecol 2003;189:364–71.

32. Abbasy S, Lowenstein L, Pham T, et al. Urinary retention is uncommon after colpocleisis with concomitant sling. Int Urogynecol J Pelvic Floor Dysfunct 2009;20:213–6.

33. Katz PR, Grossberg GT, Potter JF, et al. Geriatric syllabus for the specialists. New York: American Geriatrics Society; 2002.
34. Roizen M, Cohn S. Preoperative evaluation for elective surgery: what laboratory tests are needed? In: Stoelting R, editor. Advances in anesthesia, vol. 10. Chicago: Mosby-Year Book; 1993. p. 25–43.
35. Williams-Russo P, Sharrock NE, Mattis S, et al. Cognitive effects after epidural vs general anesthesia in older adults. JAMA 1995;274:44–50.
36. Segal JL, Owens G, Silva WA, et al. A randomized trial of local anesthesia with intravenous sedation vs general anesthesia for the vaginal correction of pelvic organ prolapse. Int Urogynecol J Pelvic Floor Dysfunct 2007;18:807–82.
37. ACOG practice bulletin No. 104: antibiotic prophylaxis for gynecologic procedures. Obstet Gynecol 2009;113(5):1180–9.
38. Toglia MR, Fagan MJ. Pyometra complicating Le Fort colpocleisis. Int Urogynecol J Pelvic Floor Dysfunct 2009;20:361–2.
39. Shayya RF, Weinstein MM, Lukacz ES. Pyometra after Le Fort colpocleis resolved with interventional radiology. AM J Obstet Gynecol 2009;113:566–8.
40. Bradbury WC. Subtotal vaginectomy. Am J Obstet Gynecol 1963;86:663–70 [discussion: 671].
41. Masson JC, Knepper PA. Vaginectomy. Am J Obstet Gynecol 1938;36:94–9.
42. Williams JT. Vaginal hysterectomy and colpectomy for prolapse of the uterus and bladder. Am J Obstet Gynecol 1950;59:365–70.
43. Adams HD. Total colpocleisis for pelvic eventration. Surg Gynecol Obstet 1951; 92:321–4.
44. Anderson GV, Deasy PP. Hysterocolpectomy. Obstet Gynecol 1960;16:344–9.
45. Percy NM, Perl JI. Total colpectomy. Surg Gynecol Obstet 1961;113:174–84.
46. Thompson HG, Murphy CJ Jr, Picot H. Hysterocolpectomy for the treatment of uterine procidentia. Am J Obstet Gynecol 1961;82:748–51.
47. Johnson CG. Vaginal hysterectomy and vaginectomy in personal retrospect. Am J Obstet Gynecol 1969;105:14–9.
48. Baer JL, Reis RA. Immediate and remote results in two hundred twelve cases of prolapse of the uterus. Am J Obstet Gynecol 1928;16:646–55.
49. Collins CG, Lock FR. The Le Fort colpocleisis. Am J Surg 1941;53:202.
50. Wolf W. The Le Fort operation. Am J Obstet Gynecol 1952;63:1346–8.
51. Massoudnia N. Kahr colpocleisis. Int Surg 1974;59:45–6.
52. Ardekany MS, Rafee R. A new modification of colpocleisis for treatment of total procidentia in old age. Int J Gynaecol Obstet 1978;25:358–60.
53. Ahranjani M, Nora E, Rezai P, et al. Neugebauer-Le Fort operation for vaginal prolapse. J Reprod Med 1992;37:959–64.
54. Ridley JH. Evaluation of the colpocleisis operation: a report of fifty-eight cases. Am J Obstet Gynecol 1972;113:1114–9.
55. Goldman J, Ovadia J, Feldberg D. The Neugebauer-Le Fort operation: a review of 118 partial colpocleises. Eur J Obstet Gynecol Reprod Biol 1981;12:31–5.
56. Denehy TR, Choe JY, Gregori CA, et al. Modified Le Fort partial colpocleisis with Kelly urethral plication and posterior colpoperineoplasty in the medically compromised elderly: a comparison with vaginal hysterectomy, anterior colporrhaphy, and posterior colpoperineoplasty. Am J Obstet Gynecol 1995;173:1697–701 [discussion: 1701–2].
57. Phaneuf LE. The place of colpectomy in the treatment of uterine and vaginal prolapse. Trans Am Gynecol Soc 1935;60:143–56.
58. Rubovitz W, Litt S. Colpocleisis in the treatment of uterine and vaginal prolapse. Am J Obstet Gynecol 1935;29:222–30.

59. Langmade CF, Oliver JA Jr. Partial colpocleisis. Am J Obstet Gynecol 1986;154: 1200–5.
60. Murphy M, Sternschuss G, Haff R, et al. Quality of life and surgical satisfaction after vaginal reconstructive vs obliterative surgery for the treatment of advanced pelvic organ prolapse. Am J Obstet Gynecol 2008;198:573.

Pathophysiology of Anal Incontinence, Constipation, and Defecatory Dysfunction

Marc R. Toglia, MD[a,b,c,*]

KEYWORDS

- Anal incontinence • Anorectal disorders • Constipation
- Defecatory dysfunction • Fecal incontinence

Anorectal dysfunction, including anal incontinence, constipation, and obstructive defecation, is common among adult women. The onset typically follows pregnancy and childbirth and becomes more common with increasing age. Women are frequently too embarrassed by their symptoms to bring them to the attention of their health care providers. Often, these providers have an inadequate understanding of diagnostic and therapeutic options.

Anorectal dysfunction may occur as the result of structural abnormalities (eg, anal sphincter rupture or rectal prolapse), or functional abnormalities (eg, constipation or irritable bowel syndrome), or both. In addition, bowel symptoms may coexist with other pelvic floor disorders, such as pelvic organ prolapse, urinary incontinence, or retention. Therefore, clinicians caring for women with pelvic floor disorders should possess an adequate understanding of these conditions, as early recognition and evaluation will facilitate care and appropriate referral in a timely manner.

ANAL INCONTINENCE

Anal incontinence refers to the involuntary loss of gas, liquid stool, or solid stool, and the symptoms of fecal urgency and soiling. In the literature, the terms *anal*

[a] Department of Obstetrics and Gynecology, Thomas Jefferson University School of Medicine, Philadelphia, PA 19063, USA
[b] Division of Urogynecology and Reconstructive Pelvic Surgery, Mainline Health System, Wynnewood, PA, USA
[c] Urogynecology Associates of Philadelphia, Suite 3404, Outpatient Pavilion, 1098 West Baltimore Pike, Media, PA 19063, USA
* Corresponding author.
E-mail address: m.toglia@att.net

Obstet Gynecol Clin N Am 36 (2009) 659–671
doi:10.1016/j.ogc.2009.08.004
0889-8545/09/$ – see front matter © 2009 Elsevier Inc. All rights reserved.

incontinence and *fecal incontinence* are used interchangeably. Anal incontinence occurs more frequently than previously thought.[1-3] Recent studies have estimated that 7% to 16% of healthy adults will admit to incontinence of gas or feces.[4,5] Two thirds of affected individuals are women, typically multiparous. Anal incontinence may affect up to 10% of women following an uncomplicated vaginal delivery. Anal incontinence is a significant burden in the geriatric population. In a survey of 249 female residents in three extended-care facilities in the Indianapolis area, 50% admitted to incontinence of stool.[6] Similar to urinary incontinence, the emotional, psychological, and social problems created by this condition can be both devastating and debilitating.

The most common cause of anal incontinence in healthy women is currently believed to be obstetrical trauma. As many as 10% of all women may experience new defecatory symptoms following an uncomplicated vaginal delivery.[7] The most common symptoms experienced postpartum are incontinence to flatus and fecal urgency. Symptoms are more common and more severe in women who suffered anal sphincter rupture (ie, third- or fourth-degree laceration) at the time of delivery. Damage to the anal continence mechanism at the time of vaginal delivery is thought to occur by either mechanical disruption of the anterior sphincter complex,[8] or by damage to the innervation of the anal sphincters and pelvic floor muscles,[9] or a combination of both.[10] Recent studies have reported that injury to the anal continence mechanism occurs more commonly following a routine vaginal delivery than previously recognized. In a prospective study of 200 pregnant women evaluated both before and after delivery, Sultan and colleagues[8] reported that 13% of women develop incontinence or urgency following their first vaginal delivery with 30% of all women having evidence of structural injury to the internal and external anal sphincter detected by anal endosonography postpartum. All women with symptoms of anal incontinence had structural defects and there was no correlation between nerve latency studies and the development of symptoms in this study, suggesting that mechanical disruption rather than neurologic injury is the most important cause for anal incontinence.

Women who suffered a traumatic rupture of the anal sphincter at the time of vaginal delivery also appear to have a greater risk of anal incontinence than previously recognized. Several investigators have reported that 36% to 63% of women develop symptoms of incontinence following primary sphincter repair.[11-14] Sultan and colleagues[15] evaluated 50 women who had undergone a primary repair of a third-degree perineal laceration at the time of vaginal delivery. Half of the women in this study admitted to symptoms related to anal incontinence following delivery. Anal endosonography demonstrated that 85% of women had evidence of a persistent sphincter defect. The investigators concluded that primary sphincter repair may be inadequate in women who sustain a third-degree laceration and that most have residual sphincter defects. Symptomatology seemed to be related to the persistent mechanical defect rather than nerve injury in this study. Studies from other centers support these high rates of structural injury following vaginal delivery.[16,17]

There is also strong evidence to suggest that vaginal delivery results in significant injury to the innervation of the pelvic floor muscles. Snooks[18] noted a significant increase in the mean pudendal nerve motor latencies (PNTMLs) 48 hours after delivery in primiparous women who had a forceps delivery compared with controls and with multiparous patients. In a study of 128 women in whom PNTMLs were measured both during pregnancy and after delivery, PNTMLs were significantly prolonged 6 weeks postpartum in 32% of women who delivered vaginally.[19] Two thirds of those women with an abnormally prolonged PNTML had a PNTML within the normal range when restudied after 6 months, suggesting that nerve damage is permanent in a minority of women.

Rectovaginal and anovaginal fistulae represent another important cause of anal incontinence in women. These fistulae can occur anywhere along the length of the rectovaginal septum. If the fistulous tract originates distal to the dentate line, the fistulae should be considered anovaginal fistulae; defects above this landmark are rectovaginal.

Obstetric injuries account for the majority of these fistulae in most published series. Most of these occur following a vaginal delivery complicated by a third- or fourth-degree perineal laceration.[20] Others may be the result of unrecognized injury to the anorectum at the time of vaginal delivery. Episiotomy infections, though uncommon, can also result in the formation of a fistulous tract. Concomitant sphincter injury has been reported to exist in only 8.3%[21] and 32%[22] of women presenting with rectovaginal fistulae. However, it is likely that sphincter injuries exist far more frequently when the location of the fistula is within the distal 3 cm of the anal canal since anatomic studies have demonstrated that this is the normal length of the sphincter complex.[23] Failure to recognize and repair such a sphincter injury may result in continued incontinence following a successful fistulectomy.

Nonobstetrical Causes of Anal Incontinence

Although obstetrical trauma is a leading cause of anal incontinence in women, it can also result from a variety of other conditions (**Box 1**). Sphincter trauma leading to anal incontinence may be related to operative or accidental injuries, such as impalement or pelvic fractures. Surgical procedures such as posterior colporrhaphy, rectovaginal fistula and anal fissure repair, hemorrhoidectomy, and therapeutic anal dilation can all cause subsequent anal incontinence. A significant number of women with urinary incontinence and pelvic organ prolapse also have anal incontinence.[24] Among the elderly and institutionalized individuals, fecal impaction is a leading cause of incontinence.[25,26] Cognitive dysfunction and rectal prolapse are other important causes of anal incontinence in the geriatric population. Diabetes can be associated with an autonomic neuropathy that can affect the internal anal sphincter and can produce incontinence, particularly with diarrheal states.[27] Radiation therapy and ulcerative colitis can be associated with rectovaginal fistula formation and radiation proctitis may result in neurologic or mechanical damage to the rectum, including a reduction in rectal compliance. Occult spinal cord injury or disease is another important cause of incontinence and is typically associated with an intact but weak external anal sphincter.

RECTAL PROLAPSE

Rectal prolapse represents a full-thickness inversion of the rectum through the anal orifice (**Fig. 1**). It is commonly associated with functional disturbances, including anal incontinence, constipation, and obstructed defecation.

Rectal prolapse is typically classified according to the extent of displacement of the rectum. Complete rectal prolapse or procedentia represents a full-thickness eversion of the rectum through the anal orifice. Prolapse of the rectum into the anal canal but not beyond the sphincters is termed *internal rectal prolapse* or *occult prolapse* (**Fig. 2**). Many believe that internal rectal prolapse is a precursor to complete rectal prolapse.

Internal or occult prolapse may represent an early stage of complete prolapse and is best diagnosed by defecation studies. Mucosal prolapse results from a disruption of the submucosa from the underlying muscularis propria and is considered to be part of

---

Box 1
Causes of anal incontinence

Anal sphincter weakness

    Obstetrical rupture of anal sphincter (chronic third- or fourth-degree perineal tears)

    Injury related to surgical procedures

        Internal sphincterotomy

        Fistulotomy

        Low anterior colorectal resection

        Hemorrhoidectomy

Neuropathy stretch injury

    Obstetric trauma

    Chronic straining

    Fecal impaction

Anatomic disturbances of the pelvic floor

    Fistula

    Rectal prolapse

    Descending perineum syndrome

Inflammatory conditions

    Inflammatory bowel disease

    Radiation enteritis

    Infectious enteritis

Neurologic conditions

    Congenital anomalies

    Multiple sclerosis

    Parkinson disease

    Systemic sclerosis

    Spinal cord injury

    Stroke

    Dementia

    Diabetic neuropathy

Diarrheal states

---

the spectrum of hemorrhoidal disease. Mucosal prolapse does not predispose to rectal prolapse.

In adults, rectal prolapse occurs much more frequently in women than men, with a peak incidence in the sixth and seventh decades of life. The overall prevalence is approximately 4 per 1000 population in the United States, and increases to 10 per 1000 in persons older than 65 years. Multiparity and a history of obstetric trauma have been implicated as risk factors in some studies.[28,29] Constipation and chronic straining with defecation may also contribute to the development of rectal prolapse. Up to 25% of women with rectal prolapse present with concomitant uterine prolapse

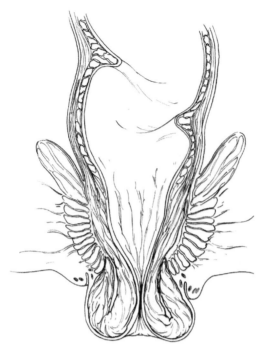

Fig. 1. Rectal prolapse. The full thickness of the rectal wall folds into itself and protrudes through the anal orifice. (*From* Weber AM, Brubaker L, Schaffer J, et al. Office urogynecology. New York: McGraw-Hill; 2004. p. 404; with permission.)

and up to 35% with a cystocele.[30,31] This suggests that an anatomic abnormality of the pelvic floor may exist that predisposes to both conditions.

The etiology of rectal prolapse is incompletely understood. Patients suffering from rectal prolapse share several anatomic features: an abnormally deep pelvic cul-de-sac, redundant rectosigmoid colon, weakness of the levator ani and anal sphincters, and lack of normal sacral fixation of the rectum. Observing that many patients with prolapse had a deep cul-de-sac, Moschcowitz,[32] in 1912, suggested that the prolapse represented a sliding hernia. His procedure for obliterating the cul-de-sac with concentric purse-string sutures remained popular for the first half of the twentieth century, despite reported failure rates of over 50%. Devadhar,[33] in 1965, was the first to propose that rectal prolapse was an intussusception of the colon. Subsequent investigators have confirmed this theory based upon videodefecography studies. Broden and Snellman[34] proposed in 1968 that rectal prolapse represented progressive intussusception of the midrectum, beginning at the level of the peritoneal reflection that develops as the result of straining at defecation. Others suggest that the intussusception begins at the level of the rectosigmoid junction, where repeated straining at defecation causes the rectum to loosen from its mesenteric connections.[35] As the intussusception progresses, the supporting structures of the rectum are stretched, including the pudendal nerves. Ultimately, a pelvic floor neuropathy develops, which significantly weakens the levator ani and anal sphincter musculature, further allowing the prolapse to progress. Eventually, the intussusception is exteriorized, resulting in prolapse of the rectal walls through the anal orifice. Constipation and obstructive defecatory symptoms are thought to occur early in the disease state, whereas anal

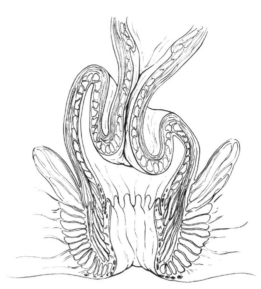

Fig. 2. Intrarectal prolapse. Note how the rectum folds inwards and enters the upper anal canal. (*From* Weber AM, Brubaker L, Schaffer J, et al. Office urogynecology. New York: McGraw-Hill; 2004. p. 405; with permission.)

incontinence, as a result of pelvic floor neuropathy and weakening of the sphincteric mechanism, is thought to develop late in the course of this disorder.

CONSTIPATION

Chronic constipation in adults, a common and sometimes debilitating problem, accounts for approximately 2 to 3 million physician visits per year.[36] Women are three times more likely than men to suffer from constipation and are more likely to have pelvic floor dysfunction. The incidence of constipation increases with age, and up to one third of elderly patients complain of constipation.[37] Constipation is the most common digestive complaint in the United States. One systematic review in North America found an average prevalence of 12% to 19%, and the incidence was observed to increase with age.[38] The prevalence of self-reported constipation in a large-population survey in Spain was 29.5%.[39] The study also found a higher incidence in females than males, and that both physical exercise and high fiber were protective. It is more prevalent in African Americans, in the southern United States, and among families with low incomes and low educational levels.[40,41]

Constipation as a symptom is difficult to define precisely. Bowel habits have a broad range of what is considered normal. Many individuals define constipation based upon stool frequency. Numerous surveys of adult populations have revealed that the great majority of women have at least one bowel movement every other day. This led early investigators to define constipation as infrequent stools, such as less than three stools per week or more than three days without stooling. Other patients complain of passing stools that are too hard or too small or that the act of defecation is prolonged or difficult, often requiring excessive straining or use of manual assistance. Some patients equate a sensation of rectal fullness or incomplete evacuation with constipation. Abdominal pain and bloating are often the primary complaint in constipated patients.

The most recent Rome criteria provide a useful resource for defining the condition (**Box 2**).[42]

The cause of constipation is usually multifactorial (**Box 3**). From a clinician's standpoint, constipation may be broadly classified into five categories: primary colonic motor dysfunction, anorectal outlet obstruction, pharmacologic causes, systemic disorders that affect normal colorectal function, and primary psychological factors. A deficiency in dietary fiber, inadequate fluid intake, and inadequate physical activity are also important contributors. A deficiency in dietary fiber has long been thought to be an important cause of constipation. Fiber may shorten whole-gut transit and increase stool weight. However, increasing dietary fiber for the treatment of constipation has had limited success and a number of studies have demonstrated a strong placebo effect.[43,44]

Diagnostic testing for screening purposes is seldom necessary in the initial approach to constipation. A recent systemic review did not support the routine use of blood tests or radiologic studies.[45] A complete blood count may be indicated to exclude anemia, especially in the elderly and in those with alarm symptoms, such as bloody stools or recent onset of constipation symptoms or abdominal pain. Thyroid function assessment to exclude hypothyroidism should be considered when clinically appropriate. Age-appropriate screening for colorectal cancer should be recommended.

Referral for dynamic assessment of the gastrointestinal tract may be considered in cases refractory to conservative medical management, such as dietary fiber, exercise, and changes in medications. Clinical testing includes colorectal transit studies, videodefecography, and evacuation proctography. Colonic transit studies were developed to better understand the pathophysiology of constipation.[46,47] On the basis of colorectal transit studies, constipated patients can be divided into those with delayed colonic transit time (colonic inertia), those with delay in rectosigmoid transit only, and those with normal colorectal transit time. Colonic inertia, also referred to as slow-transit constipation, is a condition of chronic idiopathic constipation in which patients are found to have diffuse, pan-colonic marker delay on transit studies. Although these patients typically have no organic cause for their symptoms, some investigators suggest that these individuals have a disorder of the myenteric plexus,

---

Box 2
Rome II criteria for constipation

At least 12 weeks, which need not be consecutive, in the preceding 12 months of two or more of the following symptoms:

Straining during at least 25% of defecations

Lumpy or hard stools in at least 25% of defecations

Sensation of incomplete evacuation for at least 25% of defecations

Sensation of anorectal obstruction/blockade for at least 25% of defecations

Manual maneuvers to facilitate defecations (eg, digital evacuation, support of the pelvic floor) in at least 25% of defecations

Fewer than three bowel movements a week

Rare loose stools without the use of laxatives

Adapted from Weber AM, Brubaker L, Schaffer J, et al. Office urogynecology. New York: McGraw-Hill; 2004.

Box 3
Causes of constipation

Primary colonic motor dysfunction

    Slow-transit constipation (colonic inertia)

    Irritable bowel syndrome

    Hirschsprung disease

Anorectal outlet obstruction

    Levator ani syndrome

    Idiopathic megacolon

    Rectal prolapse

    Posterior vaginal compartment defects (rectocele, sigmoidocele, enterocele)

    Painful anorectal conditions (anal fissures, hemorrhoids)

Dietary

    Low fiber intake

    Inadequate fluid intake

Pharmacologic therapy

Metabolic disorders

    Hypothyroidism

    Diabetes mellitus

    Amyloidosis

    Hypercalcemia

    Hypokalemia

Pregnancy

Neurologic disorders

    Parkinson disease

    Multiple sclerosis

    Cerebral vascular accidents

    Autonomic neuropathy

    Spinal cord pathology

Psychologic/personality factors

---

which plays an important role in the regulation of colonic motor function.[48] This disorder is found almost exclusively in women and some studies suggest that there is an unusually high incidence of psychiatric disturbances among this group.[49]

Anorectal outlet obstruction is a form of chronic constipation in which pan-colonic transit time is normal but there is delayed transit in the rectosigmoid segment. Some of these patients have dilatation of the rectum and/or colon (megacolon), while others suffer from a spasm of the pelvic floor muscles, resulting in resistance to defecation (anismus). Patients with megacolon may have loss of the normal myenteric plexus ganglion cells (Hirschsprung disease) or have idiopathic megacolon. Anismus is a condition in which the anal sphincter paradoxically contracts rather than relaxes on attempted defecation. Anismus is also known as *spastic pelvic floor syndrome*, *levator ani syndrome, paradoxical puborectalis contraction*, and *anorectal dyssynergia*. This disorder can be demonstrated on dynamic studies, such as evacuation proctography, electromyography, and anal manometry.[50,51] Clinical studies suggest that up to 38% of patients with constipation have evidence of impaired rectal emptying by evacuation proctography.[52,53] Painful anorectal conditions, such as anal fissures and hemorrhoids, can also be a cause of anorectal outlet obstruction.

Obstructed defecation can also be the result of anatomic changes, such as rectocele, enterocele, sigmoidocele, or internal rectal prolapse (intussusception). Symptoms include a feeling of incomplete evacuation, excessive straining, or the need to splint digitally against the vagina, rectum, or perineum. It is not unusual for these patients to use enemas or to self-disimpact to relieve their symptoms. Rectocele represents a herniation of the posterior vaginal wall and possibly the anterior rectal wall into the vaginal lumen, and may extend beyond the introitus. Most rectoceles are asymptomatic, but some are associated with defecatory symptoms. The relationship between rectocele and constipation is currently uncertain. Arnold and colleagues[54] reported a series in which constipation persisted in the majority of patients following rectocele repair. Sarles and colleagues[55] have stated that three factors should be demonstrated to delineate a cause-and-effect relationship between a rectocele and anorectal outlet obstruction: (1) the necessity for a digital vaginal maneuver to assist defecation, (2) defecography demonstrating the rectocele with evidence of retained stool, (3) defecography permitting the recognition of associated lesions, such as rectal intussusception.

Constipation is among the most common side effects of pharmacologic therapy (**Box 4**). Opiates and iron supplementation are perhaps the most well known pharmacologic causes of constipation. Anticholinergic medications and antidepressants are

---

Box 4
Drugs commonly associated with constipation

Over-the-counter medications

Aluminum-containing antacids

Calcium carbonate

Iron supplements

Loperamide

Pseudoephedrine

Prescription medications

Anticholinergics

Antidepressants

Beta-blockers

Calcium channel blockers

Cholestyramine

Diuretics

Narcotic analgesics

Nonsteroidal anti-inflammatory drugs

Data from Toglia MR. Pathophysiology of anorectal dysfunction. Obstet Gynecol Clin of North America 1998;25:771–81.

also commonly associated with constipation. Many antihypertensive agents, including calcium channel blockers, beta-blockers, and diuretics, are another common group of drugs that can produce severe constipation. Constipation is also a common side effect associated with nonsteroidal anti-inflammatory drugs. Clinicians may not be aware that many over-the-counter preparations can also produce constipation, including antacids containing aluminum hydrazide, calcium carbonate, and pseudoephedrine. Calcium carbonate is frequently used daily by postmenopausal women for the prevention and treatment of osteoporosis.

Constipation may be associated with many metabolic and endocrine disorders, including hypothyroidism, diabetes, and hyperparathyroidism. Severe electrolyte abnormalities, such as hypercalcemia or hypokalemia, may also produce constipation. The prevalence of constipation during pregnancy is well recognized among clinicians. Central nervous system diseases, such as Parkinson disease and multiple sclerosis, are frequently associated with constipation. There is also evidence that injury to the somatic pelvic nerves, such as the pudendal nerve, or sacral parasympathetic neuropathy can also result in constipation.

A growing body of evidence suggests that constipation is directly attributable to psychological factors. Personality factors, self-esteem, psychologic distress, and anxiety have all been linked to stool frequency and constipation.[56,57] Studies that suggest that constipation is responsive to psychological intervention give further proof to the theory that not all constipation has an organic etiology.[56]

SUMMARY

Anorectal dysfunction causes significant discomfort and embarrassment to women. Such dysfunctions are associated with diverse symptoms, including abdominal pain, constipation, incomplete defecation, and anal incontinence. Anorectal dysfunction can occur as the result of both anatomic and functional abnormalities, and are often associated with other pelvic floor disorders discussed in this issue. Clinicians caring for women with pelvic floor dysfunction should be familiar with these conditions and the initial empiric therapies so as to facilitate appropriate referral in a timely manner.

REFERENCES

1. Toglia MR, DeLancey JOL. Anal incontinence and the obstetrician-gynecologist. Obstet Gynecol 1994;84:731–40.
2. Kamm M. Obstetric damage and faecal incontinence. Lancet 1994;344:730–3.
3. Madoff RD, Williams JG, Caushaj PF. Fecal incontinence. N Engl J Med 1992;326: 1002–7.
4. Talley NJ, O'Keefe EA, Zinsmeister AR, et al. Prevalance of gastrointestinal symptoms in the elderly: a population based study. Gastroenterology 1992;102: 895–901.
5. Denis P, Bercoff E, Bizien MF, et al. Etude de la prevalance de l'incontinence anale chez l'adulte. Gastroenterol Clin Biol 1992;16:344–50 [in French].
6. McClellan E. Fecal incontinence: social and economic factors. In: Benson JT, editor. Female pelvic floor disorders—investigation and management. New York: W.W. Norton & Company; 1992. p. 326–31.
7. Sultan AH, Kamm MA. Faecal incontinence after childbirth. Br J Obstet Gynaecol 1997;104:979–82.
8. Sultan AH, Kamm MA, Hudson CN, et al. Anal sphincter disruption during vaginal delivery. N Engl J Med 1993;329:1905–11.

9. Snooks SJ, Setchell M, Swash M, et al. Injury to innervation of pelvic floor sphincter musculature in childbirth. Lancet 1984;2:546–50.

10. Snooks SJ, Henry MM, Swash M. Faecal incontinence due to external sphincter division in childbirth is associated with damage to the innervation of the pelvic floor musculature: a double pathology. Br J Obstet Gynaecol 1985;92:824–8.

11. Sorenson M, Tetzschner T, Rasmussen OO, et al. Sphincter rupture in childbirth. Br J Surg 1993;80:393–4.

12. Bek KM, Laurberg S. Risks of anal incontinence from subsequent vaginal delivery after a complete obstetric anal sphincter tear. Br J Obstet Gynaecol 1992;99: 724–6.

13. Haadem K, Dahlstrom JA, Ling L, et al. Anal sphincter function after delivery rupture. Obstet Gynecol 1987;70:53–6.

14. Haadem K, Ohrlander S, Lingman G. Long-term ailments due to anal sphincter rupture caused by delivery—a hidden problem. Eur J Obstet Gynecol Reprod Biol 1988;27:27–32.

15. Sultan AH, Kamm MA, Bartram CI, et al. Third degree obstetric anal sphincter tears: risk factors and outcome of primary repair. BMJ 1994;308:887–91.

16. Burnett SJD, Speakman CTM, Kamm MA, et al. Confirmation of endosonographic detection of external anal sphincter defects by simultaneous electromyographic mapping. Br J Surg 1991;7:448–50.

17. Deen KI, Kumar D, Williams JG, et al. The prevalence of anal sphincter defects in faecal incontinence: a prospective endosonic study. Gut 1993;34:685–8.

18. Snooks SJ, Swash M, Henry MM, et al. Risk factors in childbirth causing damage to the pelvic floor innervation. Int J Colorectal Dis 1986;1:20–4.

19. Sultan AH, Kamm MA, Hudson CN. Pudendal nerve damage during labour: prospective study before and after childbirth. Br J Obstet Gynaecol 1994;101:22–8.

20. Goldaber KG, Wendel PJ, McIntire DD, et al. Pospartum perineal morbidity after fourth-degree perineal repair. Am J Obstet Gynecol 1993;168:489–93.

21. Hibbard LT. Surgical management of rectovaginal fistulas and complete perineal tears. Am J Obstet Gynecol 1978;130:139–41.

22. Corman ML. Anal incontinence following obstetrical injury. Dis Colon Rectum 1985;28:86–9.

23. DeLancey JOL, Toglia MR, Perucchini D. Internal and external anal sphincter anatomy as it relates to midline obstetric lacerations. Obstet Gynecol 1997;90: 924–7.

24. Jackson SL, Weber AM, Hull TL, et al. Fecal incontinence in women with urinary incontinence and pelvic organ prolapse. Obstet Gynecol 1997;89:423–7.

25. Barrett JA, Brocklehurst JC, Kiff ES, et al. Anal function in geriatric patients with faecal incontinence. Gut 1989;30:1244–51.

26. Wrenn K. Fecal impaction. N Engl J Med 1989;321:658–62.

27. Schiller LR, Santa Ana CA, Schmulen AC, et al. Pathogenesis of fecal incontinence in diabetes mellitus: evidence for internal-anal-sphincter dysfunction. N Engl J Med 1982;307:1666–71.

28. Nigro ND. An evaluation of the cause and mechanism of complete rectal prolapse. Dis Colon Rectum 1966;9:391–8.

29. Parks AG, Swash M, Urich H. Sphincter denervation in anorectal incontinence and rectal prolapse. Gut 1977;18:656–65.

30. Lehtola A, Salo JA, Fraki O, et al. Treatment of rectal prolapse. A clinical study of 50 consecutive patients. Ann Chir Gynaecol 1987;76:150–4.

31. Kupfer CA, Goligher JC. One hundred consecutive cases of complete prolapse of the rectum treated by operation. Br J Surg 1970;57:481–7.

32. Moschcowitz AV. The pathogenesis, anatomy, and cure of prolapse of the rectum. Surg Gynecol Obstet 1912;15:7–21.
33. Devadhar DSC. A new concept of mechanism and treatment of rectal procedentia. Dis Colon Rectum 1965;8:75–7.
34. Broden B, Snellman B. Procidentia of the rectum studied with cineradiography: a contribution to the discussion of causative mechanism. Dis Colon Rectum 1968;11:330–47.
35. Theuerkauf FJ, Beahrs OH, Hill JR. Rectal prolapse: causation and surgical treatment. Ann Surg 1970;171:819–35.
36. Collins JG. Prevalence of selected chronic digestive conditions, United States—1979–1981. US Public Health Service (Vital and Health Statistics; series 10, no. 155). Hyattsville (MD): National Center for Health Statistics; 1986.
37. Whitehead WE, Drinkwater D, Cheskin LJ, et al. Constipation in the elderly living at home. Definition, prevalance, and relationship to lifestyle and health status. J Am Geriatr Soc 1989;37:423–9.
38. Higgins PD, Johanson JF. Epidemiology of constipation in North America: a systematic review. Am J Gastroenterol 2004;99:750–9.
39. Garrigues V, Gálvez C, Ortiz V, et al. Prevalence of constipation: agreement among several criteria and evaluation of the diagnostic accuracy of qualifying symptoms and self-reported definition in a population-based survey in Spain. Am J Epidemiol 2004;159:520–6.
40. Johanson JF, Sonnenberg A, Koch TR. Clinical epidemiology of chronic constipation. J Clin Gastroenterol 1989;11:525–36.
41. Sandler RS, Jordan MC, Shelton BJ. Demographic and dietary determinants of constipation in the US population. Am J Public Health 1990;80:185–9.
42. Longstreth GF, Thompson WG, Chey WD, et al. Functional bowel disorders. Gastroenterology 2006;130:480–91.
43. Graham DY, Moser SE, Estes MK. The effect of bran on bowel function in constipation. Am J Gastroenterol 1982;77:599–603.
44. Cook IJ, Irvine EJ, Campbell D, et al. Effect of dietary fiber on symptoms and rectosigmoid motility in patients with irritable bowel syndrome. Gastroenterology 1990;98:66–72.
45. Rao SS, Ozturk R, Laine L. Clinical utility of diagnostic tests for constipation in adults: a systematic review. Am J Gastroenterol 2005;100:1605–15.
46. Chaussade S, Khyari A, Roche H, et al. Determination of total and segmental colonic transit time in constipated patients. Results in 91 patients with a new simplified method. Dig Dis Sci 1989;34:1168–72.
47. Ducrotte P, Rodomanska B, Weber J, et al. Colonic transit time of radiopaque markers and rectoanal manometry in patients complaining of constipation. Dis Colon Rectum 1986;29:630–4.
48. Preston DM, Lennard-Jones JE. Pelvic motility and response to intraluminal bisacodyl in slow-transit constipation. Dig Dis Sci 1985;30:289–94.
49. Varma JS, Smith AM. Neurophysiological dysfunction in young women with intractable constipation. Gut 1988;29:963–8.
50. Kuijpers HC, Bleijenberg G. The spastic pelvic floor syndrome: a cause of constipation. Dis Colon Rectum 1985;28:669–72.
51. Read NW, Timms JM, Barfield LJ, et al. Impairment of defecation in young women with severe constipation. Gastroenterology 1986;90:53–60.
52. Wald A, Caruana BJ, Freimanis MG, et al. Contributions of evacuation proctography and anorectal manometry to evaluation of adults with constipation and defecatory difficulty. Dig Dis Sci 1990;35:481–7.

53. Jones PN, Lubowski DZ, Swash M, et al. Is paradoxical contraction of puborectalis muscle of functional importance? Dis Colon Rectum 1987;30:667–70.

54. Arnold MW, Stewart WRC, Aguilar PS. Rectocele repair: four years' experience. Dis Colon Rectum 1990;33:684–7.

55. Sarles JC, Arnaud A, Selezneff I, et al. Endorectal repair of rectocele. Int J Colorectal Dis 1989;4:167–71.

56. Wald A, Hinds JP, Camana BJ. Psychological and physiological characteristics of patients with severe idiopathic constipation. Gastroenterology 1989;97:932–7.

57. Tucker DM, Sandstead HH, Logan GM Jr, et al. Dietary fiber and personality factors as determinants of stool output. Gastroenterology 1981;81:879–83.

Evaluation and Treatment of Anal Incontinence, Constipation, and Defecatory Dysfunction

Tola B. Omotosho, MD[a],*, Rebecca G. Rogers, MD[b]

KEYWORDS

- Anal incontinence • Fecal incontinence • Constipation
- Defecatory dysfunction

Pelvic floor disorders are common, and 1 in 9 women with pelvic floor problems will have symptoms severe enough that they will undergo surgery.[1] While significant advances have been made in the evaluation and treatment of lower urinary tract dysfunction, anorectal functional disorders have not fared as well. Posterior compartment disorders include anal incontinence, constipation, and defecatory dysfunction. These disorders cause considerable morbidity, and are typically underreported by patients and undertreated by providers. Barriers to identification and treatment are many; patients are reluctant to report symptoms because of embarrassment, and providers are reluctant to treat because of limited effective treatment options. Despite limitations in the ability to cure these disorders, most patients benefit from treatment and deserve evaluation. This article outlines the approach to diagnosis and treatment of anal incontinence, constipation, and defecatory dysfunction with a brief description of the nature of the problem, approaches to evaluation and diagnosis, as well as medical and surgical management. The aim is to provide the clinician with an approach to the management of patients who present with these problems in the clinical setting.

[a] Johns Hopkins University School of Medicine, Women's Center for Pelvic Health, Department of Gynecology and Obstetrics, 4940 Eastern Avenue, Room 121, Baltimore, Maryland 21224-2780, USA
[b] Division of Female Pelvic Medicine and Reconstructive Surgery, Department of Obstetrics and Gynecology, MSC 10 5580, University of New Mexico, Albuquerque, NM, 87131-0001, USA
* Corresponding author.
E-mail address: tomotos1@jhmi.edu. (T.B. Omotosho).

Obstet Gynecol Clin N Am 36 (2009) 673–697
doi:10.1016/j.ogc.2009.08.008
0889-8545/09/$ – see front matter © 2009 Elsevier Inc. All rights reserved.

obgyn.theclinics.com

ANAL INCONTINENCE

The plight of a patient with frank fecal incontinence is a very unhappy one indeed. There is obvious association with uncleanliness and the feeling of being a social outcast. Such a person will not meet people, will not leave the house, or be able to do any shopping. If the situation is known to the family the patient may well be rejected as a result, especially in old age. It is indeed a very grave social problem, particularly with the elderly, and anything that will improve it is highly desirable. —Dr. AG Parks, President's Address, Royal Society of Medicine, Section of Proctology, 1974

Anal incontinence is defined as the involuntary loss of flatus, liquid, or solid stool that causes a social or hygienic problem.[2] True prevalence is unknown; however, published population-based anal incontinence rates range from 0.5% to 28% and are 6 to 8 times more common in women than men.[2,3] Reported rates of fecal incontinence, which excludes the loss of flatus, are lower. A recent survey using the validated Fecal Incontinence Severity Index (FISI) found a weighted prevalence of at least monthly loss of solid, liquid, or mucus stool of 9.0% in a population of United States women.[4] Providers who care for women with urinary incontinence or pelvic organ prolapse should routinely screen for anal incontinence symptoms; 1 in 3 women with these disorders is also anally incontinent.[5] The costs of anal incontinence are substantial. A recent estimate of the out-of-pocket expenses for anal incontinence per patient per year in the United Kingdom is $3000, the majority of which pays for indirect nonmedical costs.[6] Additional financial burden is experienced for patients who go on to have surgery. Approximately 3500 inpatient procedures for anal incontinence are performed annually in the United States at a yearly total estimated cost of $24.5 million.[7]

Anatomy

Although many patients and providers think of the anal canal as a simple tube with a plug at the end, anorectal anatomy and physiology is complex. The anal sphincter complex is remarkably able to distinguish between gas, liquids, and solids, and allow the passage of one without the others. In brief, the anorectal canal is surrounded by a complex tube of muscle fibers composed of the internal and external sphincters. The external sphincter is made of striated muscle, which is under voluntary control and is responsible for 10% to 20% of the resting tone of the anal canal. The internal sphincter is responsible for the remainder of the resting tone, and consists of smooth muscle that is an extension of the colonic muscularis. This smooth muscle sphincter is under involuntary control. These 2 sphincters overlap and extend up the anal canal for a distance of 3 to 4 cm. Anteriorly, the external anal sphincter is attached to the perineal body and laterally to the pubovisceralis (**Fig. 1**). The anal sphincter complex is attached through the rectovaginal septum to the uterosacral cardinal ligament complex, and ultimately to the sacrum. Loss of support along these attachments can result in descent of the perineum with defecation or Valsalva. Although recent descriptions of subdivisions of the external anal sphincter on magnetic resonance imaging (MRI) have been described, the relevance of these divisions to function has yet to be determined.[8,9] The anorectal complex is innervated by branches of the pudendal nerve and sacral nerves.[9] Neurologic injury may result in loss of the ability to differentiate gas from liquid or solid stool, with subsequent incontinence.

Diagnosis of Anal Incontinence

The pathophysiology of anal continence is complex, and requires normal stool delivery and consistency, intact sensation and motor innervation, an intact anal sphincter

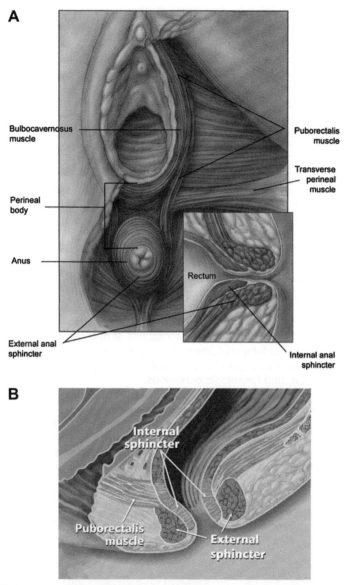

Fig. 1. (*A, B*) Anatomy of the anal sphincter complex. (*From* Rogers RG, Kammerer-Doak N. Obstetric anal sphincter lacerations; an evidence-based review, part 2: repair techniques. Female Patient 2002; May suppl: 32; with permission.)

complex, and a functioning puborectalis muscle. Loss of anal continence can result from damage to a single part of the continence mechanism or may result from multiple insults over time. Diagnosis and treatment of anal incontinence must include an evaluation of each part of the continence mechanism, and treatment should be tailored to findings.

Anal incontinence, unlike urinary incontinence, is not easily observed in the clinical setting. Most affected individuals do not voluntarily report symptoms and must be asked about it directly.[10] Women at high risk for incontinence should be given the opportunity to volunteer symptoms. In young women, the most common cause of anal incontinence is childbirth, particularly after overt laceration of the anal sphincters, a prolonged second stage of labor, or instrumented delivery. Low-risk birth in healthy women is unlikely to affect anal continence. A secondary analysis of 240 women randomized to perineal massage and self-paced or directed pushing in the second stage of labor found low rates of fecal incontinence during and after pregnancy.[11] These results are corroborated in a similar study of 576 women; although rates of any anal incontinence were high at 24% at 3 months postpartum, fecal incontinence symptoms were much lower at 6%, and few women reported significant bother from their symptoms.[12] Some anal incontinence symptoms may be due to pregnancy itself; 8% to 42% of women have mild anal incontinence symptoms before their first vaginal delivery during pregnancy.[13,14] Laceration of the anal sphincter complex at the time of vaginal delivery occurs in up to 6% of women (**Fig. 2**).[15–21] Despite repair of obstetric lacerations, 20% to 50% of women report involuntary loss of flatus or stool postpartum.[15–21] Institutions where operative delivery and episiotomy rates are very low also report very low rates of anal sphincter laceration, ranging from 1% to 2%.[22] Some lacerations are missed in the delivery room. A study of 254 women found that the diagnosis of anal sphincter laceration increased significantly from 11% to 24.5% with the addition of another trained observer.[23] Careful examination of perineal laceration at the time of birth should help to mitigate the problem of symptomatic unrecognized and unrepaired lacerations postpartum. Women with recognized anal sphincter damage at childbirth may benefit from referral to a perineal clinic postpartum for close follow-up of symptoms. Other populations at high risk for anal incontinence who should be screened for symptoms include those who have undergone surgery or radiation for other anorectal problems, irritable bowel syndrome, chronic diarrhea, chronic constipation, and neurologic conditions.

Several validated questionnaires evaluate symptoms, distress, and quality of life changes in patients with anal incontinence. Unfortunately, none of them are Grade A or "highly recommended" by the International Continence Society (ICS) because they lack rigor in their validation.[24] Symptom severity scales measure the frequency and severity of symptoms whereas quality of life measures evaluate the impact of symptoms on quality of life. **Table 1** lists some commonly used questionnaires. Although the questionnaires are helpful to quantify symptoms, a simple question on an intake form will also help to identify women with these problems.

In addition to a medical, surgical, and obstetric history, a bowel history should be obtained. Bowel movement frequency and consistency information is important to

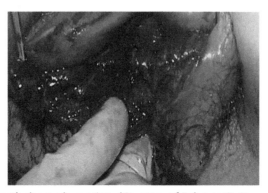

Fig. 2. Obstetric fourth-degree laceration. (*Courtesy of* Rebecca G. Rogers, MD.)

Table 1
Commonly used symptom severity and quality of life scales for anal incontinence

Scale (Abbreviation)	Number Questions	ICS Grade
Symptom Severity		
Wexner Fecal Incontinence Scale (FIS)[25]	5	C
St Mark's Score[26]	7	C
Fecal Incontinence Severity Index (FISI)[27]	5	NR
Distress Inventory and Quality of Life		
Colo-Rectal-Anal Impact Questionnaire (CRAIQ)[28]	Short form: 7 Long form: 31	B
Fecal Incontinence Quality of Life Scale (FIQOL)[29]	29	B
Combined Quality of Life and Symptom Scales		
Manchester Health Questionnaire (MHQ)[30]	31	B
Modified Manchester Health Questionnaire(MMHQ)[31]	38	B

generate a treatment plan. Normal bowel frequency varies between thrice daily and thrice weekly, and women who have bowel movements within these general parameters should be reassured that their bowel movement frequency is normal. The Bristol Stool Index is a pictorial depiction of different stool consistencies, and may aid in patient descriptions.[32] Many women report significant fecal urgency even though they may not be overtly incontinent. Urgency can significantly affect quality of life secondary to its unpredictable nature. In addition to bowel habits, women should be screened for significant straining or constipation, sexual abuse, or regular anal intercourse. For women with constipation or loose stools a review of medications, diet, and fluid patterns should also be obtained.

Physical examination includes both an abdominal examination to exclude palpable masses and a pelvic examination. A brief pelvic neurologic examination will assess sensory and motor function, including anocutaneous reflex, sacral reflexes, and perineal sensation. Perineal inspection for scarring, skin breakdown, fissures, and mucosal or rectal prolapse is performed. Observation of fecal material on the perineum should prompt questions regarding bowel control even in low-risk women. Separation of the anal sphincter as assessed by the "dovetail sign," and perianal dimpling should also be noted.[33] Digital anorectal examinations determine sphincter tone as well as the patient's ability to contract their pelvic floor musculature. Care should be taken to exclude the presence of a rectovaginal fistula or rectal prolapse. Although validated measures of pelvic floor exercise strength exist, there is no standard measure of rectal tone and strength.[34] Rectal examinations have proven as reliable as manometry in assessing rectal resting and squeeze tone,[35] and the positive and negative predictive value of digital examinations in identifying low resting pressure and squeeze pressure was 67% and 81%, respectively.[36] Digital examination can also assess whether the anal sphincter complex is intact as well as detect the presence of fecal impaction, masses, or hemorrhoids.

Diagnostic Testing

Although commonly employed, the use of diagnostic testing in the treatment of anal incontinence is limited by lack of normative data, poor standardization of testing and reporting of results, or information regarding the negative and positive predictive value of test results for either diagnosis or clinical outcomes of therapeutic interventions.[37] Nonsurgical treatment can be initiated after history and physical examination without further testing. In women who do not respond to conservative measures, further evaluation may be warranted.

Ultrasound and Magnetic Resonance Imaging

Ultrasound imaging of the anal sphincter complex can be performed endoanally, endovaginally, or translabially. Both 2D and 3D imaging has been described. The current gold standard is endoanal imaging with assessment of the anal sphincter complex at 3 levels: proximally, the internal anal sphincter can be visualized, at the mid level both the internal anal sphincter and puborectalis is seen, and distally the external anal sphincter can be seen.[38] The external anal sphincter appears as a hyperechoic ring whereas the internal anal sphincter appears as a hypoechoic ring. Disruptions of the sphincter result in a "U" rather than circle shape, and are graded by degrees. Large defects of greater than 90° of disruption are associated with higher rates of anal incontinence. Endoanal ultrasonography correlates well with anal manometry,[39] electromyographic (EMG) activity,[40] MRI,[41] and surgical findings.[42,43] Translabial imaging uses 8- to 10-MHz vaginal probes, which are readily available in most diagnostic centers; however, the reliability and validity of this imaging method is less well established (**Fig. 3**). MRI has been used to determine the anatomy of the levator ani and anal sphincter complex, but these studies are more costly and have limited clinical use. Recently, 3-dimensional ultrasound has been used to identify lesions both in the levator ani and anal sphincter complex, with resolution comparable with that of MRI, but whether this modality will offer additional diagnostic capabilities to the practicing clinician remains to be proven.[37,44–46]

Defecography

Defecography is performed by filling the rectum with a radiopaque paste, illuminating the small bowel with a radiopaque liquid, and placing a radiopaque tampon in the vagina. The patient then attempts defecation on a radiolucent toilet while a series of images are obtained with straining and contraction of the pelvic floor. Standardization both of testing and interpretation is not established.[47] Nonetheless, for women whose diagnosis is unclear despite a thorough history and physical examination,

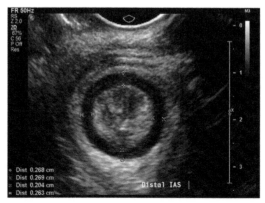

Fig. 3. Translabial ultrasound images of the anal sphincter complex showing a lacerated sphincter and an intact sphincter. (*Courtesy of* Rebecca G. Rogers, MD.)

defecography can confirm presence of an enterocele not readily apparent on vaginal examination, or stool trapping in someone without an obvious rectocele. A recent study determined that clinicians found defecography the most helpful adjunctive test compared with MRI, urodynamics, defecography, and anal sonography, when formulating a treatment plan for patients presenting with primary pelvic organ prolapse.[48]

Anorectal Manometry

Anorectal manometry provides functional information about anal resting and squeeze tone, and can also document anal sensation. Most commonly, a balloon is introduced in the rectum and filled with either air or water. Normative data from healthy individuals or predictive value for clinical symptoms is lacking.[33,49]

Neurodiagnostic Studies

Needle electromyography (EMG) was originally used to document anal sphincter disruption by mapping areas of absent electrical activity. Since the development of reliable ultrasound techniques, needle EMG is not recommended for routine clinical evaluation. Some clinicians still use EMG data to differentiate muscle versus nerve damage when evaluating the anal sphincter complex. Pudendal nerve latency measures the conduction time through the terminal portion of the pudendal nerve to the external anal sphincter. Nerve latencies were thought to provide prognostic value for outcomes of surgical interventions for anal incontinence, but have largely been abandoned because they does not provide reliable information about nerve damage. Despite prolonged latencies, patients undergoing anterior sphincteroplasty were proven to have significant improvement in continence with minimum morbidity, under-lying its limited use in determining who should have a surgical intervention for anal incontinence.[50]

Management

A variety of surgical and nonsurgical management options exist for the treatment of anal incontinence. Although difficult to cure, most women report improvement in symptoms with treatment, and many adopt adaptive behaviors that make resumption of a more normal lifestyle possible. Because surgical treatment carries significant morbidity with poor long-term results, all patients should be offered a trial of medical management before undergoing surgical management. For patients with rectovaginal fistula or rectal prolapse, nonsurgical management has limited use; these patients will have to undergo surgical repair to alleviate their symptoms.

Nonsurgical Management

Nonsurgical management options for anal incontinence include dietary and fluid manipulation, medications, enemas, behavioral and physical therapy, biofeedback, and use of plugs and pads.

Absorbent products

Absorbent products for fecal incontinence enable women and caregivers to manage symptoms in a dignified fashion. Costs of pads are significant; approximately $2 billion are spent annually on pads for both urinary and anal incontinence in the United States.[51] Two randomized trials compared a variety of disposable and nondisposable products, and found that disposable pull-ups were the most preferred but most expensive options for women.[52]

Dietary and fluid management

Increasing dietary fiber with diet changes, or bulking agents or fiber supplements such as methylcellulose or psyllium, helps to increase stool size and is a reasonable first-line therapy for fecal incontinence, particularly in women with mild constipation or diarrhea.[53] For many women, a larger, more formed stool may improve rectal sensation and emptying. Increasing fiber should not be promoted for women with isolated flatal incontinence as increasing fiber will often increase gas production, with resultant worsening of incontinence symptoms. Increased fiber may adequately treat constipation with resolution of overflow incontinence. Laxatives may be beneficial in cases of anal incontinence that are associated with constipation and fecal impaction.

Pharmacotherapy

Pharmacotherapies for anal incontinence can be divided into constipating agents and drugs that enhance anal sphincter tone. The most commonly used constipating agents used for anal incontinence are loperamide and atropine sulfate. In the United States, loperamide is available without a prescription whereas atropine sulfate requires a doctor's approval. Both medications have been proven effective in randomized trials in women with loose stools; however, they have not been helpful in women with normal stool consistency. Side effects include constipation, abdominal pain, diarrhea, headache, and nausea.[54] Recommended doses of loperamide for fecal incontinence start at 2 to 4 mg daily, with doses of 16 mg daily sufficient for most patients.[53] To titrate very small doses, loperamide comes in a liquid form. Drugs that enhance anal sphincter tone include phenylepinephrine gel, sodium valproate, and loperamide. Four trials of these agents with limited numbers of patients have shown limited improvement in patients.[53]

Physical therapy, biofeedback, and electrical stimulation

Pelvic floor exercises have proven effectiveness in the treatment of urinary incontinence, and are commonly recommended for the treatment of anal incontinence despite lack of evidence.[55] Most studies of pelvic floor exercises for the treatment of fecal incontinence also included biofeedback or electrical stimulation in their design, so extracting the independent effect of individual therapies is difficult. Biofeedback involves the use of mechanical or electrical devices to provide sensory feedback to the patient about the efficacy of voluntary control of continence. Three main modalities are described including rectal sensitivity training, strength training, and coordination training. Electrical stimulation can be delivered by surface electrodes, intra-anal plugs, or intra vaginal plugs, and usually involves the high-frequency stimulation at 50 Hz for 15 to 20 minutes daily. Cochrane reviews in 2006 and 2007 concluded that the limited numbers of trials with significant methodological flaws do not allow a definitive assessment of the role of any of these treatments in people with fecal incontinence.[56,57]

Sacral nerve stimulation

First described in 1995, sacral nerve stimulation (SNS) has emerged as a viable treatment option for patients with anal incontinence.[58,59] SNS involves placement of an electrical lead that is placed in the S3 sacral foramen and then attached to a pacemaker that provides current. Although the precise mechanism remains speculative, various theories have been postulated that the stimulation has a direct effect on the external anal sphincter, autonomic nervous system, anorectal reflexes, modulation of the corticospinal pathway, and changes in rectal sensitivity and motility. A recent randomized trial of 120 patients revealed that mean incontinence episodes decreased from 9.5 to 3.1, and that perfect continence was accomplished in 47% of patients with corresponding improvement in validated quality of life measures compared with a group randomized to best supportive therapy. Response to stimulation was best predicted by response to the test period, with all patients who responded to the test period responding to permanent lead placement.[59] This trial establishes SNS as a viable option for the treatment of fecal incontinence with low morbidity. Another study has suggested that SNS results may be durable; 60 patients followed for at least 5 years revealed that 74% of patients continued to report a 50% improvement in symptoms.[60]

Anal plugs

Anal plugs were first designed for patients who had major neurologic disorders, and are specially developed devices for containing fecal incontinence. In studies up to half of the patients discontinued the use of plugs because of discomfort. In patients able to tolerate their use, they can diminish incontinence symptoms.[61]

Surgical Management

Common surgical management of anal incontinence in patients without fistula or rectal prolapse includes sphincteroplasty, neosphincters, and bulking agents. Other procedures such as postanal repair or posterior levatorplasty have not been shown to be effective in the treatment of fecal incontinence in most patients, and are not discussed here. Radiofrequency ablation is no longer commercially available in the United States and is also not discussed.

Sphincteroplasty

In women with an anterior anal sphincter defect on clinical or ultrasound examination who are symptomatic, sphincteroplasty is the most commonly performed surgical option. For gynecologists, the traditional repair of the anal sphincter was informed by repair of third- and fourth-degree obstetric lacerations where the torn ends of the sphincter are brought together with interrupted sutures in an end-to-end fashion. Because of what was thought to be unsatisfactory success rates with end-to-end repairs, Parks first introduced the overlapping repair in 1971 (**Fig. 4**).[62] Initially, results with overlapping sphincteroplasty were good, with 60% to 82% of patients reporting symptom improvement with short-term follow-up.[2] More recently, 5 articles have reported less promising longer-term results, with mean follow-up of 3 to 10 years. Cure rates in these studies range from 0% to 28% after overlapping repair (**Table 2**).[37,63–67] Nonetheless, most patients report improvement and that they would undergo the repair again given the option.[1,64]

The majority of research comparing overlapping to end-to-end sphincteroplasty has been conducted in obstetric trials. Three obstetric randomized trials have been reviewed in a meta-analysis that compared the 2 repair methods, with a total of 279 women with follow-up ranging from 3 months to 1 year. The conclusion of the meta-analysis was that overlapping repair, at least in the hands of experienced surgeons, may result in reduced risk of fecal urgency, anal incontinence scores, and deterioration of anal incontinence symptoms.[68] If an experienced person is not available to perform the repair immediately, a delay of 8 to 12 hours was not found to be harmful regarding functional results at 1 year.[69] Patients who undergo third- or fourth-degree repair should be given a single dose of a second-generation cephalosporin; a trial of 147 women after laceration found that women who were given antibiotics reported fewer perineal wound complications than those who were not given antibiotics.[70] Two trials have looked at postpartum bowel regimens. The first trial randomized women to lactulose or codeine phosphate for 3 days following their repair.

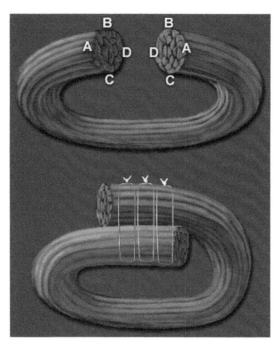

Fig. 4. Overlapping versus end-to-end sphincteroplasty. (*From* Rogers RG, Kammerer-Doak N. Obstetric anal sphincter lacerations; an evidence-based review, part 2: repair techniques. Female Patient 2002; May suppl: 32; with permission.)

Women who were on the constipating regimen reported more painful first evacuations, longer hospital stays, and more long-term troublesome constipation.[71] Addition of a bulking agent (ispaghula husk) to the laxative was not shown to be beneficial in a follow-up trial of 147 women.[72] One trial compared braided polyglactin with poly-dioxanone for repair of obstetric anal sphincter lacerations and found no differences in suture-related complications or continence, although patient follow-up in the trial was poor.[73] Internal sphincter repair is controversial but has been identified in one study as a predictor of postpartum anal incontinence.[74]

For repair remote from delivery, fewer trials have been conducted. A small trial that compared overlapping to end-to-end repair in 23 patients found no differences between groups in success at 18 months.[75] Another small trial found that opening incisions closer to the posterior forchette had fewer wound complications than incisions made in the line of the vaginal mucocutaneous junction.[76] For repairs remote from delivery, traditionally an extensive mechanical and antibiotic bowel preparation has been performed, with restriction of solid food intake before surgery. These bowel preparations are very challenging for patients who are incontinent, and have often resulted in perineal breakdown and diarrhea on the operative field. Mechanical bowel preparation in patients undergoing bowel anastomosis does not decrease wound infection rates in 6 randomized trials, and it is the authors' practice to no longer do extensive bowel preparations.[77] Likewise, food restriction or low residual diets are commonly proscribed following repair to delay time until first bowel movement; data from the obstetric literature regarding constipating agents postpartum infer that this practice may not be beneficial.[71] Fecal diversion before repair has not been found to be beneficial in a trial of 27 women, and the stoma was the source of considerable morbidity.[78]

Table 2
Long-term results following overlapping sphincteroplasty

First Author, year	Patients with Follow-up/Total (%)	Length of Follow-up, Mean (Range)	Outcomes
Malouf, 2000[63]	46/55 (84)	77 mo (60–96)	0% continent 10% incontinent flatus 79% soiling 21% incontinent stool
Karoui, 2000[64]	74/86 (86)	40 mo	28% continent 23% incontinent flatus 49% incontinent stool
Halverson, 2002[65]	49/71 (69)	69 mo (48–141)	14% continent 54% incontinent stool
Bravo Gutierrez, 2004[66]	135/191 (71)	10 y (7–16)	6% continent 16% incontinent flatus 19% soiling 57% incontinent stool
Barisic, 2006[67]	56/65 (86)	80 mo (26–154)	27% continent 21% incontinent flatus 13% soiling 39% incontinent stool

From Rogers RG, Abed H, Fenner DE. Current diagnosis and treatment algorithms for anal incontinence. BJU Int 2006;98(suppl 1):97–106a; with permission.

Because sphincteroplasty rarely cures anal incontinence, detailed preoperative counseling is important so that women and their providers can accurately weigh the advantages and disadvantages of surgical management.

Neosphincters, injectable bulking agents, and colostomy

Creation of a new sphincter using either a muscle flap such as a graciloplasty or artificial cuffs have been used to restore bowel control in some patients. These procedures are associated with significant morbidity, with nearly half of the patients requiring repeat or revision procedures. Gracilis muscle transposition without electrical stimulation has poor results, and because the pacemakers are no longer on the market this repair method has less utility. Even with electrical stimulation, the complication rate is greater than 50% and the success rate less than 35%.[79]

Artificial anal sphincters are composed of a cuff that encircles the anal canal below the plane of the levator ani muscle (**Fig. 5**). Long-term improvement in continence has been reported in patients who did not need to have the implant removed secondary to infection or erosion; however, no long-term data with intention to treat analyses has been reported, and the use of the artificial sphincter should be considered experimental until better data are published.[79]

A variety of substances have been injected into the anal sphincter to improve continence, including polytetrafluoroethylene, autologous fat, glutaraldehyde cross-linked

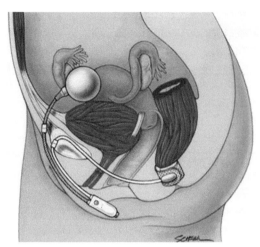

Fig. 5. Artificial anal sphincter. (*Courtesy of* American Medical Systems Inc. Minnetonka, MN; with permission.)

collagen, or carbon-coated zirconium oxide beads. Injections are either trans-sphincteric or proctoscopically guided through the rectal mucosa above the dentate line, and can be performed under ultrasound guidance.[79] Pilot data following patients injected with carbon-coated zirconium oxide beads at 1 year found that 15 of 21 patients reported subjective improvement.[80]

Colostomy

Fecal diversion is a last choice for the majority of patients with significant psychosocial impact, despite improvement in incontinence symptoms.[81]

Rectal Prolapse

Rectal prolapse can also cause anal incontinence, and is a distressing condition in which there is circumferential protrusion through the anus of all layers of the rectal wall. Causes are unclear; however, the condition occurs most commonly in elderly women. Surgical treatments include anal encirclement operations, perineal resections, and abdominal rectopexy. A recent meta-analysis examined 12 randomized trials with a total of 380 participants undergoing varying techniques, and was unable to determine whether perineal or abdominal approaches have better results.[82]

Rectovaginal Fistula

Rectovaginal fistulas are a communicating tract from the rectum to the vagina, and result in anal incontinence (**Fig. 6**). Although causes can be varied, the most common cause is secondary to obstetric trauma, followed by inflammatory and neoplastic disorders. Repair of obstetric fistula follows the tenets of vesicovaginal fistula repair; wide dissection and repair without tension. Closure rates are high, and most women report resolution of their incontinence.[83] Women with rectovaginal fistula should be screened for concurrent sphincter disruption. Repair of the fistula without repair of the sphincter has resulted in lower continence rates in at least one study.[84]

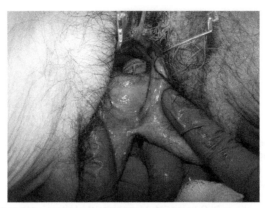

Fig. 6. Rectovaginal fistula. (*Courtesy of* Rebecca G. Rogers, MD.)

CONSTIPATION
Epidemiology

Constipation is the most common digestive complaint in the United States, accounting for 2.5 million physician visits a year.[85] A federal data set review revealed that constipation is more common in women than men, with a prevalence of 21% women and 8% in men.[86,87] Epidemiologic studies confirm that women report less frequent bowel movements than men and are more likely to have pelvic floor dysfunction that may result in impaired defecation. Population prevalence estimates, based on householder surveys or questionnaires, show a wide range in rates of constipation, varying from 2% to 28%. Estimates of the prevalence of this condition may vary considerably because there are different yet acceptable definitions for constipation.[86] Constipation is also associated with increasing age, but prevalence rates in the elderly vary as much as the prevalence in the general population.

Definition of Constipation

A commonly used definition of constipation is based on surveys that reveal that greater than 90% of people in the Western world have bowel movements between 3 times a day and 3 times a week. Based on this normal range, many clinicians define constipation as a decrease in bowel movement frequency to less than 3 bowel movements per week.[88,89] A constipation definition that is solely based on the frequency of bowel movements may not provide a complete and accurate assessment of this condition, because many patients often underestimate their stool frequency and the perception of constipation is not based only on the quantity of stools, but qualitative symptoms.[89,90] Qualitative symptoms include excessive straining, prolonged time to defecate, passage of hard stools, need for manual removal of hard stools, feeling of incomplete evacuation, and abdominal bloating; these symptoms have a negative impact on quality of life and may be more common than complaints pertaining to the frequency of bowel movements.[90,91,93,94]

In an effort to standardize the definition of constipation and ensure accurate diagnoses, consensus diagnostic criteria have been proposed by several panels of experts. The most widely recognized definition is based on the Rome III criteria (**Table 3**). Although the evidence-based Rome criteria are useful for clinical research, expert opinion suggests that these criteria may not be practical for use in everyday clinical practice.[91,92,95] Therefore, the American College of Gastroenterology (ACG)

Table 3
Rome III chronic criteria for functional constipation

Presence of 2 or more of the following:
  a. Straining during ≥25% of defecations
  b. Lumpy or hard stools in ≥25% of defecations
  c. Sensation of incomplete evacuation for ≥25% of defecations
  d. Sensation of anorectal obstruction/blockage for ≥25% of defecations
  e. Manual maneuvers to facilitate ≥25% of defecations (digital manipulations, pelvic floor support)
  f. Fewer than 3 evacuations per week
  g. Loose stools are rarely present without the use of laxatives

Insufficient criteria for irritable bowel syndrome
Criteria fulfilled for the last 3 months and symptom onset ≥6 months before the diagnosis

From Gallagher PF, O'Mahony D, Quigley EM. Management of chronic constipation in the elderly. Drugs Aging 2008:25(10):807–21; with permission.

Chronic Constipation Task Force and the American Gastroenterological Association have recommended the use of broader definitions for constipation that are less restrictive and incorporate the symptoms commonly reported by patients (**Table 4**).[89,91,93,96]

Pathophysiology and Complications of Constipation

Constipation is a multifactorial condition that may result from metabolic, structural, mechanical, pharmacologic, or functional disorders that affect the colon or anorectum directly or indirectly. These causes can be classified into the broad categories listed in **Table 5**.[85,89] Endocrine and metabolic disorders, including diabetes, hypothyroidism, and hyperparathyroidism, may cause constipation. Electrolyte abnormalities such as hypercalcemia and hypokalemia have also been associated with constipation. Constipation is also a side effect of many commonly used medications including narcotics, iron supplements, and even over-the-counter preparations such as nonsteroidal anti-inflammatory medications and antacids containing calcium carbonate or aluminum hydrazide. Neurologic diseases that are associated with constipation include multiple sclerosis and Parkinson disease, as well as spinal cord injuries. Psychological factors have also been associated with this condition. Complications associated with chronic

Table 4
Definitions of chronic constipation
American College of Gastroenterology definition of chronic functional constipation   Symptom-based disorder defined as unsatisfactory defecation and characterized by infrequent bowel movements, difficult stool passage, or both. Difficult stool passage includes straining, sense of difficulty passing stool, incomplete evacuation, hard/lumpy stool, prolonged time to defecation or passage of stool, or need for manual maneuvers to pass stool. Chronic constipation is defined as the presence of these symptoms for ≥3 months
American Gastroenterological Association definition of constipation   Symptom-based disorder defined as unsatisfactory defecation and characterized by infrequent bowel movement, difficult stool passage, or both. Difficult stool passage includes straining, sense of incomplete evacuation, hard/lumpy stool, prolonged time to defecate or pass stool, or need for manual maneuvers to pass stool

From Gallagher PF, O'Mahony D, Quigley EM. Management of chronic constipation in the elderly. Drugs Aging 2008:25(10):807–21; with permission.

Table 5
Disorders and medications associated with nonidiopathic and idiopathic constipation

Nonidiopathic constipation	
Endocrine and Metabolic Disorders	Pharmacologic Agents
Chronic kidney disease	Analgesics (NSAIDs, narcotics)
Dehydration	Antacids
Diabetes Mellitus	Anticholinergics
Hypothyroidism	Antidepressants
Hyperparathyroidism	Calcium channel blockers
Hypokalemia	Cholestyramine
Hypermagnesmia	Diuretics
Panhypopituitarism	Iron supplements
Hypercalcemia	
Myopathic disorders	Neurologic disorders
Amyloidosis	Autonomic neuropathy
Dermatamyositis	Systemic sclerosis
	Cerebrovascular disease
	Dementia
	Spinal cord lesion
	Multiple sclerosis
	Parkinson disease
	Pudendal neuropathy
Psychological factors	
Idiopathic constipation	
Primary colonic motor dysfunction	Anorectal outlet obstruction
Colonic inertia	Anismus
Irritable bowel syndrome	Enterocele, rectocele
Megacolon	Rectal prolapse
Megarectum	Rectal intussusception

Abbreviation: NSAID, nonsteroidal anti-inflammatory drug
From Toglia MR. Pathophysiology of anorectal dysfunction. Obstet Gynecol Clin North Am 1998;25(4):776–7; with permission.

constipation include fecal impaction and fecal incontinence. Severe fecal impaction may lead to intestinal obstruction or even colonic ulcerations, especially in elderly patients.[89] Difficulty passing stool with excessive straining may contribute to hemorrhoids, fissures, and rectal prolapse.

Clinical Evaluation

History
Constipated patients often present with a compilation of symptoms that include complaints of abdominal pain and bloating, feeling of incomplete evacuation, excessive straining, passage of hard stools, and the need for digital disimpaction or vaginal splinting. Patients may also report a decrease in the frequency of their bowel movements (less than 3 a week) or a change in the consistency of their stools (hard pelletlike stools). It is important that clinicians clarify the duration and onset of these symptoms, through detailed questioning about the severity of the problem as well as any alleviating or exacerbating factors such as laxative use, changes in medications, or recent surgery. Chronic or recurring symptoms of constipation that have not responded to dietary or medical interventions may suggest a functional bowel disorder, whereas acute onset or short duration of severe symptoms might suggest an organic or

neoplastic origin. A thorough history should also include an assessment of stool consistency and size; one of the tools that may help in this assessment is The Bristol Stool Scale. This scale illustrates 7 common stool forms and their consistency; not only is it the best descriptor of stool form, it also correlates with gut transit time.[97,98] A detailed dietary and bowel history should be obtained with specific information about fiber and fluid intake , number of meals consumed, and number of bowel movements. A bowel/food diary may be useful in gathering this information from patients. In addition to stool diaries, standardized symptom questionnaires may prove useful in the assessment of patients who are unable or reluctant to describe their symptoms completely. The Patient Assessment of Constipation (PAC) is a validated questionnaire that was developed to provide a brief, easily administered measurement tool for symptoms and quality of life aspects of constipation based on the patient's experience of the disorder. The PAC was designed to capture both baseline disorder status and response to treatment. This questionnaire consists of 2 separate scales, the PAC-SYM, a 12 item measure of symptom severity, and the PAC-QOL, a 28-item measure of the health-related quality of life associated with constipation. The PAC has been validated in young community-dwelling adults as well as in an older population residing in a long-term care facility.[99,100] A thorough history is important, but for complete evaluation and diagnosis of constipation objective measures should also be considered.

Physical examination

A thorough physical examination should be performed to exclude systemic and anatomic conditions that may cause constipation. Examination of the abdomen may reveal presence of distension and stool in the lower quadrants in patients with severe constipation. Neurologic examination of the perineum, including assessment of perineal sensation by using a cotton swab to assess "touch" discrimination, and evaluation of the anocutaneous reflex (reflex contraction of the external anal sphincter) by gently stroking the perineal skin can provide useful clinical information. Absence of the anocutaneous reflex or impaired sensation may indicate an underlying neuropathy.[84] A complete pelvic examination that evaluates the severity and location of any pelvic organ prolapse that may contribute to symptoms of constipation and incomplete evacuation should be performed. A digital rectal examination may identify the presence of a rectal stricture or impacted stool; during this examination it is important to ask the patient to bear down to simulate defecation. The examiner should observe relaxation of the external anal sphincter together with perineal descent with Valsalva maneuvers; if the sphincter does not relax or the perineum does not descend then the clinician should suspect functional obstruction or dyssynergic defecation.[86]

Diagnostic procedures

Historically, extensive diagnostic evaluation has been reserved for patients who have not responded to traditional therapies, including dietary changes and medical management, or when an obvious cause for the constipation cannot be identified. It is important that the diagnostic evaluation of patients with chronic constipation exclude any underlying metabolic or neoplastic condition, including colorectal cancer. It may be of clinical value to obtain screening serum tests to evaluate for endocrine and metabolic disorders such as hypothyroidism, diabetes, and hypercalcemia. If one suspects a colorectal carcinoma, based on the patient's age, duration of symptoms, and other clinical signs and symptoms (eg, rectal bleeding, anorexia), a colonoscopy would also be warranted. The yield from such invasive tests in an otherwise uncomplicated and long-standing complication is likely to be very low.[96] Several methods may be used to assess the function of the colorectal tract. The diagnostic method chosen is generally based on the clinical suspicion for the underlying cause of the condition.

Radiographic studies
Radiographic studies may be useful in patients in which an obstructive pathology is suspected. A plain radiograph of the abdomen may detect evidence of excessive stool in the colon and megacolon. A barium enema may also be useful for the evaluation of obstructive lesions or pathology if a colonoscopy or sigmoidoscopy has not been performed. Hirschsprung disease, which is rarely diagnosed in adults, can also be detected by barium enema, although confirmation of this diagnosis requires manometry and histology.[96]

Colonic transit evaluation (Sitzmark study)
A colonic transit study is a radiographic study that evaluates colonic transit time, which provides the clinician a more accurate assessment of stool frequency, because patients may have an inability to accurately recall the frequency of their bowel movements.[90] The test is performed by having a patient swallow a Sitzmark capsule (Konsyl Pharmaceuticals), which contains 24 radiopaque markers, on day 1 and then obtain a plain abdominal radiograph on day 6, 120 hours later. The results of the study are based on the number of markers that remain. Normal transit is defined as less than 5 markers remaining in the colon; slow transit is defined as greater than 5 markers scattered throughout the colon; and obstructive defecation is defined as greater than 5 markers in the rectosigmoid region with a near normal transit of markers throughout the rest of the colon.[86] Of note, some patients with chronic constipation may have a normal colon transit evaluation, and a clinician should consider the possibility of pelvic floor dysfunction in these individuals.

Defecography
Defecography is a radiographic test that may be useful in assessing pelvic floor dysfunction in patients with chronic constipation, and is previously described in this article (see Anal incontinence).

Anorectal manometry
Anorectal manometry is described earlier in this article (see Diagnostic testing for anal incontinence) and provides a comprehensive evaluation of pressure and sensation in the rectum and anal sphincter complex. Manometry is useful in the evaluation of abnormalities that occur during attempted defecation. In a normal situation, when defecation occurs there is an increase in rectal pressure that is coordinated with a decrease in anal sphincter pressure, which is attributed to the relaxation of the external anal sphincter. The inability to synchronize this maneuver can be detected on anorectal manometry, and is characteristic of patients with dyssynergic defecation (see Defecatory dysfunction).[86,101]

Management of constipation
The goals of treatment for patients with chronic constipation are to restore normal bowel function with regular formed stools at least 3 times weekly, eliminate the need for straining, and relieve symptoms such as abdominal bloating and pain with defecation. The ideal treatment for constipation should improve the quality of life for these patients without the addition of any adverse side effects.

Dietary management

Deficiency in dietary fiber is often erroneously attributed to be the cause of chronic constipation.[102] A diet containing high-fiber food such as whole grains, vegetables, and nuts is often considered first-line therapy for patients with chronic constipation. Fiber may decrease whole gut transit and increase stool weight; however, increasing fiber in patients with chronic constipation has had limited success, and some studies have shown a strong placebo effect.[85,103] The benefits from fiber may be based on the underlying etiology for the constipation; constipated patients who had either pelvic floor dysfunction or slow colonic transit times responded poorly to dietary fiber supplementation with 30 g of fiber daily, whereas patients without an underlying colonic motility disorder improved or became symptom-free.[104] The ideal regimen for fiber increase is to make subtle and gradual changes in the diet to avoid side effects of abdominal pain, bloating, and excess gas as a result of a dramatic and rapid increase in fiber intake.[89]

Pharmacotherapy

Laxatives are the most popular treatment option for patients with chronic constipation. Millions of dollars are spent on over-the-counter laxatives and stool softeners in the United States annually.[86] Laxatives can be divided into 4 main categories: bulk laxatives, osmotic laxatives, stimulant laxatives, and stool softeners.

Common bulk laxatives contain psyllium (ispaghula), bran, and methyl cellulose. This category of laxatives may take several days to have an effect, and it is often recommended that patients increase their fluid intake to avoid mechanical obstruction. Unfortunately, the amount of fluid needed to avoid obstruction has not been proven.[89] Some studies have shown that psyllium may increase stool frequency compared with placebo; however, there are still conflicting reports about the effectiveness of this category of laxatives.

Osmotic laxatives work by increasing secretion of water in the intestinal lumen by osmotic activity that leads to softer stools. These laxatives include magnesium citrate, magnesium hydroxide, and magnesium phosphate, sugars such as sorbitol and lactulose, and glycerin (glycerol) suppositories. There are no formal recommendations for the use of magnesium hydroxide (milk of magnesia) by the ACG Chronic Constipation Task Force because of the poor study design of the single trial investigating its effectiveness.[93,96] However, several studies have assessed the effectiveness of lactulose, and have confirmed that this treatment is superior to placebo with increased stool frequency, reduction in number of fecal impactions, and need for fewer enemas.[89,105]

Stimulant laxatives, such as senna, aloe, and cascara, work by increasing intestinal motility and secretions by stimulating the colonic myenteric plexus and altering fluid and electrolyte transport. Caution with these laxatives should be taken, given the potential increased risk of dehydration and electrolyte imbalance.[106] Although commonly used, there is still insufficient evidence based on the 2005 review of the ACG chronic Constipation Task Force to make a recommendation about the effectiveness of stimulant laxatives for the management of chronic constipation.[93]

Stool softeners such as docusate sodium and docusate calcium are not recommended for use in this patient population.[107]

Surgical management

Surgery may be a viable option for patients with constipation that is refractory to dietary and medical therapy, but should be considered a treatment of last resort. Generalized neuromuscular dysfunction of the gut should be excluded, and the problem should be confined to the colon in patients considering surgical treatment for their chronic constipation.[84] Surgical options available for these patients include total and subtotal colectomy, and ileostomy or ileorectal anastomosis. A large series of carefully selected surgical patients showed favorable results.[108]

Constipation caused by obstructive defecation resulting from pelvic floor dysfunction such as rectocele, enterocele, or rectal prolapse is not improved by colectomy with ileorectal anastomosis unless the dyssynergia has also been corrected.[84] The management for these particular patients with constipation is discussed in the next section.

DEFECATORY DYSFUNCTION

Defecatory dysfunction is a broad term used to describe the condition of patients who complain of symptoms associated with obstructed defecation and constipation. Symptoms of obstructed defecation include an inability to initiate rectal emptying, an inability to complete evacuation, excessive straining of stools, a need to splint the posterior vagina or perineum, and rectal digitalization.[108]

Known causes of obstructed defecation include rectocele, enterocele, sigmoidocele, anismus, perineal descent, rectal intussusception, and rectal prolapse.[109] Patients with these conditions will often complain of constipation, and on examination are found to have a clinical rectocele. These patients traditionally have been treated with posterior colporrhaphy. Despite repair of the bulge, some patients have persistent or recurrent defecatory symptoms. Cundiff and colleagues[110] studied patients who underwent defect-directed rectocele repair and reported improved constipation in 84% of patients, tenesmus in 66% of patients, and splinting in 44% of patients. Despite significant improvement in defecatory symptoms, many patients had persistent symptoms; 18% of the patients had recurrent rectoceles at 1 year.[109,110] Recent evidence suggests that these patients had other underlying causes, such as colonic dysmotility, anismus, or intussusceptions, which contributed or caused persistent symptoms and recurrences. Thompson and colleagues[109] reported a 33% incidence of occult rectal prolapse in patients with clinical rectoceles and defecatory dysfunction. This is highly clinically significant because one-third of patients in this study who were examined for defecatory dysfunction and rectocele may also require sigmoid resection rectopexy along with other reconstructive procedures to restore pelvic floor function and prevent symptomatic recurrence. Pelvic imaging must be performed to diagnose many of these conditions, and should be considered in patients who have defecatory dysfunction. Fluoroscopic defecography is one of the most common imaging modalities used to assess dynamic pelvic floor function, including defecation.[109] Information from this radiographic study can help to not only identify conditions that require surgical interventions such as rectoceles, enteroceles, and occult rectal prolapse, but also can identify patients with dyssynergic defecation.[86]

Dyssynergic defecation is an acquired behavioral disorder of defecation in approximately two-thirds of patients, and in the rest of this population the process of defecation may have not been correctly learned in childhood.[86] The treatment of dyssynergic defecation consists of standard treatment used for the management of constipation including dietary changes, medications, timed toilet training, and biofeedback techniques.[86] The purpose of biofeedback therapy is to restore a normal pattern of defecation by correcting the underlying dyssynergia that affects the abdominal, rectal, and anal sphincter muscles, and to improve the rectal sensory perception.[86]

SUMMARY

Anorectal dysfunction, including anal incontinence, chronic constipation, and defecatory dysfunction, is a prevalent group of conditions that may adversely affect quality of life. Given the multiple causes of anorectal dysfunction and the treatment options available, the clinician must manage these patients using a systematic and comprehensive approach.

REFERENCES

1. Olsen AL, Smith VJ, Bergstrom JO, et al. Epidemiology of surgically managed pelvic organ prolapse and urinary incontinence. Obstet Gynecol 1997;89(4): 501–6.
2. Norton C, Christianson I, Butler U, et al. Anal incontinence. International consultation on incontinence. In: Abrams P, Cardozo L, Khoury S, editors. Incontinence. 2nd edition. Paris: Health publications, Ltd; 2001. p. 2002.
3. Boreham MK, Richter HE, Kenton KS, et al. Anal incontinence in women presenting for gynecologic care: prevalence, risk factors, and impact upon quality of life. Am J Obstet Gynecol 2005;192(5):1637–42.
4. Nygaard I, Barber MD, Burgio KL, et al. Prevalence of symptomatic pelvic floor disorders in US women. JAMA 2009;300(11):1311–6.
5. Davis K, Kumar D. Posterior pelvic floor compartment disorders. Best Pract Res Clin Obstet Gynaecol 2005;19(6):941–58.
6. Deutekom M, Dobben AC, Dijkgraaf MGW, et al. Costs of outpatients with fecal incontinence. Scand J Gastroenterol 2005;40:552–8.
7. Sung VW, Rogers ML, Myers DL, et al. National trends and costs of surgical treatment for female fecal incontinence. Am J Obstet Gynecol 2007;197:652 e1–5.
8. Hsu Y, Fenner D, Weadock WJ, et al. Magnetic resonance imaging and 3-dimensional analysis of external anal sphincter anatomy. Obstet Gynecol 2005;106(6): 1259–65.
9. Delancey JO, Toglia MR, Perucchini D. Internal and external anal sphincter anatomy as it relates to midline obstetric lacerations. Obstet Gynecol 1997; 90(6):924–7.
10. Whitehead WE, Norton NJ, Wald A. Advancing the treatment of fecal and urinary incontinence through research. Gastroenterology 2004;126(Suppl 1):S1–2.
11. Brincat D, Lewicky-Gaupp C, Patel D, et al. Fecal Incontinence in pregnancy and postpartum. Int J Gynaecol Obstet 2009;doi:10.1016/j.ijgo.2009.04.018.
12. Rogers RG, Leeman LM, Migliaccio L, et al. Does the severity of spontaneous genital tract trauma affect postpartum pelvic floor function? Int Urogynecol J Pelvic Floor Dysfunct 2008;19:429–35.
13. Lal M, H Mann C, Callender R, et al. Does cesarean delivery prevent anal incontinence? Obstet Gynecol 2003;101:305–12.
14. van Brummen HJ, Bruinse HW, van de Pol G, et al. Defecatory symptoms during and after the first pregnancy: Prevalence and associated factors. Int Urogynecol J Pelvic Floor Dysfunct 2006;17(3):224–30.
15. Sultan AH, Kamm MA, Hudson CN, et al. Anal sphincter disruption during vaginal delivery. N Engl J Med 1993;329:1905–11.
16. Eason E, Labrecque M, Marcoux S, et al. Anal incontinence after childbirth. CMAJ 2002;166:326–30.
17. Handa VL, Danielson BH, Gilbert WM. Obstetric anal sphincter lacerations. Obstet Gynecol 2001;98:225–30.
18. Zetterstrom J, Lopez A, Anzen B, et al. Anal sphincter tears at vaginal delivery: Risk factors and clinical outcome of primary repair. Obstet Gynecol 1999;94: 21–8.

19. Fitzpatrick M, Behan M, O'Connell PR, et al. A randomized clinical trial comparing primary overlap with approximation repair of third-degree obstetric tears. Am J Obstet Gynecol 2000;183:1220–4.
20. Varma A, Gunn J, Gardiner A, et al. Obstetrical anal sphincter injury: Prospective evaluation and incidence. Dis Colon Rectum 1999;42:1537–43.
21. Fenner DE, Genberg B, Brahma P, et al. Fecal and urinary incontinence after vaginal delivery with anal sphincter disruption in an obstetrics unit in the United States. Am J Obstet Gynecol 2003;189:1543–9.
22. Albers LL, Sedler KD, Bedrick EJ, et al. Midwifery care measures in the second stage of labor and reduction of genital tract trauma at birth a randomized trial. J Midwifery Womens Health 2005;50(5):365–72.
23. Andrews V, Sultan AH, Thakar R, et al. Occult anal sphincter injuries—myth or reality? BJOG 2006;113:195–200.
24. Avery KNL, Bosch JLHR, Naughton M, et al. Questionnaires to assess urinary and anal incontinence: Review and recommendations. J Urol 2005;177:39–49.
25. Jorge JMN, Wexner SD. Etiology and management of fecal incontinence. Dis Colon Rectum 1993;36:77–97.
26. Vaizey CJ, Carapeti E, Cahill JA, et al. Prospective comparison of faecal incontinence grading systems. Gut 1999;44:77–80.
27. Rockwood TH, Church JM, Fleshman JW, et al. Patient and surgeon ranking of the severity of symptoms associated with fecal incontinence: the fecal incontinence severity index. Dis Colon Rectum 1999;42:1525–31.
28. Barber MD, Walters MD, Bump RC. Short forms of two condition-specific quality-of-life questionnaires for women with pelvic floor disorders (PFDI-20 and PFIQ-7). Am J Obstet Gynecol 2005;193(1):103–13.
29. Rockwood TH, Church JM, Fleshman JW, et al. Fecal incontinence quality of life scale: quality of life instrument for patients with fecal incontinence. Dis Colon Rectum 2000;43:9–16.
30. Bug GJ, Kiff ES, Hosker G. A new condition specific health related quality of life questionnaire for the assessment of women with anal incontinence. BJOG 2001;108:1057–67.
31. Kwon S, Visco AG, Fitzgerald MP, et al. Validity and reliability of the modified Manchester health questionnaire in assessing patients with fecal incontinence. Dis Colon Rectum 2005;48:323–34.
32. Heaton KW, Thompson WG. Diagnosis. In: Heaton KW, Thompson WG, editors. Irritable bowel syndrome. Oxford: Health Press; 1999. p. 27.
33. Rotholtz NA, Wexner SD. Surgical treatment of constipation and fecal incontinence. Gastroenterol Clin North Am 2001;30(1):131–66.
34. Brink CA, Wells TJ, Sampselle CM, et al. A digital test for pelvic floor muscle strength in women with urinary incontinence. Nurse Res 1994;43(6):352–6.
35. Hallan RI, Marzouk DE, Waldron DJ, et al. Comparison of digital and manometric assessment of anal sphincter function. Br J Surg 1989;76:973–5.
36. Hill J, Corson RJ, Brandon H, et al. History and examination in the assessment of patients with idiopathic fecal incontinence. Dis Colon Rectum 1994;37:473–7.
37. Rogers RG, Abed H, Fenner DE. Current diagnosis and treatment algorithms for anal incontinence. BJU Int 2006;98(Suppl 1):97–106.
38. Hall RJ, Rogers RG, Saiz L, et al. Translabial ultrasound assessment of the anal sphincter complex: normal measurements of the internal and external anal sphincters at the proximal, mid and distal levels. Int Urogynecol J 2007;18:881–8.

39. Falk PM, Bltchford GJ, Cali RL, et al. Transanal ultrasound and manometry in the evaluation of fecal incontinence. Dis Colon Rectum 1994;37(5):468–72.
40. Burnett SJD, Speakman CTM, Kamm MA, et al. Confirmation of endosonographic detection of external anal sphincter defects by simultaneous electromyographic mapping. Br J Surg 1991;78:448–50.
41. Rociu E, Stoker J, Eijkemans MJC, et al. Fecal incontinence: endoanal US versus endoanal MR imaging. Radiology 1999;212(2):453–8.
42. Deen KI, Kuar D, Williams JG, et al. Anal sphincter defects; correlation between endoanal ultrasound and surgery. Ann Surg 1993;218(2):201–5.
43. Meyenberger C, Bertschinger P, Zala GF, et al. Anal sphincter defects in fecal incontinence: correlation between endosonography and surgery. Endoscopy 1996;28:217–24.
44. Kleinubing H Jr, Jannini JF, Malafaia O, et al. Transperineal ultrasonography: a new method to image the anorectal region. Dis Colon Rectum 2000;43:1572–4.
45. Dietz HP, Lanzarone V. Levator trauma after vaginal delivery. Obstet Gynecol 2005;106(4):707–12.
46. Dietz HP, Shek C, Clarke B. Biometry of the pubovisceral muscle and levator hiatus by three dimensional pelvic floor ultrasound. Ultrasound Obstet Gynecol 2005;25(6):580–5.
47. Dobben AC, Wiersma TG, Janssen LWM, et al. Prospective assessment of interobserver agreement for defecography in fecal incontinence. AJR Am J Roentgenol 2005;185:1166–72.
48. Groenendijk G, Birnie E, Blok S, et al. Clinical decision taking in primary pelvic organ prolapse; the effects of diagnostic tests on treatment selection in comparison with a consensus meeting. Int Urogynecol J 2009;20:711–9.
49. Azpiroz F, Ench P, Whitehead WE. Anorectal functional testing: review of collective experience. Am J Gastroenterol 2001;97:232–40.
50. Chen AS, Luchtefeld MA, Senagore AJ, et al. Pudendal nerve latency: does it predict outcome of anal sphincter repair? Dis Colon Rectum 1998;41(8):1005–9.
51. Hu T, Wagner TH, Bentkver JD, et al. Costs of urinary incontinence and overactive bladder in the United States: a comparative study. Urology 2004;63:461–5.
52. Fader M, Cottenden AM, Getliffe K. Absorbent products for moderate-heavy urinary and/or faecal incontinence in women and men. Art. No.: CD007408. Cochrane Database Syst Rev 2008;(Issue 4). doi:10.1002/14651858:CD007408.
53. Ehrenpreis ED, Chang D, Eichenwald E. Pharmacotherapy for fecal incontinence: a review. Dis Colon Rectum 2006;50:641–9.
54. Cheetam M, Brazzelli M, Norton C, et al. Drug treatment for faecal incontinence in adults. Cochrane Database Syst Rev 2002;(Issue 3). Art No.:CD002116. doi:10.1002/14651858:CD002116.
55. Berghmans LC, Hendriks HJ, Hay-Smith EJ, et al. Conservative treatment of stress urinary incontinence in women: a systematic review of randomized clinical trials. BJU Int 1998;82(2):181–91.
56. Norton CC, Cody JD, Hoskar G. Biofeedback and/or sphincter exercises for the treatment of faecal incontinence in adults. Art. No.: CD 002111. Cochrane Database Syst Rev 2006;(Issue 3). doi:10.1002/14652858:CD002111.pub2.
57. Hoskar G, Cody JD, Norton DD. Electrical stimulation for fecal incontinence in adults. Art. No.:CD 001310. Cochrane Database Syst Rev 2007;(Issue 3)10.1002/1451858. CD001310. pub2.
58. Matzel KE, Stadelmaier U, Hohenfellner M, et al. Electrical stimulation of sacral spinal nerves for treatment of faecal incontinence. Lancet 1995;346(8983):1124–7.

59. Tjandra JJ, Chan MKY, Yeh CH, et al. Sacral nerve stimulation is more effective than optimal medical therapy for severe fecal incontinence: a randomized, controlled study. Dis Colon Rectum 2008;51:494–502.
60. Altomare DF, Ratto C, Ganio E, et al. Long term outcome of sacral nerve stimulation for fecal incontinence. Dis Colon Rectum 2009;52:11–7.
61. Bond C, Youngson G, MacPherson I, et al. Anal plugs for the management of fecal incontinence in children and adults; a randomized control trial. J Clin Gastroenterol 2007;41:45–53.
62. Parks AG. Royal Society of Medicine, Section of Proctology; Meeting 27 November 1974. President's Address. Anorectal incontinence. Proc R Soc Med 1975;68(11):681–90.
63. Malouf AJ, Norton CS, Engel AF, et al. Long-term results of overlapping anterior anal-sphincter repair for obstetric trauma. Lancet 2000;355(9200):260–5.
64. Karoui S, Leroi AM, Koning E, et al. Results of sphincteroplasty in 86 patients with anal incontinence. Dis Colon Rectum 2000;43(6):813–20.
65. Halverson AL, Hull TL. Long-term outcome of overlapping anal sphincter repair. Dis Colon Rectum 2002;45(3):345–8.
66. Bravo Gutierrez A, Madoff RD, Lowry AC, et al. Long-term results of anterior sphincteroplasty. Dis Colon Rectum 2004;47(5):727–31.
67. Barisic GI, Krivokapic ZV, Markovic VA, et al. Outcome of overlapping anal sphincter repair after 3 months and after a mean of 80 months. Int J Colorectal Dis 2006;21(1):52–6.
68. Fernando RJ, Sultan AHH, Kettle C, et al. Methods of repair for obstetric anal sphincter injury. Art. No.: CD002866. Cochrane Database Syst Rev 2006;(Issue 3). doi:10.1002/14651858:CD002866.pub2.
69. Nordenstam J, Mellgren A, Altman D, et al. Immediate or delayed repair of obstetric anal sphincter tears—a randomized controlled trial. BJOG 2008;115:857–65.
70. Duggal N, Mercado D, Daniels K, et al. Antibiotic prophylaxis for prevention of postpartum perineal wound complications, a randomized controlled trial. Obstet Gynecol 2008;111(6):1268–73.
71. Mahoney R, Behan M, O'Herlihy C, et al. Randomized, clinical trial of bowel confinement vs laxative use after primary repair of a third-degree obstetrics anal sphincter tear. Dis Colon Rectum 2004;47:12–7.
72. Eogan M, Daly L, Behan M, et al. Randomised clinical trial of a laxative alone versus a laxative and a bulking agent after primary repair of obstetric anal sphincter injury. BJOG 2007;114:736–40.
73. Williams A, Adams EJ, Tincello DG, et al. How to repair an anal sphincter injury after vaginal delivery: results of a randomized controlled trial. BJOG 2006;113:201–7.
74. Kammerer-Doak DN, Wesol AB, Rogers RG, et al. A prospective cohort study of women after primary repair of obstetric anal sphincter laceration. Am J Obstet Gynecol 1999;181(6):1317–22.
75. Tjandra JJ, Han WR, Goh J, et al. Direct repair vs. overlapping sphincter repair: a randomized, controlled trial. Dis Colon Rectum 2003;46(7):937–42.
76. Tan M, O'Hanlon DM, Cassidy M, et al. Advantages of a posterior fourchette incision in anal sphincter repair. Dis Colon Rectum 2001;44(11):1624–9.
77. Guenaga K, Atallah AN, Castro AA, et al. Mechanical bowel preparation for elective colorectal surgery. Art. No.: CD001544. Cochrane Database Syst Rev 2005;(Issue 1). doi:10.1002/14651858:CD001544.pub2.

78. Hasegawa H, Yoshioka K, Keighley MR. Randomized trial of fecal diversion for sphincter repair. Dis Colon Rectum 2000;43(7):961–4.

79. Muller C, Belyaev O, Deska R, et al. Fecal incontinence: an up to date critical overview of surgical treatment options. Langenbecks Arch Surg 2005;390: 544–52.

80. Beggs AD, Irukulla S, Sultan AH, et al. A pilot study of ultrasound guided durasphere injection in the treatment of Faecal Incontinence. Accepted article Colorectal Dis doi:10.1111/j.1463–1318.2009.01927.x.

81. Norton C, Burch J, Kamm MA. Patients' views of a colostomy for fecal incontinence. Dis Colon Rectum 2005;48(5):1062–9.

82. Tou S, Brown SR, Malik AI et al. Surgery for complete rectal prolapse in adults. Cochrane Database Syst Rev 2008, (Issue 4). Art No.: CD001758. doi:10.1002/14651858:CD001758.pub2.

83. Rogers RG, Fenner DE. Rectovaginal fistulas. In: Sultan AH, Thakar R, Fenner DE, editors. Perineal and anal sphincter trauma. London: Springer-Verlag; 2007. p. 166–77.

84. Tsang CBS, Madoff RD, Wong WD, et al. Anal sphincter integrity and function influences outcome in rectovaginal fistula repair. Dis Colon Rectum 1998; 41(9):1141–6.

85. Toglia MR. Pathophysiology of anorectal dysfunction. Obstet Gynecol Clin North Am 1998;25(4):771–81.

86. Rao SS. Constipation: evaluation and treatment. Gastroenterol Clin North Am 2003;32(2):659–83.

87. Everhart JE, Go VLW, Hohannes RS, et al. A longitudinal study o f self-reported bowel habits in the United States. Dig Dis Sci 1989;34:1153–62.

88. Pare P, Ferrazzi S, Thompson WG, et al. An epidemiological survey of constipation in Canada: definitions, rates, demographics, and predictors of health care seeking. Am J Gastroenterol 2001;96:3130–7.

89. Gallagher PF, O'Mahony D, Quigley EM. Management of chronic constipation in the elderly. Drugs Aging 2008;25(10):807–21.

90. Harari D, Gurwitz JH, Avorn J, et al. How do other persons define constipation? Implications for therapeutic management. J Gen Intern Med 1997;12(1): 63–6.

91. Locke GR 3rd, Pemberton JH, Phillips SE. AGA technical review on constipation. American Gastroenterological Association. Gastroenterology 2000;119(6): 1766–78.

92. Longstreth GF, Thompson WG, Chey WD, et al. Functional bowel disorders. Gastroenterology 2006;130(5):1480–91.

93. American College of Gastroenterology Chronic Constipation Task Force. An evidence-based approach to the management of chronic constipation in North America. Am J Gastroenterol 2005;100(Suppl 1):S1–4.

94. O'Keefe EA, Talley NJ, Ainsmeister AR, et al. Bowel disorders impair functional status and quality of life in the elderly: a population-based study. J Gerontol A Biol Sci Med Sci 1995;50(4):184–9.

95. Talley NJ. Definitions, epidemiology, and impact of chronic constipation. Rev Gastroenterol Disord 2004;4(suppl 2):S3–10.

96. Bradnt LJ, Pranther CM, Quigley EMM, et al. Systematic review on the management of chronic constipation in North America. Am J Gastroenterol 2005; 100(Suppl 1):S5–22.

97. Heaton KW, Radvan J, Cripps H, et al. Defecation frequency and timing and stool form in the general population: a prospective study. Gut 1992;33:818–23.

98. O'Donnell LJ, Virjee J, Heaton K. Detection of pseudodiarrhea by simple clinical assessment of intestinal transit rate. BMJ 1990;300:439–40.

99. Frank L, Kleinman L, Farup C, et al. Psychometric validation of a constipation symptom assessment questionnaire. Scand J Gastroenterol 1999;34(0):870–7.

100. Frank L, Flynn J, Rothman M. Use of a self-report constipation questionnaire with older adults in long-term care. Gerontologist 2001;41(6):778–86.

101. Rao SSC, Hatfield R, Soffer E, et al. Manometric tests of anorectal function in healthy adults. Am J Gastroenterol 1999;94:773–83.

102. Muller –Lissner SA, Kamm MA, Scarpignato C, et al. Myths and misconceptions about chronic constipation. Am J Gastroenterol 2005;100:232–42.

103. Cook IJ, Irvine EJ, Campbell D, et al. Effect of dietary fiber on symptoms and rectosigmoid motility in patients with irritable bowel syndrome. Gastroenterology 1990;98:66.

104. Vonderholzer WA, Schtke W, Mihldorfer BE, et al. Clinical response to dietary fiber treatment for chronic constipation. Am J Gastroenterol 1997;92:95–8.

105. Sanders JF. Lactulose syrup assessed in a double blind study of elderly constipated patients. J Am Geriatr Soc 1978;26:236–9.

106. Xing JH, Soffer E. Adverse effects of laxative. Dis Colon Rectum 2001;44:1201–9.

107. Castle SC, Cantrell M, Israel DS, et al. Constipation prevention: empiric use of stool softeners questioned. Geriatrics 1991;46:84–6.

108. Sun WM. Obstructed defecation. J Gastroenterol Hepatol 1993;8:383–9.

109. Thompson JR, Chen AH, Pettit PDM, et al. Incidence of occult rectal prolapse in patients with clinical rectoceles and defecatory dysfunction. Am J Obstet Gynecol 2002;187:1494–500.

110. Cundiff GW, Weidner AC, Visco AG, et al. An anatomic and functional assessment of the discrete defect rectocele repair. Am J Obstet Gynecol 1998;179:1451–7.

Pathophysiology of Pelvic Floor Hypertonic Disorders

Charles W. Butrick, MD[a,b,*]

KEYWORDS

- Pelvic floor • Hypertonic dysfunction • Myofascial pain
- Visceral pain disorders • Trigger points

The pelvic floor represents the neuromuscular unit that provides support and functional control for the pelvic viscera. Its integrity, both anatomic and functional, is the key in some of the basic functions of life: storage of urine and feces, evacuation of urine and feces, support of pelvic organs, and sexual function. When this integrity is compromised, the results lead to many of the problems seen by clinicians. Pelvic floor dysfunction can involve weakness and result in stress incontinence, fecal incontinence, and pelvic organ prolapse. Pelvic floor dysfunction can also involve the development of hypertonic, dysfunctional muscles. This article discusses the pathophysiology of hypertonic disorders that often result in elimination problems, chronic pelvic pain, and bladder disorders that include bladder pain syndromes, retention, and incontinence. The hypertonic disorders are very common and are often not considered in the evaluation and management of patients with these problems.

NEUROPATHOLOGY OF MYOFASCIAL PAIN

When muscle fiber trauma occurs, inflammatory mediators such as bradykinin, serotonin, prostaglandins, adenosine triphosphate, and histamine are released locally. This sensitizes muscle nociceptors (group III and IV afferents) and reduces their mechanical threshold. This results in muscle hyperalgesia and mechanical allodynia. This causes innocuous pressure or normal muscle contraction to be perceived as painful. This process results in peripheral sensitization (**Fig. 1**).[1]

Central sensitization involves a series of neuroplastic changes that occur in the central nervous system because of prolonged noxious stimuli. These biochemical, neuroinflammatory changes in the spinal cord result in pain impulses becoming

[a] The Urogynecology Center, 12200 W. 106th Street Suite 130, Overland Park, KS 66215, USA
[b] Department of Obstetrics and Gynecology, Kansas University Medical School, 3901 Rainbow Blvd., Kansas City, Kansas 66160, USA
* Corresponding author. The Urogynecology Center, 12200 W. 106th Street Suite 130, Overland Park, Kansas 66215, USA.
E-mail address: cwbutrick@gmail.com

Obstet Gynecol Clin N Am 36 (2009) 699–705
doi:10.1016/j.ogc.2009.08.006
0889-8545/09/$ – see front matter © 2009 Elsevier Inc. All rights reserved.

obgyn.theclinics.com

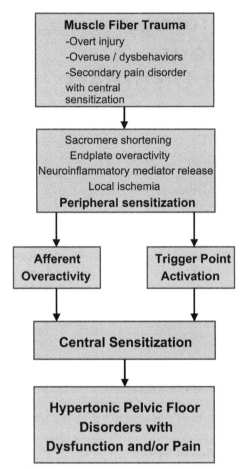

Fig. 1. Neuropathology of myofascial pain.

amplified, in generation of spontaneous pain impulses, in the expansion of the area of perceived pain and in non-noxious stimuli being perceived as painful.[2] This wind-up or upregulation is best studied as it relates to neuropathic pain, but animal studies suggest that deep myofascial pain actually is more effective at inducing central sensitization.[3,4]

WHAT CAUSES PELVIC FLOOR HYPERTONIC DYSFUNCTION?

Pelvic floor control begins as part of potty training in early childhood. As children attempt to voluntarily suppress accidents, they learn to squeeze and then relax their pelvic floor muscles in order to void or pass stool when socially appropriate. During these formative years, the brain and sacral reflexes are very plastic and, therefore, susceptible to being disrupted by abnormal behaviors. At times, a child can develop a hypervigilance with holding urine and not be able to relax to void. Approximately 7% of all children present to their clinicians with various elimination disorders, typically between the ages of three and seven. As has been demonstrated by many authors, the dysbehaviors of childhood can continue into adulthood.[5] A childhood history of recurrent urinary tract infections, ureteral reflux, vulvar pain, and constipation are very common in adults who are found to have pelvic floor hypertonic disorders.[6]

Dysbehaviors of the pelvic floor can also be acquired in adults because of holding patterns such as in nurses who must hold urine for hours while working. Asymmetric overload or postural circumstances can occur in certain vocations that can also result in development or worsening of hypertonic disorders. Prolonged lack of motion such as long car rides can also trigger the same problems in certain individuals. Postural abnormalities such as short leg syndrome or gait disturbances often trigger pelvic floor muscle imbalance that can result in muscle dysfunction and pain. Certainly, there can be an emotional component to some patients' pelvic floor dysbehaviors. This is seen in patients with severe anxiety disorders or patients who have been sexually abused— especially at a young age.[7]

Direct neuromuscular injury to the pelvic floor commonly induces pelvic floor muscle spasm with resultant dysfunction or pain. This type of injury occurs in patients who have suffered a traumatic vaginal delivery especially if forceps or vacuum extractors were involved.[8] Levator injuries have been associated with stress urinary incontinence and pelvic organ prolapse because of lack of support, but in some patients these levator avulsion injuries can result in postpartum pain syndromes, urinary frequency syndromes, and voiding dysfunction that can persist for years after the delivery.[9] Surgery can also trigger the development of pelvic floor hypertonic disorders and can cause postoperative voiding dysfunction, urinary frequency, urgency, and pain syndromes. In particular, surgical procedures that involve fixation to muscle sites are at great risk to induce or worsen pelvic muscle hypertonic dysfunction. Examples would include sacrospinous vaginal vault suspensions, mesh kits that use levator muscle sites to anchor the repair,[10] and levator plications done for correction of rectoceles.

The most common cause of pelvic floor hypertonic disorders are those that develop secondary to other pelvic pain disorders. Any pelvic pain disorder that is prolonged or particularly intense can result in such a barrage of noxious stimuli to the dorsal horn that it could result in upregulation of the dorsal horn. Examples include interstitial cystitis/bladder pain syndrome (IC/BPS), irritable bowel syndrome, vulvodynia, and endometriosis. These disorders can lead to prolonged noxious stimuli that cause metabolic, biochemical and electrophysiologic changes in the dorsal horn that results in the upregulation or wind up of the dorsal horn. This results in neuropathic changes that involve a decrease in the sensory threshold of afferent nerves that leads to the finding of allodynia (stimuli that would normally not be painful are perceived as painful). Additionally, this neuroplasticity of the dorsal horn results in neuropathic reflexes, including neurogenic inflammation in the periphery, which results in viscerovisceral hyperalgesia (also called pelvic organ cross talk).[11] One of the more common neuropathic reflexes that occur is visceromuscular hyperalgesia. This results in muscular instability and a hypertonic contractile state within the muscles of the pelvic floor. This hypertonicity not only induces voiding and defecatory problems, it is a major contributor to the self-perpetuation of visceral pain disorders (**Fig. 2**).[12] Pelvic muscle dysfunction is seen in 50% to 85% of patients with IC/BPS. Voiding dysfunction and urethral symptoms are often seen in many of these patients.[13] It is because of the hypertonic pelvic floor dysfunction that urethral dilation was, in the past, often chosen as part of an ill-conceived management plan for patients. This pelvic floor hypertonic disorder is also why urethral pressures are found to be abnormally elevated in patients with chronic pelvic pain disorders.[6,14] Bilateral pudendal blocks make these elevated pressures resolve and urethral instability disappear. These are all manifestations of the myofascial component to IC/BPS and are found in many patients with irritable bowel syndrome, chronic pelvic pain, and vulvodynia.

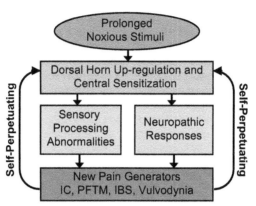

Fig. 2. Etiology of visceral pain syndromes. IC, Interstitial cystitis; PFTM, Pelvic floor tension myalgia; IBS, Irritable bowel syndrome.

MYOFASCIAL PAIN SYNDROMES

When a patient develops a hypertonic pelvic floor disorder, it could result in dysfunction of the viscera such as an elimination disorder with constipation or recurrent urinary tract infections. It also could result in a pain disorder secondary to a myofascial pain syndrome. Many patients with chronic pelvic pain disorders have more than one pain generator and clinicians must always be diligent in attempts to identify each of those pain generators. The myofascial component of pain cannot be overlooked. Patients often present with pelvic muscle dysfunction and a myofascial pain disorder.

Myofascial pain syndromes involve the development of a trigger point (TP). A TP is a hypersensitive spot located within a taut band of skeletal muscle. Characteristics of an active TP include a referral of pain that often reproduces the distribution of pain that the patient typically experiences. Active TPs also demonstrate a twitching response: the patient experiences a muscle twitch when the TP is stroked or manipulated.[15] Myofascial pain syndromes can be regional or diffuse. When diffuse it can often be confused with fibromyalgia but one must remember that patients with fibromyalgia have multiple and unique areas of tenderness to palpation; but there are no taut bands or TPs, just areas of diffuse tenderness.

Myofascial pain is often a chronic and a progressive disorder. Thirty percent of patients with regional pain seen in primary care settings and 85% in dedicated pain centers are diagnosed to have a myofascial pain syndrome. Early identification and treatment are the keys. There are two specific stages to myofascial pain syndromes.[16] The first is the neuromuscular stage, which involves fiber injury with release of neurotransmitters, trophic agents, and various inflammatory and immune chemotactic products. Local muscle ischemia and spontaneous electrical activity are characteristic of an active TP. This results in overactivity of the afferent nociceptors and central sensitization (windup), which results in self-perpetuation and the generation of new TPs. The second is the musculodystrophic stage, which results in fibrosis of muscle fibers due to the prolonged and sustained contractile activity, and the continued release, of the noxious byproducts mentioned above.

The natural history of myofascial pain involves periods of quiescence and periods of flares. There are many factors to reactivation of a latent TP. These perpetuating factors act clinically to potentially make an acute myofascial pain episode turn into a chronic myofascial pain disorder. Systemic perpetuating factors include chronic stress and anxiety, sleep disorders, hypothyroidism, hypokalemia, and malnutrition with associated vitamin deficiencies, especially B-complex and vitamin D.[17] Mechanical factors are often behavioral, such as holding patterns, occupational positional triggers, or postural factors. Skeletal asymmetry leads to muscular imbalance, which causes muscle overload. Enrolling the help of a well-trained physical therapist who specializes in pelvic floor dysfunction is the key to identifying and correcting these skeletal and postural factors.

TREATMENT OF PELVIC FLOOR HYPERTONIC DISORDERS: THE BIG PICTURE

Specific recommendations for each of the varied manifestations of pelvic floor hypertonic dysfunction are covered in detail elsewhere in this issue. This article discusses the basic strategies that need to be employed to successfully treat these disorders. With the understanding of the pathophysiology and, in particular, the concepts of upregulation, central sensitization, and self-perpetuation, the importance of these general treatment guidelines becomes evident.

The first step is to determine the underlying cause of the patient's pelvic floor symptoms. Did it begin with childhood symptoms or a history that was compatible with childhood pelvic floor dysfunction, such as recurrent urinary tract infections, lifelong chronic constipation, or bed-wetting past the age of six? Or did it start after a surgery for pelvic organ prolapse involving a muscle fixation point? It is also important to verify that the patient in fact had significant prolapse[18]—a prolapsed organ at the introitus or beyond—because many patients with pelvic floor hypertonic dysfunction have complaints of pelvic pressure or heaviness that is often quite severe that is misdiagnosed as prolapse. If the trigger is a visceral pain disorder like IC/BPS or endometriosis, verify which symptom came first. History often points the clinician toward the original precipitating factor and, therefore, guides the clinician in the correct direction for therapy. The initial trigger may have already been removed (eg, endometriosis treated with a total abdominal hysterectomy or bilateral salpingo-oophorectomy with complete removal of endometriosis and no signs of recurrence) but the myofascial component induced by the endometriosis is persistent. If the initiating trigger is still present (eg, vulvodynia), it is now a perpetuating factor and, therefore, must be treated aggressively or the myofascial component does not typically respond. The clinician should look for systemic perpetuating factors such as sleep disorders, hypothyroidism, or anxiety; and these must be treated.

Treatment for pelvic floor myofascial dysfunction involves retraining or rehabilitation of the dysfunctional pelvic floor. This typically involves biofeedback techniques, teaching relaxation, or reverse Kegels. Soft-tissue work is also one of the keys to success and typically involves localized heat, massage, and myofascial release techniques. These techniques require the care of a physical therapist with advanced training. The American Physical Therapy Association Web site (http://www.womenshealthapta.org) can assist in locating physical therapists that specialize in pelvic floor hypertonic dysfunctions. Additional local therapies may involve TP injections and the use of botulinum toxin (Botox) injections. These steps are be covered in detail elsewhere in this issue.

Since the perpetuation of pelvic floor hypertonic disorders involves central sensitization and neuropathic upregulation, especially if pain is a component of the patient's symptoms, then down-regulation of these neuropathic changes is typically required. Drugs to assist in decreasing muscle tone and spasticity, and the allodynia that is often part of their symptoms, are required. Drugs often used for this include amitriptyline, gabapentin, pregabalin, and baclofen. Neuromodulation can also be used to down-regulate the neuropathic changes that are often major factors in patients' elimination disorders and pain.

The more prolonged the symptoms before the initiation of therapy, the worse the prognosis and, therefore, the more aggressive the therapy must be. Once significant benefit to this multimodal approach is seen (as defined by at least 6 months of approximately 80% resolution in symptoms), then, and only then, should clinicians consider slowly tapering off the interventions that have helped. Since TPs never go away—they just become latent—reoccurrence is common and an ongoing home program that involves avoidance of myofascial triggers and a liberal policy toward reinstitution of drug therapy, physical therapy, and behavioral modification needs to be reviewed with patients. The concept of muscle memory in these cases is very helpful in explaining to patients why myofascial dysfunction and pain disorders are often managed and controlled but not totally eradicated.

SUMMARY

The pelvic floor is instrumental in the proper function and support of all pelvic viscera. Hypertonic disorders are very common and are a major component in the symptom complex for most patients who suffer with pelvic pain and various bladder dysfunctional states. The pelvic floor dysfunction that is commonly seen in many patients can be easily identified and treated, but the clinician must look for it.

REFERENCES

1. Graven-Nielsen T, Mense S. The peripheral apparatus of muscle pain: evidence from animal and human studies. Clin J Pain 2001;17(1):2–10.
2. Butrick CW. Interstitial cystitis and chronic pelvic pain: new insights in neuropathology, diagnosis, and treatment. Clin Obstet Gynecol 2003;46(4):811–23.
3. DeSantana JM, Sluka KA. Central mechanisms in the maintenance of chronic widespread noninflammatory muscle pain. Curr Pain Headache Rep 2008; 12(5):338–43.
4. Jensen R. Pathophysiological mechanisms of tension-type headache: a review of epidemiological and experimental studies. Cephalalgia 1999;19(6):602–21.
5. Minassian VA, Lovatsis D, Pascali D, et al. Effect of childhood dysfunctional voiding on urinary incontinence in adult women. Obstet Gynecol 2006;107(6): 1247–51.
6. Butrick CW, Sanford D, Hou Q, et al. Chronic pelvic pain syndromes: clinical, urodynamic, and urothelial observations. Int Urogynecol J Pelvic Floor Dysfunct 2009;20:1047–53.
7. Peters KM, Carrico DJ. Frequency, urgency, and pelvic pain: treating the pelvic floor versus the epithelium. Curr Urol Rep 2006;7(6):450–5.
8. Dietz HP. Pelvic floor trauma following vaginal delivery. Curr Opin Obstet Gynecol 2006;18(5):528–37.
9. Quinn M. Injuries to the levator ani in unexplained, chronic pelvic pain. J Obstet Gynaecol 2007;27(8):828–31.
10. Hurtado EA, Appell RA. Management of complications arising from transvaginal mesh kit procedures: a tertiary referral center's experience. Int Urogynecol J Pelvic Floor Dysfunct 2009;20(1):11–7.
11. Ustinova EE, Fraser MO, Pezzone MA. Colonic irritation in the rat sensitizes urinary bladder afferents to mechanical and chemical stimuli: an afferent origin of pelvic organ cross-sensitization. Am J Physiol Renal Physiol 2006;290(6): F1478–87.

12. Doggweiler-Wiygul R. Urologic myofascial pain syndromes. Curr Pain Headache Rep 2004;8(6):445–51.

13. van Os-Bossagh P, P Pols, T Hop WC, et al. Voiding symptoms in chronic pelvic pain (CPP). Eur J Obstet Gynecol Reprod Biol 2003;107(2):185–90.

14. Cameron AP, Gajewski JB. Bladder outlet obstruction in painful bladder syndrome/interstitial cystitis. Neurourol Urodyn 2009 [Epup ahead of print].

15. Simons DG, Travell JG, Simons LS. In: Travell JG, Simons DG, editors. Myofascial pain and dysfunction: the trigger point manual, vol. 1 and 2. Baltimore (MD): Williams and Wilkins; 1999: Chaper 1.

16. Cantu R, Grodin A. Myofascial pain syndromes. In: Lewis C, editor. Myofascial manipulation—therory and clinical application. New York: Aspen Publishers; 1992.

17. Howard FM, Perry CP, Carter JE, et al. Abdominal wall and pelvic myofascial trigger points. In: Carter JE, editor. Pelvic pain: diagnosis and management. Philadelphia: Lippincott Williams and Wilkins; 2000.

18. Gutman RE, Ford DE, Quiroz LH, et al. Is there a pelvic organ prolapse threshold that predicts pelvic floor symptoms? Am J Obstet Gynecol 2008;199(6):683, e1–7.

Pelvic Floor Hypertonic Disorders: Identification and Management

Charles W. Butrick, MD[a,b,]*

KEYWORDS

- Pelvic floor hypertonic disorder • Myofascial pain
- Elimination disorder • Interstitial cystitis • Vaginismus
- Vulvodynia • Trigger point • Botulinum toxin

In the previous article titled, "Pathophysiology of Pelvic Floor Hypertonic Disorders", the pathophysiologic mechanisms of pelvic floor hypertonic dysfunction and pain were reviewed. The importance of triggers and perpetuating factors that can result in years of symptoms that often go undiagnosed and untreated are emphasized. The various syndromes that are associated with these pelvic floor hypertonic (PFH) disorders and how to identify and treat them are now reviewed with this article. The importance of identifying and treating the pelvic floor hypertonic component of the patient's symptoms cannot be overstated. The PFH dysfunction can be the primary symptom generator, or it can be just a component of the patient's symptoms and it often is a perpetuating factor in the ongoing dysfunction and chronic pain. If not identified and treated, symptoms will often persist or re-occur after traditional therapy.

CLINICAL SYNDROMES ASSOCIATED WITH PELVIC FLOOR HYPERTONIC DYSFUNCTION

As stated in the previous article, pelvic floor hypertonic dysfunction can present with dysfunction of the viscera that are controlled by the pelvic floor or it may present as a primary pain generator or just as a component of a chronic pain syndrome. We will first discuss syndromes and symptoms caused by the hypertonic dysfunction of the pelvic floor.

Childhood Eliminating Disorders

Approximately 40% of the visits to a pediatric urologist involve caring for children with dysfunctional voiding.[1] Dysfunctional voiding is associated with recurrent urinary tract infections, urinary retention, and vesicoureteral reflux. Childhood eliminating disorders also include children with constipation, incomplete bowel emptying, and fecal soiling.

[a] The Urogynecology Center, Overland Park, KS 66215, USA
[b] Department of Obstetrics and Gynecology, Kansas University Medical Center, Kansas City, KS 66160, USA
* The Urogynecology Center, Overland Park, KS 66215.
E-mail address: cwbutrick@gmail.com

Obstet Gynecol Clin N Am 36 (2009) 707–722
doi:10.1016/j.ogc.2009.08.011
0889-8545/09/$ – see front matter © 2009 Elsevier Inc. All rights reserved.

The vast majority of these children are found to have high tone pelvic floor dysfunction.[2] These children often wake up in the middle of the night with lower abdominal pain or perineal pain related to the increased bladder volume and the pain of the hypertonic pelvic floor. This symptom is sometimes reported by adults with this disorder as well. When the pelvic floor hypertonic dysfunction is treated with biofeedback, the ureteral reflux resolves in 63% of patients and improves in another 29%. The symptoms of urinary urgency/frequency and urinary tract infections as well as constipation are resolved in more than 70% of these patients.[3] Adults with a history of childhood elimination disorders have a marked increased risk for bladder, bowel, and sexual dysfunction as well as pain disorders such as interstitial cystitis and vulvodynia.[4,5]

Idiopathic Urinary Retention

Although dysfunctional voiding (also called discordant voiding) is common in our patients with various pelvic pain disorders, it is frequently seen in children with elimination disorders and was called Hinman syndrome in 1971 or "non-neurogenic neurogenic bladder."[6] We now know this represents an up-regulated guarding or "holding" reflex and is referred to as idiopathic urinary retention. Fowler and colleagues[7] described a unique type of urinary retention associated with abnormal urethral sphincteric electromyography (EMG) activity and polycystic ovaries. The symptom of urinary retention is often triggered by a significant life event that may have been emotional or surgical. Sacral nerve stimulation has been found to be very beneficial for these patients with urinary retention and has a long-term success rate of 68%.[8]

Vaginismus

Vaginismus is one of the most common causes of entry dyspareunia affecting more than 1% of all women. It is characterized by persistent involuntary contractions of the pelvic floor. Vaginismus typically is primary (a woman who has never been able to have completed intercourse) or secondary (acquired dyspareunia). When identified in patients with other medical conditions such as interstitial cystitis (IC) or endometriosis, it could be a primary trigger or a secondary pelvic floor hypertonic disorder rather than primary vaginismus. Therapy should therefore be directed toward both the pain disorder as well as the myofascial dysfunction. The perpetuation of vaginismus is closely tied to the dyspareunia cycle. This conditioned response is initiated by an unpleasant experience such as past sexual abuse, or painful first pelvic examination or first sexual attempt. The dyspareunia cycle is often initiated by this unpleasant experience, which then causes fear of pain with the next attempt at intercourse. This causes anxiety with poor sexual response and leads to involuntary pelvic floor contractions resulting in entry dyspareunia and continuation of the cycle[9] (Fig. 1).

Constipation/Pelvic Floor Dyssynergia

Constipation is a symptom complex with many different causes. It affects over 18% of Americans and is more common in women and the elderly. Many symptoms can be described when patients report constipation: 9% report bowel movements fewer than three times per week, 30% report incomplete emptying, 29% report hard stools, 24% report a feeling of blockage with attempts at stool passage. When evaluated by simple radiologic techniques, 20% of patients are found to have colonic inertia and the rest have some form of outlet dysfunction.[10] Outlet obstruction can be anatomic (eg, rectocele) or functional (eg, dyssynergic defecation). Another study involved 179 patients with severe chronic constipation who failed traditional therapy and

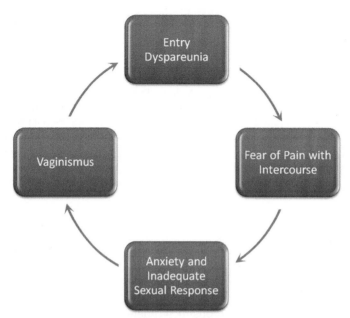

Fig. 1. Dyspareunia cycle. (*Data from* Howard FM, editor. Pelvic pain: Diagnosis and Management. Baltimore: Lippincott Williams and Wilkins; 2000. p. 288.)

underwent extensive evaluation including colonic transit time, defecography, anorectal manometry and anal sphincter EMGs. Outlet dysfunction was found in 43.3%, irritable bowel disease (IBS)/idiopathic constipation in 33.3%, megacolon in 12.5%, and colonic inertia in 11%. Patients with outlet dysfunction were then divided into two groups—those with anatomic problems (63%) and those with functional problems (37%).[11] It is therefore important to realize that pelvic floor dysfunction is certainly a common cause of constipation and symptoms of lifelong constipation should alert the clinician to the possibility of lifelong pelvic floor dysfunction.

PAIN SYNDROMES ASSOCIATED WITH PELVIC FLOOR HYPERTONIC DISORDERS
Bladder Pain Syndrome/Interstitial Cystitis

Bladder pain syndrome/interstitial cystitis (BPS/IC) is characterized by urinary frequency, urgency, irritable voiding dysfunction, and pelvic pain. It is associated with a number of other pain disorders including vulvodynia, irritable bowel syndrome, endometriosis, fibromyalgia, and chronic fatigue syndrome. The prevalence of PFH dysfunction is thought to be 50% to 87% in patients with BPS/IC.[12] Patients with fibromyalgia, IBS, and vulvodynia are all found to have a high prevalence of pelvic floor hypertonic dysfunction and myofascial pain. Seventy-six percent of patients with BPS/IC are also found to have voiding dysfunction and very high urethral pressures,[5] which are both manifestations of the pelvic floor hypertonic component of their symptoms. Patients with a significant myofascial component to their pain will often report leg or groin pain that occurs with bladder filling and urinary frequency that is severe during the day but not at night. The "pressure" arising from the pelvic floor hypertonicity is perceived as a need to void but during sleep the pelvic floor relaxes, therefore the need to void is generated only by bladder volume and not by the pelvic floor. As documented by many authors including Weiss,[13] and Peters and Carrico[14] when pelvic floor therapy is used in patients with BPS/IC the response to therapy is much improved as compared with bladder-directed therapy.

Vulvodynia

Vulvodynia is a vulvar pain disorder associated with sensations of burning, irritation, and rawness located typically at the introitus. These symptoms typically flare with attempts at intercourse (provoked vulvodynia). They can also be continuous (unprovoked). Vulvodynia is associated with many other pain disorders such as fibromyalgia, IBS, and temporomandibular joint (TMJ), but is especially associated with BPS/IC. Between 12% and 68% of patients diagnosed with BPS/IC report vulvodynia symptoms.[15] Pelvic floor hypertonic dysfunction is found in 80% to 90% of patients with vulvodynia.[16] Therapy directed toward the pelvic floor alone has a success rate of greater than 50%.[17]

Colorectal Pain Disorders

There are two basic types of anal/rectal pain disorders typically seen by colorectal surgeons. Protalgia fugax is defined as sudden, severe, intermittent pain in the anal/rectal area lasting less than 5 minutes in the absence of other known pathology. The second is the levator ani syndrome—a pelvic floor hypertonic pain disorder associated with a relatively constant or frequent dull anal or rectal pain. The hypertonic pelvic floor muscles often result in obstructed defecation because of failure of the pelvic floor to relax and this is typically associated with the symptom of postdefecatory pain that is located inside the anus rather than at the anus as one would expect with hemorrhoids or fissures. The clinician must be mindful that rectoceles do not cause pain and the functioning of the pelvic floor must be considered in any patient with defecatory pain and obstructed defecation. Many of these patients will have a rectocele from years of straining but the rectocele is not the cause of the pain. IBS is a classic example of a visceral pain syndrome (as is BPS/IC) and as such it can induce central sensitization and secondary pelvic floor hypertonic disorders with dysfunctional defecation and colorectal pain.[18]

Chronic Pelvic Pain/Myofascial Pain Syndromes

Chronic pelvic pain is a very common disorder affecting 16% of women. There are many causes of chronic pelvic pain and primary myofascial causes are involved in 12% to 87% of pelvic pain patients evaluated at a tertiary pain center.[12] The symptoms of myofascial pain often erroneously lead the clinician to seek out visceral sources of pain. The clinician must always realize that myofascial pain is a very common cause of chronic pelvic pain and this explains why 25% to 40% of laparoscopies done for the evaluation of pelvic pain are found to be negative. Once the clinician has determined that symptoms are myofascial in origin then he or she must attempt to determine if this is a primary myofascial pain disorder or if it is secondary to another pain disorder such as BPS/IC, vulvodynia, or IBS. If it is a secondary myofascial pain disorder, then the primary pain generator must be treated as well as the myofascial component.

HISTORY AND SYMPTOMS

Pelvic floor hypertonic disorders can present with symptoms of pain or dysfunction. The pain symptoms are often vague and poorly localized. Pain is described as achy, throbbing, and as having a pressure or heaviness quality to it. Often this feeling is similar to the symptoms seen in patients with pelvic organ prolapse, yet on examination no significant prolapse is seen (typically the leading edge of prolapse must be at the level of the introitus to produce any symptoms or awareness[19]). Pain can be described as vaginal, rectal, suprapubic, or in either or both lower quadrants. It is this latter symptom that often is associated with the report that this is "my ovarian cyst pain." Radiation into the hip and back is also common. Pain often is worse as the day progresses and is typically worsened by pelvic floor muscle activities such as sitting, walking, exercise, intercourse, voiding, or passing stool. Like most muscular pain disorders, the pain may be worse after these activities, ie, after sex or after voiding. The reader is referred to Travell's excellent text on myofascial pain and figures from that text are included to better understand the common distributions of pelvic floor myofascial pain.[20]

Symptoms of pelvic floor dysfunction typically involve symptoms of the pelvic viscera that are controlled by the pelvic floor. Symptoms can involve the bladder such as voiding dysfunction, post void pain, urethral pain, hesitancy or "shy" bladder, or the constant or exaggerated urge to void. Symptoms can involve the lower colorectal area such as constipation, obstructed defecation, painful defecation, or sharp rectal pain-proctalgia fugax. Vaginal and introital symptoms may include vulvodynia, dyspareunia, and vaginismus. A classic symptom is post coital pain that can exacerbate symptoms for 12 to 48 hours after intercourse. This type of post coital pain is seen only in patients with pelvic floor hypertonic dysfunction and to a lesser degree pelvic congestion syndrome. Clitoral pain and pain with orgasm are also both typically caused by pelvic floor hypertonic dysfunction.

It is important to stress that myofascial pain and hypertonic dysfunction can be a primary problem and must not be missed. It also must be stressed that the myofascial pain and dysfunction can be secondary to other pelvic and systemic disorders. The history must therefore involve a careful search for visceral sources of pain such as IC, IBS, and endometriosis, which can secondarily induce the pelvic floor problem. Determining the chronology of symptom onset helps us to understand the triggers and the perpetuating factors of our patients' symptoms.

It is also important to identify factors such as job stress, constipation, or menstrual cycle triggers not only to help evaluate the true source of pain (eg, sitting for a prolonged time commonly worsens pelvic floor pain but not endometriosis pain) but also to identify targets for intervention. Cycle suppression often helps menstrual-related triggers to myofascial pain as does changes in positioning when a job requires prolonged sitting on a hard chair. These environmental factors must always be taken into consideration as you evaluate your patients with pelvic floor hypertonic disorders.

PHYSICAL EXAMINATION

Clinical evaluation of the pelvic floor begins with simple observation of pelvic floor muscle activity during the process of squeezing and relaxation. The simple observation of the perineum and introital area in the dorsal lithotomy position during the performance of a Kegel squeeze is often quite revealing. It can be compared with watching a patient walk to determine if there are any disturbances of gait. A brief lesson to help the patient understand the desired muscle action is often beneficial and using the analogy of holding urine or holding flatus is often helpful. Patients with pelvic floor hypertonic dysfunction often have so much muscle tension at "rest" that they are unable to produce more contractile strength and therefore cannot produce an effective squeeze. Often they cannot relax completely or in a continuous manner and instead will show a step-wise type of relaxation or demonstrate rebound hypertonicity, ie, the pelvic floor tightens up after they relax. Spontaneous muscle fasciculation can be seen in some patients and has the appearance of subtle twitches that occur during attempts at squeeze and relax maneuvers.

A lubricated cotton tip applicator is then used to carefully evaluate for signs of allodynia and vulvodynia. This also provides an opportunity to verify where symptoms are perceived versus where they can be reproduced. It is relatively common that patients describing urethral pain actually have reproduction of "the location" of their pain with manipulation at the anterior fourchette or the supraurethral area.

At this point the examiner should place a generously lubricated single finger in the vagina to assess pelvic floor awareness and the ability to squeeze and relax the levator ani. Many scales are available to document strength, tone, and tenderness, yet all these scales are subjective and unvalidated. Normally the vaginal vault and its under-lying levator muscles should form a smooth cylindrical configuration with complete relaxation. Often patients with hypertonic disorders will have a "V" configuration and as a finger is advanced it will drop off the shelf caused by the contracted levator muscles and drop down onto the coccygeus muscle (**Fig. 2**).

The examination thus far should have been pain-free and should have been per-formed with a very light touch. At this point in the examination determining the degree of pelvic floor muscle tenderness becomes important so the examiner can ascertain if a myofascial component to pain exists. This is done by applying gentle pressure to the levator muscles and assessing whether or not the patient's reported pain is reproduced and whether the urge to urinate is reproduced with downward pressure against the pelvic floor musculature. Many patients will be found to be most tender along the lateral border of the levator ani, which is where the levator muscles insert on to the arcus ten-dineus levator ani (**Fig. 3**). Active trigger points are often identified by the finding of an exquisitely tender area palpable as a small 3- to 6-mm nodule within a taut band that reproduces the patient's pain as well as the referral pattern of her pain (**Fig. 4**).

A general pelvic pain–directed pelvic examination should also be done that empha-sizes the location of areas of allodynia and hypersensitivity. The examiner should attempt to determine the areas of greatest tenderness and evaluate whether this

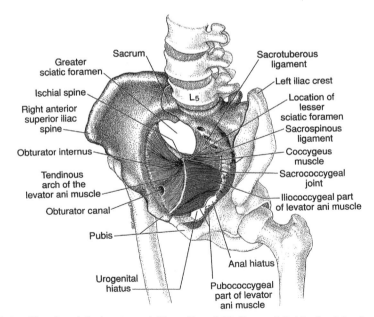

Fig. 2. Lateral border of the levater ani. (*From* Travell JG, Simons DG. Myofascial pain and dys-function: the trigger point manual. Baltimore: Williams and Wilkins, 1992; with permission.)

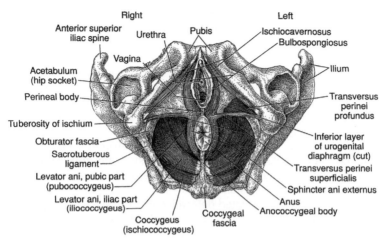

Fig. 3. Normal pelvic floor as viewed from below. (*From* Travell JG, Simons. Myofascial pain and pysfinction: the trigger point manual. Baltimore: Williams and Wilkins, 1992; with permission.)

reproduces an area associated with the patient's symptoms. This examination targets introital areas, bladder base, cervix, uterus, cul-de-sac, and adnexa. Urine and/or vaginal cultures should be obtained if abnormal findings are encountered.

DIAGNOSTIC STUDIES

Objective identification of pelvic floor hypertonic dysfunction can be obtained with various techniques. The most common is with surface EMGs, which often are done as a part of a pelvic floor evaluation by physical therapists and nurse clinicians trained in the evaluation and management of patients with pelvic floor dysfunction. Patients

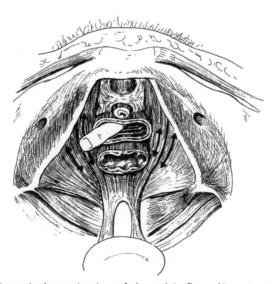

Fig. 4. Single digit vaginal examination of the pelvic floor. (*From* Laycock J. Pelvic floor re-education: principles and practice. New York: Springer-Verlag; 1994; with permission.)

with hypertonic dysfunction will have at least three of five of the following findings (listed in order of prevalence): elevated and unstable resting baseline activity, poor recovery, poor postcontraction and relaxation, spasms with sustained contractions, and poor strength.[21] Fowler and collegues[7] describe the use of concentric needle EMGs to identify a unique EMG pattern in the urethral sphincter in patients with non-relaxing pelvic floor and idiopathic urinary retention.

Characteristic findings often seen with multichannel urodynamics include abnormal voiding studies, elevated urethral pressure at rest, and urethral instability. The International Continence Society has defined urethral instability as wide fluctuation in urethral pressure measured during filling phase not associated with detrusor activity.[22] Of note is the fact that these fluctuations in urethral pressure are abolished by bilateral pudendal blocks and this demonstrates that these fluctuations originate from the levator ani/pelvic floor muscle dysfunction.[23]

When symptoms involve obstructed defecation and rectal pain, defecography can be used to identify the presence of a nonrelaxing pelvic floor or even paradoxic activity of the pelvic floor during defecation. Magnetic resonance defecography is used by some with excellent results and no radiation exposure.[24] The clinician must remember that patients can present with localized symptoms such as bladder pain or vulvodynia but may show dysfunction in other areas of the pelvis, which they downplay. Classic examples would be chronic constipation and/or obstructed defecation. Although these other problems are not always reported, the clinician must be aware that the pelvic floor dysfunction can cause symptoms to arise from any one or all of the organs of the pelvic floor.

TREATMENT OF PELVIC FLOOR HYPERTONIC DISORDERS

The clinician must always use management plans that best approach the patient's primary complaints. However, as patients' problems become more complex so do their treatment options. When the patient's myofascial pain or dysfunction is just a component of their overall syndrome of multiple pain generators and multiple organ dysfunction, the myofascial component may be a primary trigger or simply a perpetuating factor. Typically the pelvic floor must therefore be aggressively treated as part of a multimodal treatment plan. In the more complex patient, myofascial therapy alone rarely will provide a major breakthrough in symptom control. When patients appear to have an isolated myofascial symptom generator such as isolated hip pain from a piriformis muscle injury, therapy is targeted to this one pain generator. Although this section reviews the therapy of pelvic floor hypertonic disorders (**Box 1**) it assumes the clinician is also treating the other pain and dysfunction generators that these patients often possess. This includes problems such as chronic constipation, insomnia, depression, and BPS/IC, to name a few.

PELVIC FLOOR REHABILITATION

Improvement in pelvic floor function begins with patient education about the normal function of the pelvic floor at rest and during various pelvic floor activities. Teaching the patient that her pelvic floor is normally relaxed and that she should not be actively "holding her muscles" all the time can be a major breakthrough for some. Often these patients have no awareness of their pelvic floor and instructing them to "check" their pelvic floor tension throughout the day is helpful in their understanding the importance of keeping the pelvic floor relaxed. Many simple measures are very beneficial to help the pelvic floor muscles relax. Heat applied with heating pads or microwavable "rice bags" are very helpful. Dysbehaviors such as "holding urine" or positional or postural

---

Box 1
Therapeutic options for pelvic floor hypertonic disorders

Behavioral

- Education, rest, heat
- Avoidance of triggers
- Fluids and stool management

Physical Therapy

- Biofeedback/"Reverse" Kegels
- Soft tissue/myofascial therapy
- Ultrasound therapy

Pharmacologic Therapy

- Amitriptyline
- Tiazadine
- Compounded baclofen suppositories

Trigger Point Injections

- Wet trigger point injections, 3 to 5 sessions
- Botox A
- Consider caudal block, ganglion impar block

Neuromodulation

- Sacral nerve stimulation
- Posterior tibial nerve

---

problems caused by prolonged sitting can produce continued or prolonged myofascial stress. Simple measures such as providing appropriate perineal protection pads (three in cushions with central cutouts) or simply allowing that patient to stand and walk on a regular basis rather than continuously sitting can often provide great benefit. It is also important to note that postural problems (short leg syndrome) or gait disturbances owing to orthopedic problems can often trigger pelvic floor dysfunction and pain.

When patients have no muscle awareness they must be taught this skill. Using biofeedback techniques that are typically used by highly trained physical therapists is key to pelvic floor reeducation. With surface electrodes applied to the perianal area or a vaginal probe, levator ani activity can be monitored by the patient and her therapist. With careful coaching the patient is taught how to contract and then relax her pelvic floor using various protocols but generally the goal is to teach muscle awareness and relaxation or "reverse Kegels."[25,26] Excessive and prolonged contraction phase protocols are to be avoided. Typically sessions last 20 to 30 minutes and occur once per week. These exercises need to be continued at home each day. Manual therapy techniques are especially important for patients with myofascial pain disorders and include myofascial release, trigger point release, soft tissue mobilization, and massage.[13] This approach was first developed by Theile in his use of the internal massage for the management of coccydynia.[27] This internal work can be complemented by the patient being educated in the use of vaginal dilators for self massage. Sexual partners are also educated in these techniques to encourage and provide further supportive therapy at home. Myofascial manipulation can be augmented with the use of ultrasound/diathermy therapy to aid in deep muscle relaxation. Multiple studies have demonstrated excellent response with improvement of chronic pelvic pain,[28] vulvodynia,[29] BPS/IC,[13,30] sexual pain and dysfunction,[25] as well as anal rectal pain disorders.[31,32]

PHARMACOLOGIC THERAPY

The pelvic floor muscles are never totally quiescent and like all muscles they have "muscle memory." Thus, there is a tendency during and immediately after therapy for muscles to return to their original hypertonic state. Medications provide an excellent approach to maintaining muscle relaxation and stopping the continued pain that leads to the neurochemical cascade that maintains hypertonic pelvic muscles as described in the previous article. Drug therapy alone is less beneficial than combining medications with direct myofascial interventions such as physical therapy.

Tricyclic antidepressants (TCA) have been studied in many types of pain disorders and have consistently shown benefit.[33] Amitriptyline is the most commonly studied drug using doses of between 25 to 75 mg per day typically given as a single dose 1 hour before sleep. Its benefits are likely generated by improving sleep patterns and decreasing sympathetic tone. TCA have widely been advocated for the management of fibromyalgia, chronic headache, IC, and IBS. The benefit is not generated by treating depression and if depression is present this should be treated with another drug.

Myorelaxant drugs such as mataxolone/Skelaxin or cyclobenzaprine/Flexeril have not been studied for chronic pelvic pain but have generally been shown to be beneficial for myofascial pain. Tiazadine/Zanaflex has also been found by many to be very beneficial for muscle spasticity and secondarily for myofascial pain. Pregablin/Lyrica is a relatively new drug that is indicated for the treatment of both fibromyalgia and neuropathic pain disorders. It has been found to be very beneficial for many patients with a significant myofascial pain disorder as well as neuropathic symptoms (such as burning). Anecdotally, Pregablin in doses up to 600 mg per day is well tolerated and provides excellent results.

Many patients with chronic pain syndromes also have a syndrome known as "chemical hypersensitivity." These patients are generally poorly tolerant of any pharmacologic approaches and therefore nonpharmacologic and alternative approaches are often required. These patients are encouraged to aggressively use behavioral modification and physical therapy as their main approach to management. In addition, the transvaginal use of compounded baclofen suppositories (30 mg) or compounded diazepam suppositories (5 mg) every 8 hours has been very beneficial and well tolerated when placed either in the vagina or in the rectum for these patients.

TRIGGER POINT INJECTION THERAPY FOR MYOFASCIAL PAIN

If noninvasive techniques to resolve myofascial pain fail despite use of the previously mentioned therapies, trigger point injection therapy would be the next step. The main objective is to inactivate the trigger point, thereby reducing pain and restoring function to the muscle. Combining this temporary relief with continued physical therapy techniques—both manual stretching and massage at the time of the injection as well as continued soft tissue work and exercises by the patient to elongate the muscle fibers—will hopefully prolong the benefit. Trigger point injections typically require a series of injections (three to five) with each injection session demonstrating increasing sustained relief. The first often will last only 1 or 2 days but the duration of benefit should quickly progress to several weeks. If after five injections this

prolonged improvement is not seen then the clinician must again consider if perpetuating factors—both physical such as IC and vulvodynia and/or emotional/behavioral—must be addressed. Trigger point injection also provides diagnostic information. If resolution of pain is complete even though short-lived, it demonstrates that the myofascial component represents a significant etiology of the patient's pain.

Trigger point injections seem to be equally effective whether they are "dry" or "wet." Mechanical disruption of the trigger point is the likely mechanism of action. Injection of trigger points can be painful therefore most clinicians use a "wet" technique that involves a local anesthetic (1 to 3 mL without a vasoconstricting agent). This decreases the pain of the procedure as well as adds to the mechanical disruption. The technique of trigger point injection involves identification of the trigger point with digital palpation then the use of a 21- to 25-gauge needle placed into the trigger point. This may occur transvaginally or transabdominally based on the location of the trigger point. When the needle penetrates the trigger point this typically elicits a local twitch response that reproduces the patient's localized pain and the anesthetic is then injected. The needle should then be backed out of the trigger point without being totally withdrawn and then advanced 1 to 3 mm surrounding the original trigger point and its associated taught band multiple times using a "dry" needling technique and augmented with anesthetics if necessary (**Fig. 5**). The addition of corticosteroids such as 20 mg of methylprednisolone acetate/Depo-Medrol is often used in areas of the fascial insertion but randomized controlled trials do not show additional benefit with the addition of steroids.[34] This author will use steroids if pain appears to be the result of previous injury (eg, surgery), fascial insertion site, or a foreign body reaction such as pain associated with synthetic mesh placement.

Trigger point injection techniques can be applied transabdominally for rectus muscle or post surgical scar pain. It can be applied transvaginally for pelvic floor

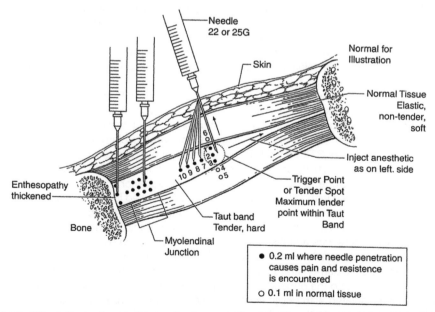

Fig. 5. Illustration of technique of trigger point injections. (*From* Fischer AA. New approaches in treatment of myofascial pain. Phys Med Rehbil Clin North Am 1997:8;158; with permission.)

trigger point management. If applied to trigger points just inside the introitus, the pubococcygeus muscle can be easily reached with a standard syringe and needle. When injections are required for the deeper muscles such as iliococcygeus or coccygeus or when the trigger point is located quite lateral or even behind the pubic symphysis (the insertion of the pubococcygeus muscle), then the use of an Iowa trumpet (from a pudendal nerve block tray) has many advantages. One of these advantages is that a gentle bend can be applied to the Iowa trumpet that allows for the safe and accurate performance of trigger point injection for an otherwise difficult to reach location. Levator ani trigger point injections in patients with chronic pelvic pain (CPP) show that at least 72% of patients report a greater than 50% improvement in symptoms[35]

Complications from trigger point injections are rare but include hematoma (attempt prevention with postinjection pressure for 1 minute), infection (attempt prevention by iodine prep), and drug reactions. These complications are rare, occurring less than 1% of the time, but must be discussed with the patient because if they do occur it will typically exacerbate pain rather than improve it.

BOTULINUM TOXIN THERAPY

If a trigger point injection provides excellent response with resolution of pain but is persistently short lived then the addition of botulinum toxin (eg, Botox A [BTX/A]) should be considered. BTX/A has been used for many of the pelvic floor hypertonic dysfunctions that we have discussed including vulvodynia, chronic pelvic pain, vaginismus, obstructed defecation, voiding dysfunction, urinary retention, perianal pain disorders, and anal fissures.[36]

The mechanism of pain relief with BTX/A was initially thought to involve the muscle relaxation induced by blockade of the release of acetylcholine at the neuromuscular junction. Pain relief is now thought to also involve the direct antinociceptive activity of blocking the release of local neurotransmitters involved in pain signaling as well as maintaining stimulation of local inflammatory mediators. This decrease in peripheral sensitization results in a secondary decrease in central sensitization by a direct reduction in neurotransmitter release in the dorsal horn.[37] Additionally, after an intramuscular injection BTX/A is transported by the axons to the central nervous system with the direct effect of a reduction in the release of substance P and glutamate within the dorsal horn. Both substance P and glutamate are involved in central sensitization and chronic pain (**Fig. 6**).[38] Clinically, the analgesic affect from a decrease in this afferent input occurs sooner than the direct effects on muscle relaxation. This dual mode of action makes BTX very attractive for many of our pain disorders and clinical experience also supports its use. When compared with injections of local anesthesia and methylprednisolone, BTX/A was shown to be far superior.[39]

Vaginismus treated with 150 to 400 units of BTX/A resulted in a 75% response rate with no recurrence with a mean follow-up of 12 months.[40] In a randomized controlled trial of Botox (80 units) versus physical therapy for chronic pelvic pain caused by levator spasm, there was a statistically significant decrease in dyspareunia and non-menstrual pelvic pain in the Botox subjects.[41] Treated with 35 units of BTX/A injected into the submucosa demonstrated a favorable outcome but in this author's experience 100 units injected into the pubococcygeus muscle has proved to be very effective for vulvodynia associated with pelvic floor pain and significant hypertonicity.

Urologic uses include the treatment of detrusor overactivity in patients with both neurogenic (200–300 units BTX/A) and idiopathic (100–200 units) detrusor overactivity. BPS/IC patients respond well to intravesical/submucosal injection of 200 units of

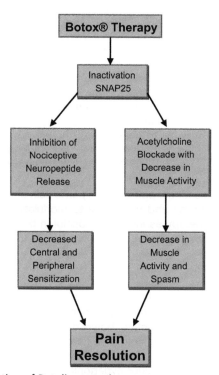

Fig. 6. Dual mode of action of Botulinum toxin.

BTX/A in case series and anecdotal experience. Urethral sphincteric injection with doses between 50 to 200 BTX/A provides marked improvement for patients with voiding dysfunction and urinary retention. This subject has been reviewed in a European consensus report by Apostolidis in 2008.[42]

Side effects are rare and include pain at the injection site, hematoma, and infection. The prevalence of side effects is similar to traditional trigger point injection therapy when used for myofascial pain. Adverse events associated with the neuromuscular affects of Botox have been rare and are dose-dependent. Urinary retention when treating patients with detrusor overactivity is dose related and can occur in as many as 30% of patients. Fecal incontinence has occurred in less than 5% of patients after perianal injections of BTX/A and is also dose related.

NEUROMODULATION

The pelvic floor is controlled by a delicately balanced set of neural reflexes that have the ability to be modified by a process known as neuroplasticity. This can be beneficial for activities like toilet training but at times can result in disruption of these neural reflexes with resultant pelvic floor dysfunction. This dysregulation is involved in the development of pelvic floor hypertonic dysfunction and pain disorders in many patients. Neurostimulation—typically of the sacral nerves—can result in correction of this dysregulation in approximately 60% to 75% of our patients with urinary retention, urge incontinence, and urinary frequency.[43] Predictors of successful neurostimulation often are linked to the findings of pelvic floor hypertonic dysfunction especially in patients with urinary frequency and retention.[44] Although not indicated for the management of chronic pelvic pain disorders, there are reports of up to 50% of patients demonstrating resolution of chronic pelvic pain[45] and 85% of patients with diagnosis of IC also demonstrating improvement in pain and quality of life.[46]

Medtronic's InterStim system is one method of sacral nerve stimulation, and other new methods have been developed and are currently being studied in patients with pain and pelvic floor dysfunction. Alternative approaches that appear promising include posterior tibial nerve stimulation (an intermittent percutaneous stimulation of the S3 nerve) and pudendal nerve stimulation (continuous stimulation of the pudendal nerve approximately 6 cm distal to where an S3 neural stimulation would typically occur). Zabihi and Raz reported the use of a bilateral quadralead placement across the entire sacral area between S2 and S4 in patients with intractable chronic pelvic pain and reported a 50% response rate.[47]

The future holds promise for our patients with pelvic pain of myofascial origin. There are new drugs on the horizon and new ways to modulate the pain. Case reports include such innovative therapy as intrathecal baclofen pain pumps and new techniques of neurolysis including selective neurolysis using pulsed radiofrequency nerve ablation techniques.

SUMMARY

Pelvic floor hypertonic disorders are very common and can present with various symptoms including bladder dysfunction, bowel dysfunction, and various pain disorders. The diagnosis is simple if you look for it. Learning how to find it and the importance of looking for it is the goal of this article. I want to emphasize to the reader that we must be more aware of pelvic floor hypertonic disorders in our daily practice of pelvic medicine. There are many therapeutic options but like many of the problems we see in medicine, the earlier the diagnosis, the easier the treatment. The treatment of these pelvic floor hypertonic dysfunction and pain disorders will markedly improve the quality of life for many of the patients you see on a regular basis.

REFERENCES

1. Farhat W, Bagli DJ, Capolicchio G, et al. The dysfunctional voiding scoring system: quantitative standardization of dysfunctional voiding symptoms in children. J Urol 2000;164(3 Pt 2):1011–5.
2. De Paepe H, Renson C, Van Laecke E, et al. Pelvic-floor therapy and toilet training in young children with dysfunctional voiding and obstipation. BJU Int 2000;85(7): 889–93.
3. Kibar Y, Ors O, Demir E, et al. Results of biofeedback treatment on reflux resolution rates in children with dysfunctional voiding and vesicoureteral reflux. Urology 2007;70(3):563–6 [discussion: 566–7].
4. Fitzgerald MP, Thom DH, Wassel-Fry C, et al. Childhood urinary symptoms predict adult overactive bladder symptoms. J Urol 2006;175(3 Pt 1):989–93.
5. Butrick CW, Sanford D, Hou Q, et al. Chronic pelvic pain syndromes: clinical, urodynamic, and urothelial observations. Int Urogynecol J Pelvic Floor Dysfunct 2009;20:1047–53.
6. Hinman F Jr. Nonneurogenic neurogenic bladder (the Hinman syndrome)—15 years later. J Urol 1986;136(4):769–77.
7. Fowler CJ, Christmas CJ, Chapple CR, et al. Abnormal electromyographic activity of the urethral sphincter, voiding dysfunction, and polycystic ovaries: a new syndrome? BMJ 1988;297(6661):1436–8.

8. Datta SN, Chaliha C, Singh A, et al. Sacral neurostimulation for urinary retention: 10-year experience from one UK centre. BJU Int 2008;101(2):192–6.
9. Crowley T, Goldmeier D, Hiller J. Diagnosing and managing vaginismus. BMJ 2009;338:b2284.
10. Rao SS. Dyssynergic defecation. Gastroenterol Clin North Am 2001;30(1):97–114.
11. Lacerda-Filho A, Lima MJ, Magalhaes MF, et al. Chronic constipation— the role of clinical assessment and colorectal physiologic tests to obtain an etiologic diagnosis. Arq Gastroenterol 2008;45(1):50–7.
12. Peters KM, Carrico DJ, Kalinowski SE, et al. Prevalence of pelvic floor dysfunction in patients with interstitial cystitis. Urology 2007;70(1):16–8.
13. Weiss JM. Pelvic floor myofascial trigger points: manual therapy for interstitial cystitis and the urgency-frequency syndrome. J Urol 2001;166(6):2226–31.
14. Peters KM, Carrico DJ. Frequency, urgency, and pelvic pain: treating the pelvic floor versus the epithelium. Curr Urol Rep 2006;7(6):450–5.
15. Kennedy CM, Nygaard IE, Bradley CS, et al. Bladder and bowel symptoms among women with vulvar disease: are they universal? J Reprod Med 2007;52(12):1073–8.
16. Reissing ED, Brown C, Lord MJ, et al. Pelvic floor muscle functioning in women with vulvar vestibulitis syndrome. J Psychosom Obstet Gynaecol 2005;26(2):107–13.
17. Glazer HI, Rodke G, Swencionis C, et al. Treatment of vulvar vestibulitis syndrome with electromyographic biofeedback of pelvic floor musculature. J Reprod Med 1995;40(4):283–90.
18. Verne GN, Price DD. Irritable bowel syndrome as a common precipitant of central sensitization. Curr Rheumatol Rep 2002;4(4):322–8.
19. Gutman RE, Ford RE, Quiroz LH, et al. Is there a pelvic organ prolapse threshold that predicts pelvic floor symptoms? Am J Obstet Gynecol 2008;199(6):e1–7, 683.
20. Travell JG, Simons DG. Myofascial Pain and Dysfunction: The Trigger Point Manual. 2nd edition; 1999. Lippincott Williams and Wilkins.
21. White G, Jantos M, Glazer H. Establishing the diagnosis of vulvar vestibulitis. J Reprod Med 1997;42(3):157–60.
22. Abrams P, Cardozo L, Fall M, et al. The standardization of terminology of lower urinary tract function: report from the standardization subcommittee of the International Continence Society. Am J Obstet Gynec 2002;187:116.
23. Raz S, Smith RB. External sphincter spasticity syndrome in female patients. J Urol 1976;115(4):443–6.
24. Fletcher JG, Busse RF, Riederer SJ, et al. Magnetic resonance imaging of anatomic and dynamic defects of the pelvic floor in defecatory disorders. Am J Gastroenterol 2003;98(2):399–411.
25. Rosenbaum TY, Owens A. The role of pelvic floor physical therapy in the treatment of pelvic and genital pain-related sexual dysfunction (CME). J Sex Med 2008;5(3):513–23 [quiz 524–5].
26. Clemens JQ, Nadler RB, Schaeffer AJ, et al. Biofeedback, pelvic floor re-education, and bladder training for male chronic pelvic pain syndrome. Urology 2000;56(6):951–5.
27. Holzberg A, Kellog-Spadt S, Lukban J, et al. Evaluation of transvaginal theile massage as a therapeutic intervention for women with interstitial cystitis. Urology 2001;57(6 Suppl 1):120.
28. Montenegro ML, Vasconcelos EC, Candido Dos Reis FJ, et al. Physical therapy in the management of women with chronic pelvic pain. Int J Clin Pract 2008;62(2):263–9.

29. Glazer HI. Dysesthetic vulvodynia. Long-term follow-up after treatment with surface electromyography-assisted pelvic floor muscle rehabilitation. J Reprod Med 2000;45(10):798–802.

30. Oyama IA, Rejba A, Lukban JC, et al. Modified Thiele massage as therapeutic intervention for female patients with interstitial cystitis and high-tone pelvic floor dysfunction. Urology 2004;64(5):862–5.

31. Markwell SJ. Physical therapy management of pelvi/perineal and perianal pain syndromes. World J Urol 2001;19(3):194–9.

32. Bharucha AE, Trabuco E. Functional and chronic anorectal and pelvic pain disorders. Gastroenterol Clin North Am 2008;37(3):685–96, ix.

33. Onghena P, Van Houdenhove B. Antidepressant-induced analgesia in chronic non-malignant pain: a meta-analysis of 39 placebo-controlled studies. Pain 1992;49(2):205–19.

34. Carter JE. Abdominal Wall and Pelvic Myofascial Trigger Points in Pelvic Pain: Diagnosis and Management. Howard FM, editor. Philadelphia: Lippincott Williams and Wilkins; 2000.

35. Langford CF, Udvari Nagy S, Ghoniem GM. Levator ani trigger point injections: an underutilized treatment for chronic pelvic pain. Neurourol Urodyn 2007;26(1): 59–62.

36. Maria G, Cadeddu F, Brisinda D, et al. Management of bladder, prostatic and pelvic floor disorders with botulinum neurotoxin. Curr Med Chem 2005;12(3): 247–65.

37. Aoki KR. Evidence for antinociceptive activity of botulinum toxin type A in pain management. Headache 2003;43(Suppl 1):S9–15.

38. Aoki R. The development of Botox: its history and pharmacology. Pain Digest 1998;8:337–41.

39. Porta M. A comparative trial of botulinum toxin type A and methylprednisolone for the treatment of myofascial pain syndrome and pain from chronic muscle spasm. Pain 2000;85(1–2):101–5.

40. Ghazizadeh S, Nikzad M. Botulinum toxin in the treatment of refractory vaginismus. Obstet Gynecol 2004;104(5 Pt 1):922–5.

41. Abbott JA, Jarvis SK, Lyons SD, et al. Botulinum toxin type A for chronic pain and pelvic floor spasm in women: a randomized controlled trial. Obstet Gynecol 2006; 108(4):915–23.

42. Apostolidis A, Dasgupta P, Denys P, et al. Recommendations on the use of botulinum toxin in the treatment of lower urinary tract disorders and pelvic floor dysfunctions: a European consensus report. Eur Urol; 2008 [epub ahead of print].

43. Chartier-Kastler E. Sacral neuromodulation for treating the symptoms of overactive bladder syndrome and non-obstructive urinary retention: >10 years of clinical experience. BJU Int 2008;101(4):417–23.

44. Koldewijn EL, Rosier PF, Meuleman EJ, et al. Predictors of success with neuromodulation in lower urinary tract dysfunction: results of trial stimulation in 100 patients. J Urol 1994;152(6 Pt 1):2071–5.

45. Mayer RD, Howard FM. Sacral nerve stimulation: neuromodulation for voiding dysfunction and pain. Neurotherapeutics 2008;5(1):107–13.

46. Peters KM. Neuromodulation for the treatment of refractory interstitial cystitis. Rev Urol 2002;4(Suppl 1):S36–43.

47. Zabihi N, Mourtzinos A, Maher MG, et al. Short-term results of bilateral S2-S4 sacral neuromodulation for the treatment of refractory interstitial cystitis, painful bladder syndrome, and chronic pelvic pain. Int Urogynecol J Pelvic Floor Dysfunct 2008;19(4):553–7.

Index

Note: Page numbers of article titles are in **boldface** type.

Obstet Gynecol Clin N Am 36 (2009) 723–735
doi:10.1016/S0889-8545(09)00098-9
0889-8545/09/$ – see front matter © 2009 Elsevier Inc. All rights reserved.

obgyn.theclinics.com

Moving?

Make sure your subscription moves with you!

To notify us of your new address, find your **Clinics Account Number** (located on your mailing label above your name), and contact customer service at:

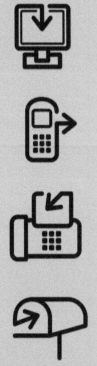

Email: journalscustomerservice-usa@elsevier.com

800-654-2452 (subscribers in the U.S. & Canada)
314-447-8871 (subscribers outside of the U.S. & Canada)

Fax number: 314-447-8029

Elsevier Health Sciences Division
Subscription Customer Service
3251 Riverport Lane
Maryland Heights, MO 63043